Cambridge Studies in Biotechnology

Editors: Sir James Baddiley, N. H. Carey, J. F. Davidson,
I. J. Higgins, W. G. Potter

2 Biotechnology and wastewater treatment

Biotechnology and wastewater treatment

C.F.FORSTER

Department of Civil Engineering, The University of Birmingham

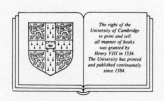
CAMBRIDGE UNIVERSITY PRESS

Cambridge

London New York New Rochelle

Melbourne Sydney

Published by the Press Syndicate of the University of Cambridge
The Pitt Building, Trumpington Street, Cambridge CB2 1RP
32 East 57th Street, New York, NY 10022, USA
10 Stamford Road, Oakleigh, Melbourne 3166, Australia

First published 1985

Printed in Great Britain by the University Press, Cambridge

Library of Congress catalogue card number: 84-22948

British Library cataloguing in publication data
Forster, C. F.
Biotechnology and wastewater treatment. –
(Cambridge studies in biotechnology; 2)
1. Sewage – Purification – Biological treatment
I. Title
628.3'51   TD755
ISBN 0 521 25723 9

To Bridget and Frances

Contents

Preface

Although the technology of sewage treatment is relatively new, the art of sanitation is several thousand years old. An examination of the historical development of sewerage and sewage treatment shows that three main epochs can be identified: the period up to the collapse of the Roman civilisation, the middle ages and finally the period since the late nineteenth century. Although one of the earliest recorded sewerage systems dates back to the Stone Age, probably the most famous pre-historic systems are those of (a) the Akkadian city of Eshnunna, situated close to what is now Baghdad, (b) the city of Mohenjo-Daro in Pakistan (both of these are dated at around 3000 BC), and (c) the Aegean civilisation of around 2000 BC typified by the palace of Minos, equipped with flushing toilets, on the island of Crete. In all these systems terra-cotta pipe work was used to convey domestic wastewater either to an early form of septic tank, or, in the Minoan case, to a combined sewerage system. It is worth noting that this latter system still functions very effectively for surface water drainage. Little is known about the treatment methods used by these early civilisations and it may well be that once outside the city boundaries the sewers discharged directly to rivers, although the Assyrians (700 BC) had strict laws to prevent their irrigation canals being polluted. The Romans were not so fastidious. Their system of sewers was not connected to houses and used primarily surface water drains. However, almost all types of domestic wastes were thrown into the streets and were flushed into the sewers by street cleaning. The result was a class III or even IV river Tiber.

Even these somewhat limited systems for sanitation disappeared with the collapse of the Roman civilisation and the next 1300 years were, in the main, a period of neglect. The main receptacles for sewage were streets, rivers, cesspits and the castle moat. Apart from the public health problems associated with these practices there were other hazards. Cesspits were frequently built beneath the floors of houses and several instances are recorded of people drowning when floors collapsed. The use of moats necessitated the toilet facilities being built out over the moat, which, whilst not necessarily hazardous, was certainly draughty! Despite this somewhat dismal situation there were occasional glimmers of sanitation sanity. One of the results of the Black

Death was the first British Act relating to sanitation which, in 1388, forbade 'the dumping of filth and garbage in rivers, ditches and streams'. The Elizabethan era saw the development in 1596 of the water closet although the U-bend was not patented until 1782. Even at this stage, discharges were still normally made to cesspits and until 1815 it was illegal to discharge foul sewage to sewers. This then was the situation which was to receive the first cholera epidemic in the early 1830s.

As the cholera epidemics rolled across Europe they left behind a greater awareness of the needs for proper sanitation, a spate of legislation and a rushed programme of sewer building. Also, although the science of microbiology is not attributable to cholera, Koch's discovery of the 'Comma Bacillus' confirmed the microbial nature of the disease and the carrier role of water. The two main Public Health Acts of this era were passed: in 1848 – making it compulsory to drain houses into sewers – and in 1875. The cost to a householder at about this time for water supply and drainage was £0.54 per year. Having at last channelled foul sewage into sewers, the first tentative steps towards treatment were made. Initially the treatment of sewage was aimed both at improving the environment and utilising the manurial value of the sewage on the land – hence the term sewage farm – although the concept was not new, having been used in Germany 400 years earlier. However, by 1865 it had been discovered that treatment, as opposed to fertilisation, could be improved by filtration prior to irrigation on the land.

Among the types of filter used at the time were upflow filters, which have recently been rediscovered, and brush wood filters, which are now being recommended by some workers for the treatment of farm effluents. By the 1880s the role of bacteria in effluent treatment had been appreciated and bio-engineering concepts started to become involved in plant design. In the case of bio-filters this was so successful that during the last 70 years little further development has been required apart from modifications to the ancillary equipment as technology has advanced.

Mechanical aeration systems took slightly longer to reach their full potential. The first use of air to purify waste water was recorded in the 1860s; a precursor to the oxidation ditch was developed in 1903; however, it remained for Ardern and Lockett to recognise that 'activated' sludge was the main purifying agent. Hence activated sludge systems have only been in widespread use since the 1920s. It is to be regretted that colloid chemists, who played a major part in the initial understanding of both bio-oxidation systems, appear to have lost interest in the science of effluent treatment.

What then of today? Plastics have arrived, in the shape of packings for high-rate bio-filters and support media in rotating disc or drum filters, and, with the increasing price of petrochemicals, may well be about to leave. Oxygen as well as air is being used both in sewers, as a form of pretreatment, and in bio-oxidation systems. Physico-chemical systems are being suggested as alternatives to microbial reactors, but this concept was suggested over 100 years ago. Certainly our ideas have a better scientific basis and our understanding of the complexities of the interactions between the various eco-systems that impinge on our society is greater. However, this is merely a natural acceleration that has accompanied our growth in technology; in our repertoire of sewerage and sewage treatment there is very little that is new.

This situation would appear to offer a challenge to the biotechnologist. However, it is unlikely that many significant process advances will result from his or her intervention. Some genetically engineered microbes may be produced that are more robust than the natural strains currently in use and marginal improvements in processes will probably be developed. Nevertheless, it is essential that the biotechnologist becomes involved in the treatment of wastewaters as a proper understanding of the biology, the chemistry and the engineering is essential for the total optimisation of the processes being used. This approach has already led to the concept of mass flux as a means for designing and operating settlement tanks and to the understanding of the significance of endogenous respiration of activated sludge in optimising aeration. The aim of this book is, therefore, to provide the biotechnologist with the essential fundamentals of wastewater treatment technology and so promote further developments of this kind.

1 Basic biology

1.1 Microbial anatomy

1.1.1 *General discussion*

Living beings on the earth can be divided into three groups: the plants (the metaphyta), the animals (metazoa) and the protists (the microbes). The microbes are generally unicellular, in contrast to the others which are always multicellular. There are, however, some multicellular microbes but these usually consist of masses of similar cells without the marked differentiation into specialised types (for example the liver, kidneys, brain cells, etc.) that is found in the higher groups. As a general rule, microbes are invisible to the naked eye. On our scale they range in size from the mouse to the elephant; in other words one of the smallest particles, the foot and mouth virus, has a size of about 10 nm (10^{-9} m), while at the other end of the scale, the giant amoeba has a size of about 300 μm (3×10^{-4} m).

Any cell is composed of two principal internal regions known as the nucleus and the cytoplasm. The nucleus carries the majority of the DNA of the cell and therefore serves as the carrier of the genetic code. The cytoplasm which surrounds the nucleus contains most of the RNA and protein of the cell. It is the primary site of the synthetic processes and is separated from the external environment by a delicate membrane which is known as the cytoplasmic membrane. This is composed of a mosaic of proteins and lipids and is the barrier through which any material must pass to enter or leave the cell. As such it is a semi-permeable membrane. As well as the differentiation between unicellular and multicellular types, microbes are further divided into two major groups on the basis of their internal structure, particularly that of the nucleus. These are;

(a) *Procaryotes* (bacteria, blue-green algae and others)
These have a single chromosome which is not organised within a discrete, membrane-bound nucleus. The cytoplasm of procaryotic cells is limited to extension by invagination of the surrounding membrane. In other words, the cells have a relatively simple internal structure which has no division of labour (i.e. a liver, a kidney etc.). Most of this group divide by simple cell division and resting stages are limited to spore formation.

(b) *Eucaryotes* (fungi, yeasts, algae, protozoa)

These cells have more than one chromosome which are organised within a membrane bound nucleus. Their cytoplasm contains specific organelles which tend to have specific job functions. For example, the mitochondria and the chloroplasts are concerned with energy production; the lysosomes and vacuoles are concerned with food absorption, digestion and excretion. The reproduction of eucaryotic cells is by asexual and/or sexual processes which may alternate in relatively complicated life cycles. The resting states of this class of cell consist of either spores or cysts.

(c) *Viruses*

It is difficult to classify this particular group of microbes. Their growth and reproduction depends absolutely on the host cells which they parasitise and they consist solely of a protein/nucleic acid mixture.

1.1.2   *The bacteria*

As well as being subdivided in terms of their structure, microbes can be classified in terms of their food sources and their methods of producing energy. This is probably most pronounced in the bacteria. Thus we can consider phototrophic and chemotrophic organisms. Phototrophic organisms rely for their energy on the reaction between light and photosynthetic pigments (i.e. chlorophyll). This classification can be further subdivided into photolithotrophy, in which the light reaction is linked to inorganic electron donors such as sulphide, and photoorganotrophy in which the light reaction is linked to an organic electron donor such as acetate or succinate. In the same way, the chemotrophic classification can be subdivided into chemolithotrophy in which the energy-rich compound adenosine triphosphate (ATP) is produced by the oxidation of an inorganic electron donor (e.g. $H_2 \rightarrow H_2O$), and chemoorganotrophy in which the ATP is produced by the oxidation of a reduced organic compound (e.g. methane or glucose). Bacteria (or Schizomycetes) are usually classified by a highly complex method in which 10 orders, 47 sub-orders, 190 genera, and 1474 species are used to specifically identify each type (e.g. Tables 1.1 and 1.2). The criteria used for classification include:

(a) The size, shape and method of grouping of individual cells
(b) The characteristics (e.g. shape, colour, surface texture) of the colony when grown on agar plates
(c) The behaviour towards stains
(d) The growth requirements
(e) The degree of motility
(f) Specific chemical reactions
(g) Antibody/antigen reactions

Table 1.1. *The orders in the class Schizomycetes*

Order	Description	Number of families
1. Pseudomonadales	Bacteria with polar flagella	10
2. Chlamydobacteriales	Filamentous iron bacteria	3
3. Hyphomicrobiales	Budding bacteria	2
4. Eubacteriales	True bacteria	13
5. Caryophanales	Filamentous sheathed bacteria	3
6. Actinomycetales	Mycelial bacteria	4
7. Beggiatoales	Filamentous sulphur bacteria	4
8. Myxobacteriales	Slime bacteria	5
9. Spirochaetales	Spirochaetes	2
10. Mycoplasmatales	Pleuropneumonia-like organisms	1

Table 1.2. *The arrangement of a typical order within the class of Schizomycetes*

Order: Actinomycetales			
Sub-order or family			
Mycobacteriaceae	Streptomycetaceae	Actinomycetaceae	Actinoplanaceae
Genus (no. of species)			
Mycobacterium (14)	Streptomyces (149)	Norcardia (45)	Actinoplanes (1)
Mycococcus (6)	Micromonospora (5)	Actinomyces (3)	Streptosporangium (1)
	Thermoactinomyces (3)		

Cell morphology. Bacterial cells have essentially four main shapes; coccus – spherical; rod – ellipsoidal; spirillum – spiral; and vibrio – 'comma' shaped. From these basic shapes chains and agglomerates can be built up. Thus, for example, in the case of the cocci it is possible to have: diplococcus – 2 cells; streptococcus – a chain; sarcina – a 3-dimensional cube-like structure; and staphylococcus – random clusters.

In considering the size of bacteria (Table 1.3) two points must be borne in mind:

(a) That in any colony, there will be a variety of sizes.
(b) That the measurements quoted in any text will have, out of necessity, been made on treated cells. In other words they will have been fixed or stained in some way and this means that in fact they will probably have shrunk or been distorted and therefore will only be an approximation to the actual size.

Table 1.3. *Typical bacterial dimensions*

	Diameter (μm)	Length (μm)	Shape
Staphylococcus aureus	0.8–1.0	—	sphere
Escherichia coli	0.4–0.7	1.0–1.3	rod
Bacillus anthracis	1.0–1.3	3.0–10	rod

Staining. Stains or dyes are frequently used to colour bacteria, not only so that they can be seen more clearly themselves, but also so that specific parts can be highlighted. Bacteria normally behave acidically so that the stains that are used are usually basic in nature; for example, crystal violet, methylene blue. In addition to this type of stain, differential staining techniques can also be used; that is to say a technique which depends on the nature of the bacterium being stained. Probably the most common of these methods is the Gram stain which depends on the ability of bacteria to retain the colour of crystal violet when treated with solvent. The cells in some bacteria (the Gram negative bacteria) are decolorised by the solvent. The cells of others (Gram positive bacteria) retain their blue/violet coloration. It is then usual to counterstain the cells with a red dye such as safranin or carbol fuschin. Under the microscope, Gram positive cells are seen as blue and Gram negative cells as red. However, not all bacterial cells give a clear-cut differentiation. Some bacteria may therefore be described as Gram indeterminate and it is not unusual for bacteria to change their Gram character depending on the age of the bacteria being examined. This difference in staining behaviour is in fact due to differences in the chemical composition of the cell wall.

Cell components. As has been mentioned earlier, somewhere at the centre of the cell is a nucleus and this is never separated from the cytoplasm by any form of membrane (Fig. 1.1). Also within the nucleus there is never any sign of the organisation of the DNA into individual chromosomes. However the DNA is structured (as a double-stranded loop) so that it is equivalent to a single chromosome. Within the cytoplasmic region there may be a variety of inclusions: for example, ribosomes, sulphur granules, volutin granules (these are usually polyphosphates), lipid droplets and polysaccharide aggregates. Surrounding all this there is a cytoplasmic membrane. This consists of two electron-dense layers sandwiching an electron-thin layer. This membrane is relatively impermeable to ionic organic molecules. Compounds of this type must therefore be transferred enzymically. The membrane is surrounded by a cell wall which is relatively rigid and can

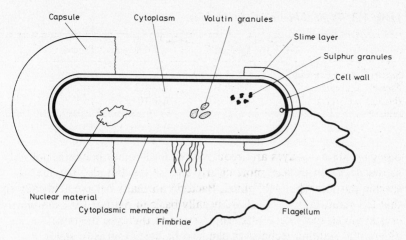

Fig. 1.1. Schematic diagram of a bacterium.

withstand quite high osmotic pressures. For example, the osmotic pressure within some bacteria can be as high as 30 atmospheres. It is the cell wall which is responsible for the shape of the cell. Basically two types of cell wall have been noted, one which is 10–25 nm thick, which is totally homogeneous, and which usually gives a Gram positive reaction. Gram negative cells on the other hand have a laminated cell wall, the innermost layer of which provides the rigidity of the wall. The cell walls of Gram negative bacteria contain a full range of amino acids and contain 10–20 per cent lipids. This contrasts with the cell walls of Gram positive bacteria in which there is only about 0.2 per cent lipids and the aryl and sulphur amino acids are absent. Beyond the cell wall there is a rather diffuse layer which is described either as a micro-capsule, a capsule or a slime layer depending on the thickness and composition of the material involved. These layers are nearly always formed of high viscosity polymeric compounds (e.g. polysaccharide, proteins, or polypeptides).

Some bacteria have a movement organ called a flagellum; this is a helically twisted fibrous protein and can be up to seven times the cell length. During movement, flagella have a sine-wave shape of a constant amplitude. This means that the movement is not of a wiggling nature as this would give a sine-wave of decreasing amplitude. Flagella movement is in fact caused by mechano-chemical contractions in which the bond energy of ATP is used to change the molecular form of the protein in such a way that the change in the molecular form is translated into the act of contraction. Most bacteria have their flagella (one or more) sited in the polar position, but some bacteria do have flagella all round the cell (these are known as peritrichous flagella). In addition to these appendages, bacteria also can have fimbriae. These are sited round the outside of the cell and in appearance look like miniature flagella (see Fig. 1.1).

Bacterial growth. In general, bacteria reproduce asexually by binary fission. Once a mature cell reaches a critical size, the nuclear material divides and the cell splits to give two daughter cells. The rate of this division can be as high as once every 20 minutes. The growth pattern of bacteria can best be considered by examining the growth of a pure culture. This is done in terms of a plot of bacterial numbers against time (Fig. 1.2). Immediately after the inoculation of a sterile medium with a pure culture there is a lag period. This can be altered by the size, age and the physical condition of the inoculum together with the nature of the medium and the temperature. One way of reducing it is to use a growing inoculum and by using an identical medium for growing the inoculum. On average, the lag period is about three to four hours. It is a period of high metabolic activity (as can be measured by the oxygen consumption or the output of carbon dioxide). The lag period is

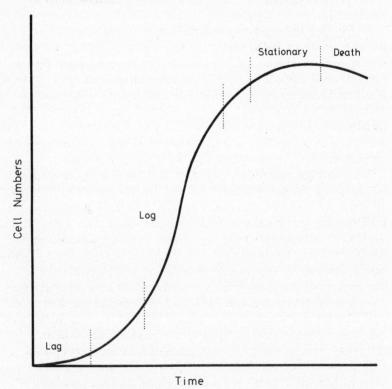

Fig. 1.2. A typical bacterial growth curve.

followed by a transition stage which then leads into a phase of logarithmic growth which occurs at a more or less constant rate by binary fission. This phase can be described mathematically:

$$x_n = x_0 2^n$$
$$\log x_n = \log x_0 + n\log 2$$
$$n = (\log x_n - \log x_0)/\log 2$$

$$\text{Mean generation time} = \varDelta t/n = \frac{\varDelta t \log 2}{\log x_n - \log x_0}$$

where x_0 = the number of bacteria at time = t_1, x_n = the number after n generations at time = t_2, $\varDelta t = (t_2 - t_1)$.

Thus the mean generation time is taken as the time for the culture to double its number. The logarithmic phase is followed by a second transition stage. During these stages bacterial cells are very susceptible to environmental conditions. This second transition phase is followed by a stationary period when the bacteria are still dividing but the rate at which the bacteria are increasing is being balanced by the rate at which cells are dying. Thus an equilibrium is established. Eventually, a death phase is reached in which the number of bacteria starts to decrease.

So far, only the vegetative cells have been considered, that is to say the cells which are in the process of growing and reproducing. Some cells have the capability of forming a resting state or spore. This is formed within the cell initially and is surrounded by a series of layers which make the spore very resistant to heat, chemical toxicity, and desiccation. Sporulation occurs when the cells are well nourished, usually at a point just after the maximum growth rate. This is in fact a survival mechanism for the species concerned. Spores once formed can germinate in any favourable environment.

What then are the environmental requirements for growth? The normal range for pH is between 5.5 and 8.5, usually with an optimum of about 7. Most bacteria require moisture for their growth and it is usually taken that a water availability of more than 0.6 is needed (water availability equals vapour pressure of solution/vapour pressure of water). As far as temperature is concerned, three main types of bacteria can be considered: *psychrophilic* which have an optimum growth temperature of less than 20 °C, *mesophilic* which have an optimum growth temperature of about 37 °C and *thermophilic* which have an optimum growth temperature of greater than 45 °C. In a similar way, the oxygen requirements of bacteria can be subdivided into four categories: *aerobic* bacteria which specifically require oxygenation for their growth; *anaerobic* bacteria which will only grow in the absence of oxygen; *facultative anaerobic* bacteria which have the capability of growing either in the presence of oxygen or in its absence; and *microaerophilic* bacteria which will tolerate only small amounts of oxygen. The nutritional requirements for bacteria are the same whatever their type. They require carbon, energy, a nitrogen source and traces of inorganics (e.g. K, Mg, Fe, PO_4, SO_4, Zn, Cu).

1.1.3   *The protozoa*

These are a complex group of eucaryotic cells which are unicellular and as a general rule motile. As far as classification is concerned one can consider subdivisions based either on the nutritional requirements or the way in which the cells move.

(a) Nutritional requirements

(i) Autotrophs – these are primary producers which use carbon dioxide and the energy of sun.
(ii) Saprozoic forms – this group uses dissolved organic material and as such must be in direct competition with the chemo-organotrophic bacteria.
(iii) Phagotrophs – this group feed on bacteria and in some cases there is a marked preference for specific bacterial types.
(iv) Predators and cannibals.

(b) Modes of movement
Flagella/ameboid
Ameboid
Parasitic – immotile.
Cilia.

Within this latter group all but parasitic forms are of interest in the wastewater treatment field but it is probably the ciliates which are of prime importance. With this in mind, it is probably best to consider the structures and functions of the protozoa by taking as an example a simple ciliate, *Tetrahymena*. This is a pear-shaped organism which is about 50 μm in length. It is enclosed by a thin pellicle which is, in effect, a specialised and thickened cytoplasmic membrane. The cilia are arranged around the surface in longitudinal rows. Each cilium is inter-linked through basal granules so that the movement of the cilia is co-ordinated. Food is ingested through the cytostome which acts as a mouth. Specialised cilia are arranged so that food can be swept into the mouth. Having entered the cell, food is kept in food vacuoles which are formed at the base of the mouth cavity. These are circulated within the cell by cytoplasmic streaming until all the food has been digested. Any residual matter is then excreted through the cytoproct. Because the osmotic pressure within the cell is considerably greater than that of the normal exterior environment, the cell water balance must be carefully maintained. This is achieved by the action of the contractile vacuole which in effect concentrates and pumps the water from the cell thus counteracting the steady flow into the cell. The other main characteristic of the ciliates is the fact that they can have two different types of nucleus: the macro-nucleus which is involved in the asexual reproductive cycle and the micro-nucleus which is used when sexual reproduction occurs.

The identification of the ciliates depends on: their size and their shape; the number, shape and position of the nuclei (this observation may be facilitated by staining); the number and arrangement of the contractile vacuoles; and the arrangement and motion of the cilia or the cirri (these are compound cilia in which a number of cilia are bound together).

1.1.4   *Viruses*

The viruses are small microbes – so small that they will pass through those filters which normally retain bacteria. For example, a typical bacterium *Serratia marcascens* has a diameter of 800 nm whereas the foot and mouth virus has a diameter of 10 nm and the polio virus has a diameter of between 25 and 30 nm. Viruses are parasites; in other words, they require a host cell for their reproduction. In general, they are very resistant to the cold, and their resistance to heat is comparable to that of non-spore-forming bacteria (see §1.3); they are also quite resistant to most chemicals although chlorine at a concentration of about 1 mg l^{-1} (available chlorine) will de-activate them. The structure of viruses is very simple: they consist of protein and nucleic acid. We can consider three types of virus: Animal viruses where the nucleic acid can be either DNA or RNA; plant viruses in which the nucleic acid is usually RNA; and the viruses which infect bacteria. The viruses in this latter group are called bacteriophages (usually abbreviated to phages) and in general the nucleic acid material is DNA.

Perhaps the best way of examining the behaviour of viruses is to examine the infective cycle of bacteriophages. A typical phage particle (T$_4$) consists of a polyhedral head which would be between 50 and 100 nm in cross section, and a short thin tail (Fig. 1.3). The head consists of a core of DNA surrounded by a protein coat and the tail, which consists solely of protein, has a hollow core. When a bacterium is attacked by a phage particle, the tail attaches to the bacterial cell surface and the DNA is injected down the hollow core of the tail into the cell cytoplasm. Having entered the cell, the phage DNA effectively takes over the metabolic processes of the bacterium so that the latter is compelled to produce phage protein and phage DNA. This stage of the cycle is known as the *vegetative* stage. Towards the end of this stage, the proteins and nucleic acid are assembled into new virion units and when this process is complete, cell lysis occurs (that is to say the cell breaks open) releasing the virion particles. This then is the *lytic cycle*

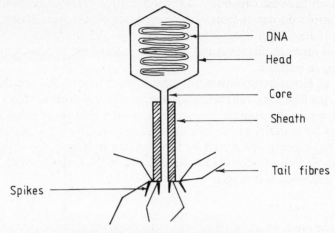

Fig. 1.3. Schematic diagram of the bacteriophage, T_4.

and is the result of infection by virulent phages. However not all phages are virulent: some can be what is termed temperate. Infection by a temperate phage gives rise to *lysogeny*. In this type of relationship the injected phage nucleic acid does not replicate to give more phage material; rather it is incorporated into the chromosome of the bacterium and in that state is reproduced together with the chromosome. In effect therefore it becomes part of the genetic material of the bacterium. This is known as the prophage state and a bacterium which carries a prophage is said to be lysogenic. A lysogenic bacterium carries an immunity to infection by the phage which has been incorporated into its genetic material. It is possible for a phage to be carried by a lysogenic bacterium for several generations and then suddenly, for no known reason, for the phage to revert to the vegetative state and to cause cell lysis. This transition is quite a rare event but it can be induced by agents which are capable of causing cell mutation (e.g. ultra-violet light and nitrogen mustards).

This brief survey leads to two questions: firstly, what is a phage? Is it the virion, the vegetative DNA or the prophage? And secondly, should a virus really be classified within the microbial world as a living organism or is it merely an assemblage of chemicals?

Viruses (that is to say those which infect plants and animals) tend to have a simpler structure than the phage particles. For example the tobacco mosaic virus is a cylinder about 280 nm in length and about 50 nm in diameter. Thus the whole virion probably acts as the infective unit and it may well be that the protein sheath plays some part in the multiplication cycle, although it has been shown that purified viral nucleic acid can infect cells. Phage virions contain enzymes in their tail unit which have the capability of penetrating the bacterial cell wall. Virus virions do not, in general, have enzymes of this type. Many viruses can establish latent infection, that is to say an infection which does not result in disease symptoms. It is comparable in some ways to lysogeny in bacteria.

Not all biological groups suffer from viral infections. Among the plants, the flowering varieties are prone to infection whereas ferns and mosses are not; in animals, the vertebrates are prone to infection whereas the majority of invertebrates are not; in the microbial world every major group of bacteria has been shown to be prone to attack, whereas no case of infection has been found in the higher protists (algae, protozoa and fungi).

1.1.5   *The algae*

The algae are a group of eucaryotic organisms that should perhaps in the strictest sense of the word be classified as plants. In attempting to subdivide the algae into their various classifications it is probably best to use five main criteria: the nature of the photosynthetic pigments; the nature of the food reserves; the nature of the cell wall components; the types of flagellae; and finally details of the cell structure. Three types of photosynthetic pigments are found in the algae; these are chlorophyll, carotenoids and the biloproteins. On the basis of their spectra five different types of chlorophyll have been identified. Of these chlorophyll-*a* is the most common, being found in all types of algae, and as such is frequently used for the quantitative determination of algae in water. The chlorophylls and carotenoids are soluble in lipid solvents and cannot be extracted in aqueous solution. However, a water soluble pigment can be extracted from certain types of algae; this is the biloprotein which is a pigment–protein complex.

The proportion of one kind of pigment to the other is variable and is responsible for the characteristic colour of the particular species of algae. For example, the *Chlorophyta* are green because they have an excess of chlorophyll in relation to the carotenoid pigment, whereas the yellow-brown colour of, for example, the *Cryptophyta* and the yellow-green colour of the *Xanthophyta* indicate an excess of carotenoid. Similarly the characteristic colours of the *Cyanophyta* (blue-green) and the *Rhodophyta* (red) are the result of an excess of biloprotein. However it must be remembered that the relative proportions of the pigments can vary with the environmental conditions which means that its use as a specific taxonomic feature can be unreliable. Similarly any attempt to classify the algae by their food storage products can lead to difficulties. The algae, like most microbes, accumulate various polymeric materials, for example, starch and other polysaccharides, fats and sterols. However, the distribution and concentration of these compounds again can vary with the environmental conditions so that their use is limited perhaps to a preliminary indicator test. The cell wall material again can only offer a broad classification: for example, into those algae which have a cell wall made up of cellulose, or of alginic acid, or mucopeptide material. Some algae have a cell wall which contains silica and when this is found it is a fairly definite indication of that particular species. The nature, number and position of the flagella are used as a fairly important indication in the primary classification of the algae. Thus, for a very generalised classification, one must rely primarily on observation of the algae's shape, colour and the arrangement of the flagella.

As far as the Water Industry is concerned, perhaps the most significant types are the unicellular and the filamentous forms together with the diatoms. The unicellular forms may be either motile, non-motile or amoeboid. A typical motile unicellular algae is *Chlamydomonas*. It is an ellipsoidal cell which moves by means of a pair of identical flagella. It can reproduce asexually by multiple fission with each cell dividing internally to produce up to eight daughter cells. It also has the capability of a sexual reproductive cycle. Two cells fuse to form a quadri-flagellate unit which eventually loses its flagella and then encysts. The cyst will eventually germinate producing four vegetative cells. A typical example of non-motile unicellular algae is *Chlorella*. This reproduces exclusively by multiple fission. Filamentous algae can be typified by *Ulothrix*. Generally the reproduction of *Ulothrix* is by the asexual formation of zoospores inside some of its cells. These are released from the filament and are biflagellate. After a period of swimming in this form they germinate into the parent plant. Not all algae have a recognisable photosynthetic mechanism. Those that do not are known as leucophytes and are colourless. The leucophytes are all unicellular and in the main are flagellates; they show very close structural affinities to particular groups of the more conventional algae. In the case of one particular species of *Euglena* the conversion from a photosynthetic flagellate to a leucophyte can be reproduced in the laboratory, for example, by treatment with ultra-violet light. Algae that have lost the photosynthetic mechanism obtain their energy either from organic substrates or by predation on smaller microbes (phagocytosis).

1.2   Microbial biochemistry
1.2.1   *Structures and functions of biologically important compounds*

In considering the chemistry of microbial cells there is a need, first of all, to identify certain key types of chemical, to examine their structure and to recognise what their main functions are within the general

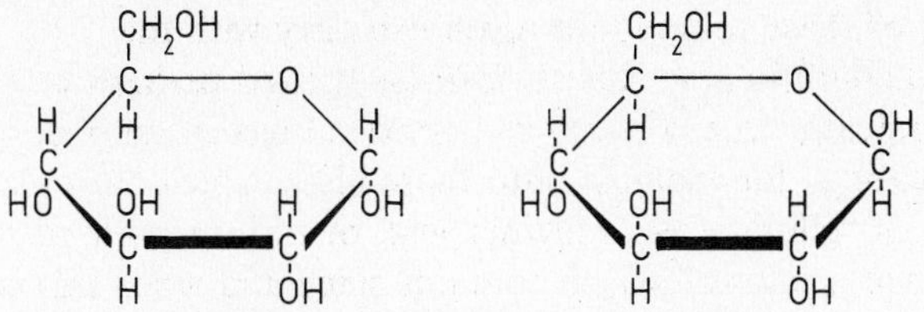

Fig. 1.4. The two types of glucose.

framework of the biochemistry of cells. However, it must also be realised that a detailed discussion of these subjects is beyond the scope of this text. Therefore if detail is required specialist books should be consulted.

The *carbohydrates* are a class of compound which occurs readily in nature and as such are a common source of food for microbes. Indeed in laboratory studies carbohydrates are frequently used as the sole carbon source. There are three main subgroups within this general class of compound: the monosaccharides, the oligosaccharides (> 1 saccharide unit) and the polysaccharides (a large number of saccharide units). The monosaccharides contain between three and seven carbon atoms per molecule, and although examples of all these are found at various stages of metabolism, the most common are the pentoses (C_5) and the hexoses (C_6). Glucose is a typical hexose and its empirical formula $C_6H_{12}O_6$ is best described by the structure shown in Fig. 1.4. This shows that glucose can exist in two forms; α- and β-glucose. The importance of this can be seen when the formation of oligosaccharides is being considered. An examination of Fig. 1.5 shows that the condensation of two molecules of glucose can produce either maltose (from two α-forms) or cellobiose (from two β-structures). By extrapolating this phenomenon to include other monosaccharides and longer chains it can be seen that a wide and varied range of carbohydrates is possible. However, the more common polysaccharides, which can contain several hundred monosaccharide units, tend to have relatively straightforward repetitive structures. Thus, for example, amylose is a linear chain of 200–3000 α-glucose units.

Proteins are essential structural components of cells. They are polymers of amino acids which have the general formula

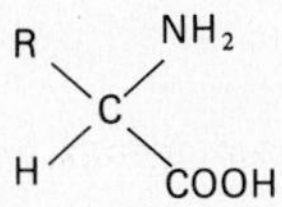

Twenty-two different amino acids can be found in proteins, the side chain (R) varying from a simple hydrogen unit to aromatic and

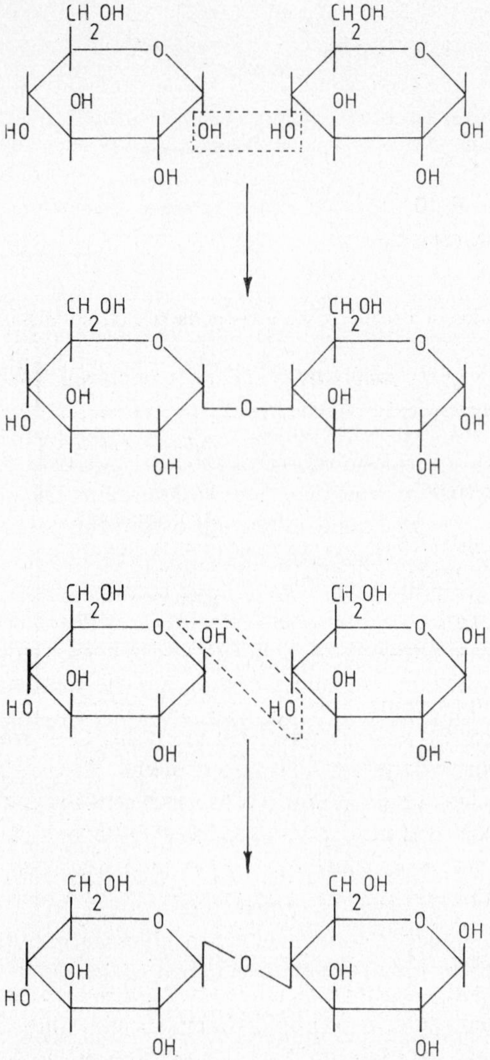

Fig. 1.5. The structure of maltose (two α-forms) and cellobiose (two β-forms).

heterocyclic ring structures. The protein chains are formed by peptide (CONH) links between adjacent amino acids (Fig. 1.6). The structure of protein molecules is complex. Not only is the amino acid sequence both specific and important but also the three-dimensional spatial arrangement is unique, with hydrogen bonding and disulphide bridges being used to define it.

In addition to the simple proteins, which are just polypeptide units, there exists a class known as conjugated proteins. These are simple

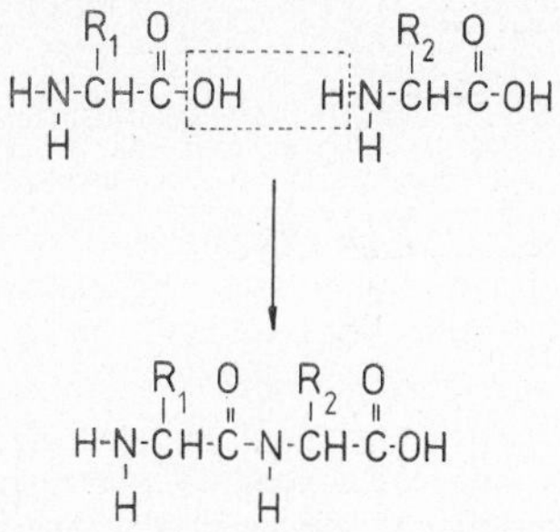

$$
\begin{array}{cc}
\underset{H}{\overset{R_1}{\underset{|}{H\text{-}N\text{-}CH\text{-}C\text{-}OH}}}\overset{O}{\overset{\|}{}} & \underset{H}{\overset{R_2}{\underset{|}{H\text{-}N\text{-}CH\text{-}C\text{-}OH}}}\overset{O}{\overset{\|}{}}
\end{array}
$$

$$
\underset{H\ \ \ \ \ H}{\overset{R_1\ \ \ O\ \ \ R_2\ \ \ O}{H\text{-}N\text{-}CH\text{-}C\text{-}N\text{-}CH\text{-}C\text{-}OH}}
$$

Fig. 1.6. Formation of a peptide bond between the two amino acids.

Table 1.4. *A summary of the functions of the more important nucleotides*

Nucleotide	Agent transferred
Adenosine triphosphate (ATP)	Energy
Coenzyme A (CoASH)	Acyl groups
Flavin adenine dinucleotide (FAD)	Electrons
Nicotinamide adenine dinucleotide (NAD)	Electrons
Guanosine triphosphate (GTP)	Energy
Uridine diphosphate (UDP)	Sugars

proteins bound to non-proteinaceous material: for example, lipoproteins (lipid/protein) and glycoproteins (carbohydrate/protein). Enzymes, the biological catalysts of cells, are proteins. Their catalytic action tends to be highly specific and it is this specificity which enables the cell to regulate its biochemical reactions. Enzymic activity can be affected by the environment in which the enzymes are operating. Each enzyme has an optimum pH range and any significant deviation from this will reduce the rate of catalysis considerably. Temperature will affect the reaction rate in two ways. An increase in temperature will increase the rate, as in any other chemical reaction; however, further increase in temperature will also eventually bring about an inactivation of the enzyme. Thermal improvement to reaction rates should therefore be considered as having an upper limit of around 50 °C. Enzymes, like any other type of catalyst, can be poisoned, and this is something which often needs to be considered when the treatment of industrial wastewaters is being assessed.

Some enzymes require the presence of other compounds to assist in the catalysis. These compounds are known as co-factors. The nucleotides are one of the most prominent type of co-factor and can be thought of as transferring agents. Table 1.4 describes the functions of the more important and the more common nucleotides. Of these adenosine triphosphate (ATP) is worthy of special mention. ATP can

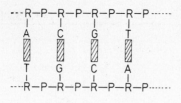

= hydrogen bonding

Fig. 1.7. Schematic representation of the DNA molecule. R = deoxyribose; P = phosphate; A = adenine; G = guanine; C = cytosine; T = thymine.

be thought of as the energy currency of the cell, in that when it is hydrolysed to adenosine diphosphate (ADP) approximately 7000 cal per mol are released and made available to drive the reactions to which the ATP hydrolysis is coupled. Therefore to ensure that there is no hindrance to reactions that require an energy input, it is essential that the cell regenerates ATP. In structural terms, the nucleotides consist of three main parts; a heterocyclic base (usually a purine or pyrimidine), a sugar (usually ribose or deoxyribose) and phosphoric acid.

Arguably the most important type of nucleotides in any cell are the polynucleotides, ribonucleic acid (RNA) and deoxyribonucleic acid (DNA). This latter compound (Fig. 1.7) consists of two strands in the form of a helix. Each strand consists of alternating units of deoxyribose and phosphate. A heterocyclic base is attached to each pentose unit, these bases being cytosine, guanine, adenine and thymine. The two strands are linked by hydrogen bonding between the bases, cytosine invariably linking with guanine and adenine with thymine. The order of the bases along a strand is the code to all the genetic characteristics of the cell and as such is what makes the DNA unique to the cell. The invariability of the hydrogen bonding is what ensures the precision of transfer of this genetic code. For all the genetic information to be encoded obviously requires that the DNA molecule be large. For example, in the bacterium *E. coli* some 3×10^6 base pairs are required to achieve the synthesis of the structural proteins and the enzymes required by the cell.

RNA is a polynucleotide in which the backbone of the chain is ribose and phosphate. The heterocyclic bases are the same as in DNA except that uracil replaces thymine. A simplistic view of the role of RNA is that it is synthesised to carry selected parts of the DNA code (cytosine being matched with guanine; uracil with adenine). The code carried by this RNA then controls the synthesis of amino acids in the precise order necessary for the formation of specific proteins. More complete descriptions of these processes can be found in most of the modern texts dealing with microbial biochemistry (e.g. Gaudy & Gaudy, 1980).

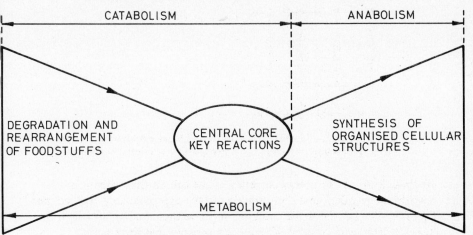

Fig. 1.8. Schematic diagram showing the various metabolic stages.

The final class of compound that needs to be mentioned is the lipids. In general these can be thought of as esters of fatty acids (usually with more than 12 carbon atoms) and alcohols (very often glycerol), although in the case of phospholipids one of the hydroxyl units in the glycerol molecule is reacted with phosphoric acid (or a substituted phosphoric acid).

1.2.2 *Metabolism*

Metabolism is the term which is used to describe the overall processing of food to new cellular material. However, it should be considered as two separate processes: catabolism and anabolism (Fig. 1.8). Catabolism itself occurs in two stages. Initially the molecules present in the feed are broken down and converted into compounds that are suitable for use in a set of key reactions. These reactions have been called the central core (Gaudy & Gaudy, 1980), and their function is to produce the basic building blocks from which the essential cellular material is eventually produced (anabolism). In addition to doing this, the central core reactions produce ATP.

Reactions in the 'central core'. The initial catabolic routes which prepare the compounds present in the feed for entry into the central core are many and varied, depending on the nature of the feed and the type of microbe involved. The central core reactions can also vary to a certain extent but in general they can be taken as being:
  (a) the Embden–Meyerhof–Parnas (EMP) pathway and
  (b) the tricarboxylic acid (TCA) cycle
together with possibly:

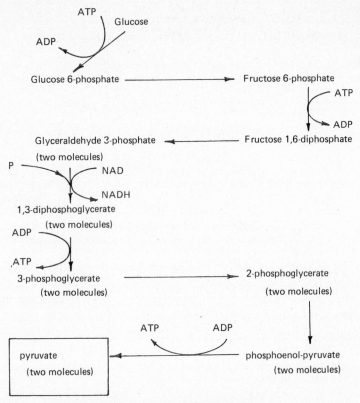

Fig. 1.9. The Embden–Meyerhof–Parnas (EMP) pathway.

(c) the hexose monophosphate (HMP) pathway and
(d) the Entner–Douderoff pathway

The EMP pathway which converts glucose to two molecules of pyruvate consists of ten enzymically catalysed reactions (Fig. 1.9). The most characteristic of these is the splitting of the six-carbon fructose 1,6-diphosphate into two molecules of triose phosphate by the enzyme aldolase. During the subsequent conversion to pyruvate, two molecules of ATP are formed for each triose phosphate – a total of four molecules of ATP per molecule of glucose. However, since two molecules of ATP have been used in the formation of the fructose diphosphate the overall gain to the cell is only two. The EMP pathway is common to both aerobic and anaerobic bacteria. The difference between the two types is the fate of the pyruvate and the two molecules of reduced NAD (NADH) that have been formed. Anaerobic systems will be discussed later. In aerobic systems the pyruvate undergoes an oxidative decarboxylation which involves the co-factor coenzyme A and which

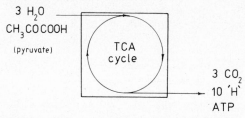

Fig. 1.10. Schematic representation of the TCA cycle showing the inputs and outputs.

results in the formation of acetyl coenzyme A. This then enters the TCA cycle.

$$CH_3 . CO . COOH + CoASH + NAD = CH_3 . CO . S\,CoA + CO_2 + NADH$$

The TCA cycle is a series of eight reactions which starts with the compound oxaloacetate condensing with the acetyl residue of the pyruvic acid and finishes with the regeneration of oxaloacetate, having achieved a complete degradation of the acetyl residue into carbon dioxide and hydrogen (Fig. 1.10). The cyclic process also generates one molecule of ATP.

Although this discussion has focussed on the degradation of carbohydrate molecules, it must be recognised that most other natural polymers are also oxidised through the TCA cycle. Long chain fatty acids and hydrocarbons eventually form acetyl CoA whilst the amino acids resulting from the breakdown of proteins form either acetyl CoA or TCA cycle intermediates For aerobic metabolism therefore the TCA cycle ought to be thought of as the core of the central core.

It must also be realised that, for carbohydrates, the EMP pathway is not the only route to pyruvate. In some cases, bacteria may not possess the key enzyme aldolase. In other cases, the monosaccharide produced by the preparatory catabolism may be a pentose rather than a hexose. In these cases other pathways are available. The most notable of these are the HMP route and the Entner–Douderoff pathway. Of these, the HMP route is perhaps of greater significance in that it provides a route for the transformation of pentose sugars to pyruvate. In its most complete mode of operation (Fig. 1.11) it transforms three molecules of the hexose, glucose, into three molecules of ribulose 5-phosphate (a pentose) (together with three molecules of carbon dioxide). The second stage of the pathway converts the three pentose molecules into two molecules of fructose 6-phosphate and one of glyceraldehyde 3-phosphate. All of these molecules can then enter the EMP pathway. Alternative reasons for the use of the HMP pathway are that it:

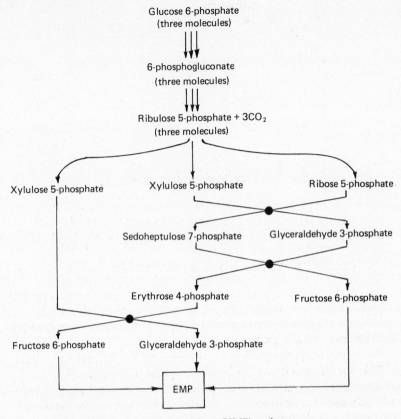

Fig. 1.11. The hexose monophosphate (HMP) pathway.

(a) generates pentose sugars which may be needed for nucleic acid synthesis and as precursors for aromatic synthesis or

(b) generates the reduced form of NAD-phosphate which is essential for reductive anabolism.

The final stage of the oxidation process involves the regeneration of the reduced nucleotides. This is accomplished by the passage of electrons along a redox chain. The compounds which transfer the electrons along these chains include flavoproteins, quinones and cytochromes. The actual sequence and the location of the chain within the cell varies with the species involved. In eucaryotic cells electron transport is sited in the mitochondria and, because it is possible to isolate these organelles and therefore to study the reactions in isolation, it is relatively well defined. In bacteria the process is located in the cytoplasmic membrane and is therefore more difficult to study. However, the current knowledge would indicate that (a) no one

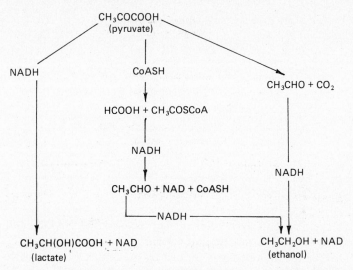

Fig. 1.12. Routes for the re-oxidation of NADH under anaerobic conditions.

bacterial species possesses an electron transport chain that can be considered as typical of procaryotic cells, and (b) the chains tend to be more complex with a greater degree of branching.

As well as transferring electrons the respiratory chain also generates ATP by the process known as oxidative phosphorylation. With mitochondrial respiration, three molecules of ATP are formed for every two hydrogens transferred from NADH. With bacteria the yields of ATP are not as well defined although in some cases it can be as high as three.

Electron transport chains can be terminated in one of three ways. In an aerobic system the terminal electron acceptor is molecular oxygen and this is in fact the only point in the overall oxidation that oxygen, as such, is used. This is the only mode of termination for mitochondrial systems. The bacterial transport systems are more flexible. A series of compounds can be used as terminal electron acceptors when anaerobic respiration is occurring. These compounds all contain inorganically bound oxygen (e.g. nitrate, sulphate) and, because they have a lower redox potential than molecular oxygen, produce a lower yield of ATP. The third process in which bacteria can participate is anaerobic fermentation. Under these circumstances the electrons associated with the reduced NAD are transferred directly to organic compounds. There is a wide variety of fermentation end-products and as such there is a range of routes for the re-oxidation of NADH. These can be found in standard text-books but examples are shown in Fig. 1.12. These are based on pyruvate, which cannot realistically be oxidised through the

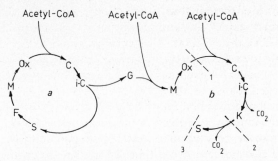

Fig. 1.13. The glyoxylate bypass. *a* TCA-cycle with 'bypass' *b* Open TCA-cycle with termination points at 1, 2 or 3.

TCA cycle since this generates further molecules of NADH, and show the formation of lactic acid and ethanol.

Most of the intermediates formed by the central core reactions can be syphoned off for biosynthesis. Whilst this does not cause any disruption to the continued operation of those pathways which have a distinct beginning and end, the withdrawal of intermediates from the TCA cycle can present problems. This is because of the cyclic nature of the reaction set. If compounds are withdrawn for anabolic reactions, it is essential that the four-carbon molecules are supplied by some other route. This is particularly true for oxaloacetate since it needs to be available to absorb acetyl CoA and thus to effect the terminal oxidation of the energy source. Two of these alternative routes are worth mentioning. The first of these allows pyruvate or phosphoenolpyruvate (EMP pathway) to react with carbon dioxide in one of several ways to form either oxaloacetate or its precursor in the TCA cycle, malate:

$$CH_3.CO.COOH + CO_2 \rightarrow HOOC.CH_2.CO.COOH.$$

The other (the glyoxylate bypass) involves the conversion of isocitrate into succinate and glyoxylic acid. This latter compound then reacts directly with acetyl CoA to form malate. As shown in Fig. 1.13, the malate then proceeds through an open TCA sequence which can be terminated after the formation of oxaloacetate, ketoglutarate or succinate, these compounds being the intermediates most likely to be needed for biosynthesis. The succinate formed along with the glyoxylate passes through a closed TCA sequence to generate more glyoxylic acid. In this way, acetyl CoA can be used both in its normal role, of producing carbon dioxide and reduced nucleotides (and therefore ATP), and for the production of cellular material.

It is the very wealth of pathways of this type, which allow such a ready manipulation both of raw materials and core intermediates, that endows the bacterial cell with such versatility. Indeed the diversity and interwoven network of these pathways can perhaps be thought of as analogous to a road map of England on which it is possible to identify the M1 (EMP/TCA), the A1 (HMP), other major routes and even B-roads. A totally inter-linked network such as this provides the facility of going from any point (or compound), *A*, to any other, provided that there are no blocked roads (lack of the specific enzymes), no lack of petrol (nutriment limitation) and no traffic police (enzyme inhibitors).

Enzymes are obviously very critical to the operation of cellular biochemistry. However, cells do not necessarily contain all their genetically coded enzymes at any one time. Those that are invariably present in significant quantities are known as *constitutive* enzymes. Those whose synthesis is either stimulated or suppressed by the demands of the cell (or more precisely by the presence of key compounds within the cell) are known as *induced* enzymes. It is because of this that the batch growth curve (Fig. 1.2) exhibits a lag phase. It is during this period that the synthesis of any necessary induced enzyme systems occurs. The way in which enzyme synthesis is induced and repressed and the way in which enzymes themselves can be activated and inhibited is complex and no attempt will be made to discuss this in detail. However, some explanation of the way in which a cell can control its metabolism is necessary. This control is facilitated by the sequential nature of the biochemical pathways. Let us consider a hypothetical sequence:

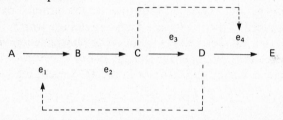

The cell can avoid the wasteful production of intermediates by the process known as feedback inhibition. Thus, for example, an excess of compound D is capable of inhibiting (reversibly) the enzyme (e_1) which catalyses the conversion of A to B. This effectively shuts down the sequence until the excess of D disappears. Conversely, to ensure that enzyme systems are ready to continue the sequential pathways, precursor activation allows an intermediate, say C, to activate an enzyme further along the chain (e.g. e_4 which converts D to E). This then is the fine-control system operated by the cell and it can be thought of as being based on the conservation of energy (ATP) principle. To understand how the control is achieved, in biochemical terms, requires an appreciation of the mechanisms involved in protein synthesis. This can be obtained from standard biochemical text-books.

What is probably of greater importance to the engineer is to know how enzymic reactions can be either quantified or expressed in mathematical terms. This is discussed in the next section.

1.2.3 *Enzyme kinetics*

The kinetic equations for enzymic reactions can be developed by considering the reaction of an enzyme (E) with a substrate (S). The first stage of the reaction is the reversible formation of an intermediate complex followed by an irreversible breakdown of the complex to produce the product and the free enzyme.

$$\text{E} + \text{S} \underset{k_2}{\overset{k_1}{\rightleftharpoons}} \text{Complex} \xrightarrow{k_3} \text{Product} + \text{E}$$

$$(e-c) \quad s \qquad\qquad c$$

The total concentration of enzyme within the reaction is e and the amount bound in the complex is c. If the substrate concentration is s, then the rate of change in the complex concentration is:

$$k_1(e-c)(s) - k_2(c) - k_3(c).$$

At equilibrium, this is zero so that

$$k_1(e-c)(s) = c(k_2+k_3)$$

$$c = \frac{es}{\left[\dfrac{k_2+k_3}{k_1}\right]+s} = \frac{es}{K_m+s}$$

The overall reaction velocity (v) is controlled by the rate at which the complex is converted to the product. Hence:

$$v = k_3 c$$

$$= \frac{k_3 es}{K_m+s}$$

The maximum velocity will occur when all the enzyme within the reaction is in the complex form. In other words:

$$v_{max} = k_3 e$$

Thus

$$v = \frac{s v_{max}}{K_m+s}$$

This is the equation of a hyperbola and K_m is the Michaelis–Menten constant. By substituting $K_m = s$, it can be seen that K_m is in fact equal to that substrate concentration which produces a reaction velocity of one-half the maximum velocity. The value of this constant can be determined experimentally by measuring the reaction velocities at a range of initial substrate concentrations. The data obtained from these experiments can be processed in several ways. The most usual is the

Lineweaver–Burk plot ($1/v$ against $1/s$) which gives an intercept on the
X-axis of $-1/K_m$. However, the accuracy of this technique has been
questioned and more rigorous techniques, which tend to use computers,
are available (see Cornish-Bowden, 1976; Clarke & Forster, 1983).

In dealing with wastewater treatment systems it is often more
important to consider microbial growth than reaction velocities. This
can be done by using the expression developed by Monod in the 1940s:

$$\mu = \mu_{max}\left[\frac{s}{K_s+s}\right]$$

together with the fact that the rate of change in any microbial
concentration will be proportional, at any given time, to the
concentration (x)

$$\text{i.e. } \frac{dx}{dt} = \mu x.$$

This proportionality constant, μ, is the specific growth rate. Combining
the two expressions gives

$$\frac{dx}{dt} = x\mu_{max}\left[\frac{s}{K_s+s}\right]$$

This can be related to the substrate removal by means of the yield
constant (Y) where

$$Y = -\frac{dx}{ds}$$

Thus

$$-\frac{ds}{dt} = \mu_{max}\left[\frac{x}{Y}\right]\left[\frac{S}{K_s+s}\right]$$

These equations, the Michaelis–Menten and the modified Monod, form
the basis for most of the mathematical models for bio-oxidation
systems (see Chapter 10).

1.3   Sterilisation

Sterility means the complete absence of microbes that are capable of
growth; it should therefore not be confused with disinfection, which is
the removal of those microbes which cause infection (together with a
good number of harmless microbes). As far as bacteria are concerned,
we can consider two types of agent: *bacteriostatic* agents which merely
inhibit the growth of bacteria and *bactericidal* agents which in fact kill
bacteria. These definitions are somewhat arbitrary as enough
bacteriostatic material will in fact kill and too little bactericidal will
merely inhibit. Although the mode of action will vary depending on the
particular agent being used, in general they can be said to act (a) on the
cell membrane, (b) on the nucleus or (c) by denaturation of the

proteins. It is generally stated that bacterial death is a logarithmic process. However, there are many deviations from this type of response, particularly when chemical agents are used. Under these circumstances, the death curve is sigmoidal in character. Having said this, it must be recognised that the concentration of a disinfectant and the temperature of the disinfection will influence the rate of death, so that as the concentration is increased there is likely to be a progression from the sigmoidal curve to one of an exponential nature. In the laboratory and in certain major industries the most reliable method of sterilisation is heat and in particular moist heat. Thermal death of microbes takes place as the result of the inactivation of cellular proteins (including enzymes). In defining sterilisation by heat, one of the most commonly used terms is the thermal death time (time to reach an acceptable level). Thermal death times for non-sporing bacteria range from a few hours at 47 °C to 60 minutes at 60 °C to 5 minutes at 70 °C. The spores of bacteria are much more resistant and to ensure that any spore-forms are killed it is necessary to use temperatures in excess of 100 °C. The most common way of doing this is to use pressurised steam. In the laboratory this means an autoclave (15 psi/15 minutes) or for very small volumes a domestic pressure cooker. Dry heat can also be used and is particularly useful for the sterilisation of laboratory glassware.

Another important means of sterilisation is ionising radiation. However, although radiation is used fairly widely the mechanism of the biocidal action is not fully understood. In general terms, radiation is thought to interfere with the cellular metabolism and it has been assumed that each cell possesses certain vulnerable 'targets' in which one or more 'hits' must be registered to bring about the inactivation of the target. When a target requires one 'hit' for the inactivation of a cell, an exponential death rate results; when a target requires two or more hits to inactivate the cell a sigmoidal death rate is the result. Most bacteria comply with the one hit mechanism although certain strains of *E. coli* indicate a two hit mechanism. There are two schools of thought as to which cellular components are the targets; one is the DNA, the other is the cell wall.

The resistance of bacteria to radiation is always greater when the bacteria are cultured in the laboratory than when they are in their natural state. These differences can be quite considerable but it is in fact not a difference in the actual resistance of the organism but is due to the different level of protection afforded by the different environments. In general terms vegetative organisms are more susceptible than spores, and Gram positive organisms are more resistant than Gram negative ones, although there is considerable overlap. Within the field of public health engineering the two most important types of radiation are ultra-violet and gamma radiation. Ultra-violet radiation has been used to disinfect water for swimming pools, water for public supply, and of course the ultra-violet radiation from the sun is relied upon to kill pathogens in sewage sludge which has been spread on the land. The main disadvantage of ultra-violet radiation is that it has a relatively low penetration, so that in the event of its being used as a disinfectant for water, the water must be irradiated as a thin film. As yet, the use of gamma radiation is still at the experimental stage, its main application being in the disinfection of sewage sludges prior to land application (see Chapter 9).

1.4 Freshwater biology

Having examined the characteristics of the more important microbial classes, together with some aspects of their biochemistry, we must now consider how the various species live and interact in the natural and man-made parts of the water cycle – in other words, their ecology.

The first hurdle that must be overcome is the meaning of the word ecology. This is the study of the interactions of different biological populations within a community which is defined either by a particular environment or by geographical or spatial restraints. Thus an anthropologist studying the behaviour of people in a remote village might be said to be examining the ecology of the village, just as a forest warden is a practising ecologist when he has to balance the requirements of trees, deer and sometimes sheep within the confines of his particular stretch of forest. Similarly, at a microbial level, the ecologist would be concerned about the way in which bacteria, protozoa and algae lived and died within, for example, a stabilisation pond, so as to achieve and maintain a steady state community. In non-human terms, it is the establishment of stable and reliable food chains which is the key factor in determining population levels and, therefore, for defining the condition of the eco-system; indeed, the same could be said for human systems if the earth were examined as a single eco-system. In a typical microbial eco-system, soluble nutriments would provide food for bacteria which would provide food for herbivorous protozoa which would provide food for carnivorous protozoa which would themselves provide food for successive levels of carnivorous organisms. Thus the number of organisms at any one level will, under steady state conditions, depend on the amount of food available for that level and the degree to which it itself is being culled by the next higher level. Some limitations are also placed on this type of food web by energy conservation principles. At each link in the food chain there is a reduction, in the amount of energy conserved, by an order of magnitude. Thus, in any food web, energy defines the number of

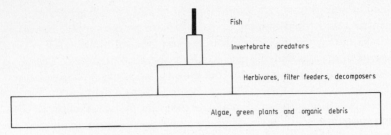

Fish

Invertebrate predators

Herbivores, filter feeders, decomposers

Algae, green plants and organic debris

Fig. 1.14. Trophic pyramid for river eco-system (based on 20 per cent energy conversion at each stage).

trophic levels, and the supply of food to the primary producers tends to define the numbers at the various levels (Fig. 1.14).

In any ecological study, there is a need to examine (a) the types of interaction that are taking place, and (b) how these vary with the different types of eco-system. The types of interaction that are most significant are:

(a) *Symbiosis* – this is where two organisms live together, both deriving some benefit from the other. For example *Paramecium bursaria* and the green algae, *Zoochlorella*. In this case, the former excretes carbon dioxide which is used by the algae which in turn produces oxygen which is used by the *Paramecium*.

(b) *Parasitism* – this is where one organism lives in or on another at the expense of the host.

(c) *Competition* – the competition most commonly found is that for nutriments. A typical example would be where bacteria and protozoans compete with each other for soluble organic matter.

(d) *Predation* – a typical example of this would be the situation where grazing ciliates and bacteria are interacting. The action of the ciliates is in effect to prevent the bacteria from reaching self-limiting numbers and as such there is a degree of stimulation of the bacterial metabolism. Whether this stimulation is due solely to the predation by the ciliates or whether some other factor is involved is not precisely clear at the moment. It may well be, therefore, that predation and stimulation should be considered as two distinct interactions.

These interrelations within a community give it stability. Indeed it is thought that the greater the diversity (i.e. the number of species in relation to the total number of individuals) of a community, the greater is the stability.

Besides the interactions between populations within a community, the community as a whole interacts with its non-living environment. This leads to the more advanced definition of an eco-system as being any area of nature including non-living material and living organisms

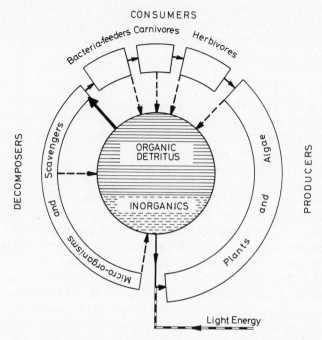

Fig. 1.15. Diagrammatic representation of an eco-system (Hawkes, 1977).

interacting to produce an exchange of material between the living and non-living.

In any aquatic eco-system therefore we have to identify three main groups within the population (Fig. 1.15): (a) the producers; (b) the consumers; and (c) the decomposers.

The producers are mainly the plants and algae which convert inorganic matter to organic matter by the process of photosynthesis. A useful side effect of this process is the production of oxygen. The consumers are mainly animals, although the protozoan population can also be considered as falling within this classification. Consumers feed directly, as herbivores, or indirectly, as carnivores, on the organic matter synthesised by the producers. Waste matter resulting from the activity and death of the producers and consumers is degraded by the decomposers. These are mainly bacteria and fungi although some scavenging animals are also significant in this classification. The decomposers are an essential part of the eco-system as they bring about the recycling of inorganics.

The balance and diversity of life within any eco-system will depend on both the physical and the chemical characteristics of the aquatic habitat.

In considering rivers and streams it must be remembered that as far as any particular point on a river is concerned, the ecology will be influenced by a gain of material from upstream and a loss of material downstream. Furthermore this material can range from soluble nutriments to microbial and animal life. Considering the river as a single unit, it can be seen that an external input of energy (in biological terms) is necessary to replenish the energy which is lost to the sea. One can identify two main types of energy-material which are inputs to a river system: soluble mineral salts (nitrates, phosphates etc.) originating from land drainage; and organic matter in the form of detritus washed from the land, particularly after heavy rains, and dead vegetation. Each of these inputs supports different populations, the mineral salts being used by primary producers and the organics by saprobic organisms. However, the relative effects will depend on the nature of the river habitat. In shallow stretches, which permit good light penetration, the photosynthetic utilisation of the mineral salts will be dominant, whereas in the deep slow stretches, where organic debris will accumulate, a dominant population of saprobic organisms will develop.

In addition to the microbial populations, the higher animals are of considerable significance in river ecology (i.e. worms, molluscs, crustaceans, insect nymphs and larvae and, of course, fish). In the same way that the different river habitats promote different dominant microbial populations, so the higher animals have different physical attributes which enable them to populate the different stretches of a river. For example, some species of Mayfly nymph are flattened, which enables them to withstand currents, whilst the larvae of other species have specific organs of attachment. Fauna of this type, which have an ability to withstand current, are characteristic of rapidly flowing stretches of the river whereas fauna without this ability tend to populate the slower reaches of a watercourse.

In addition to this differentiation of the fauna on the basis of the physical characteristics of the river, there will also be a differentiation as a result of the chemical characteristics of the water. Aquatic animals differ in their tolerance of oxygen depletion (and therefore pollution). For example, the nymphs of stone-flies and most mayflies require well aerated waters; the water louse (*Asellus aquaticus*) can withstand considerable de-oxygenation, and some mud-dwelling forms, such as the larvae of the *Chironomus riparius* group, have been found to prefer low oxygen levels. This variability in the tolerance of pollution provides a possible tool for assessing the degree of pollution within a river (see Chapter 2).

In a totally uncontaminated stream, therefore, there will be a succession of eco-systems from the source to the sea, based purely on the physical nature of the stream (e.g. its depth, its temperature, its current). However, because rivers are flowing systems, there can be a blurring of distinction with species from one eco-system being carried downstream into an alien system.

1.5   The biology of wastewater treatment systems

No assessment of the biology of wastewater treatment systems, and therefore the interactions of the component flora, can realistically cover every type of treatment without becoming a lengthy and possibly repetitive exercise. This discussion will therefore be restricted to three general types of reactor:

> activated sludge
> attached film systems (trickling filters)
> anaerobic systems.

The activated sludge system is a continuous fermentation with a solids feedback and the activated sludge itself is a flocculated mass of microbes, mainly bacteria and protozoa, which has the ability to (a) degrade the substrate and (b) settle quickly in quiescent conditions. The bacteria involved (about $10^{10}/g$ mixed liquor solids) tend in the main to be Gram negative species and include carbon oxidisers and nitrogen oxidisers; floc-formers and non floc-formers; aerobes and facultative anaerobes. It is usually not necessary either to count them or to identify them. However, specialised research needs may dictate that this be done. This is not as simple and straightforward a task as might at first be supposed. Counting, or at least viable counting, requires that the sample is diluted until a concentration of about 30–300 bacteria per ml has been achieved, and then growing the bacteria on a nutrient material so that individual colonies can be counted. The first problem is obtaining a representative sample. The second is separating the bacteria from the floc matrix of biological polymers, dead bacteria and protozoans. This can be done by some form of homogensiation, but too severe a technique will rupture viable cells, while too mild a method will not effect a complete separation. The final problem is the selection of the nutrient material. The bacteria in any sewage treatment system function in a severely nutriment limited environment, truly on the knife-edge of starvation, and their transference to a rich medium can bring about 'substrate-accelerated death'. In addition, there is no one medium that can be expected to support the growth of all the species present. These problems have been discussed in greater detail by Pike & Carrington (1972), who also offer some possible solutions.

The species which are present will be those selected by the chemical nature of the sewage or trade effluent being fed to the plant and by the conditions of operation. This latter factor is critical in maintaining an

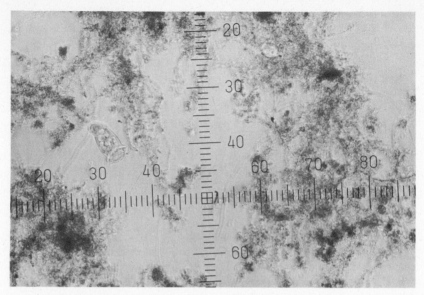

Fig. 1.16. Stalked ciliates in activated sludge.

adequately sized population of the nitrifying bacteria, *Nitrosomonas* and *Nitrobacter*. These are slow growing species and it is therefore essential to adjust the sludge wastage rate so that they are not washed-out. Although floc-formers will in the main be selected by the process of solids concentration (i.e. settlement) and feed-back, activated sludge can become dominated by filamentous bacteria. This situation is frequently associated with poor settlement characteristics. Since this is a key function of the process, the identification of these species has been examined in some detail and as a result a detailed method of identification has been developed based on the shape of the filaments, and their behaviour to the Gram stain, the Neisser stain and a sulphur storage test (Eikelboom, 1975).

The final group of bacteria that are worth mentioning are the actinomycetes, in particular *Nocardia* and *Rhodococcus* spp. These species are thought to cause the formation of stable foams ('chocolate mousse') on activated sludge tanks. The reasons for the proliferation of these species are not known and methods for their control have yet to be established.

The protozoan population of activated sludge, which can be as large as 5×10^4 ml^{-1}, will include flagellates, amoebae and ciliates. Indeed over 200 different species of protozoa have been found in activated sludges. Ciliates are the most frequently occurring type and one order has been found to constitute about a third of the species identified. This is the order to which species such as *Vorticella* and *Opercularia* belong. These are sessile types which attach themselves to the sludge flocs (see Fig. 1.16). The other significant type of ciliate in activated sludge are the species which creep over the sludge surface (e.g. *Aspidisca; Trachelophylum*). The actual balance of these species will depend, as with bacteria, on the nature of the sewage and the plant operation. It is sometimes claimed that protozoans are more susceptible than bacteria to toxic agents and heavy metals and that a common cause of poor operation is disruption of the protozoan population.

Whilst this tends to be true for pure cultures, the data from full-scale plant tends to be both variable and frequently conflicting (Curds, 1975). It is likely that this is caused by the capacity of the sludge matrix to adsorb or chelate metal ions, thus reducing their toxicity. The organic loading rate has been found to affect the number of ciliates and it has also been shown that major changes to the loading rate can disrupt the stability of the sludge and thus its balance of protozoans. Generally a sludge in poor condition is characterised by a predominance of flagellates whereas a good sludge will contain a dominant population of ciliates (Curds & Cockburn, 1970).

The role of the protozoa would appear to be one of maintaining a steady bacterial population, particularly by feeding on free-swimming bacteria which would otherwise produce a turbid effluent. However, *Trachelophylum pusillum* is a carnivorous ciliate and as such maintains a check on the bacteria-feeding population. It can be seen therefore that the protozoa have an important function in determining the quality of effluent produced and it has been suggested that this could be predicted from a knowledge of the numbers and types of protozoa present (Curds & Cockburn, 1970). However, it must be stressed that this approach can be an oversimplification and that many factors can affect the sludge ecology.

Despite this caveat it has proved possible to develop a mathematical model for the process based on a four-component sludge (Curds, 1971). These components were floc-forming and non-floc-forming bacteria together with two species of ciliated protozoa (free-swimming and attached). The results showed that this was a realistic basis for assessing the activated sludge process in terms of the cyclic succession of species. More complex models will give a still closer approximation to the actual behaviour, thus providing the biologist with a tool which will enable him to explain and possibly predict the operational idiosyncrasies of what is in fact a complex eco-system.

Although bacteria and protozoa dominate the biology of activated sludge, other organisms can be present. These include fungi, nematodes and rotifers. The fungi appear to have two possible roles: as a consumer of organic matter (particularly if the aeration tank pH is low

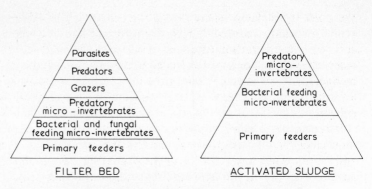

Fig. 1.17. Trophic pyramids for trickling filters and activated sludge.

and bacterial activity is therefore inhibited) or as a predator for nematodes and rotifers. The former is more common but, irrespective of the role, a proliferation of fungi usually imparts poor settlement characteristics to the sludge. The nematodes fulfil a similar role to that of the protozoa, ingesting bacteria. The rotifers also graze on the sludge flocs removing small particles that would otherwise cause turbidity. They also break up large flocs thus creating fresh adsorption sites.

Trickling filters, which, as will be seen in Chapter 3, are packed bed reactors with a counter-current flow of air and substrate, have as their active content a biological film growing on the packing material. This biofilm has a much greater diversity than activated sludge (see Fig. 1.17). However, the organisms involved are in the main the same as those described in the discussion on activated sludge. Thus, bacteria (and occasionally fungi) form the lowest trophic level and metabolise the polluting matter. Protozoans, rotifers and nematodes then graze on the bacterial film. The differences between the filter biofilm and activated sludge are seen not only in the greater numbers and frequency of occurrence of rotifers and nematodes but also in the presence of higher organisms. These include fly larvae and worms, both of which prey upon species in the lower trophic levels. Trickling filters can also support the growth of algae in their upper regions where light is available.

The species involved in this ecological pyramid are not really significant to the design of filters and although there are certain problems which stem from biological imbalances it could also be argued that detailed biological knowledge is not relevant to operational techniques.

Two of the main problems that occur are ponding and spring sloughing. Since these are primarily an operational concern, they will be discussed in Chapter 6. Nitrification in trickling filters tends to occur in the lower layers. Here, where the carbon content of the effluent has been significantly reduced, the slow growing nitrifiers are able to compete with the carbon oxidisers. However, in an overloaded filter where the carbon content remains high, the nitrifiers are less able to compete and can be forced out of the filter. If this happens, the result is an unsatisfactory (in terms of the removal of ammoniacal nitrogen) effluent.

It is possible to model the processes within a fixed film reactor. In most cases these models examine the film as a single biological entity and do not assess any variation in the populations within the film. The general basis for the models is substrate removal. Thus, under steady state conditions, the substrate input to the film (assumed to be controlled by diffusion and therefore by Fick's law) can be equated to substrate removal within the film (Michaelis/Monod kinetics) (Atkinson & Howell, 1975; Williamson & McCarty, 1976). Despite the existence of models of this type, their use for design purposes is not common.

The general heading of anaerobic reactors encompasses both sludge digestors and the more modern type of reactor used for the digestion of liquid wastes (see Chapter 3). Despite their differences in design and operational characteristics, their biology is essentially the same. The main concern in operating these systems is to ensure that various bacterial species function in a balanced and sequential way. Therefore, although other species may exist in these reactors, the attention of biologists is focussed more or less exclusively on the bacteria.

These can be thought of as falling into two generalised types: the hydrolytic species, which degrade large molecules into their component 'monomers', and the post-hydrolytic species. The way in which this latter group function is complicated and not adequately understood. Certainly it can be said that acetate, hydrogen and carbon dioxide are formed as precursors to methane. It can also be said that some 70 per cent of the methane is formed from the methyl group of the acetate by acetophilic methanogens (e.g. *Methanothrix* spp., *Methanosarcina* spp.), the remainder coming from the oxidation of hydrogen (at the expense of carbon dioxide) by the hydrogenophilic methanogens (e.g. *Methanobacterium* spp.) (Fig. 1.18). However, these steps frequently involve 'quasi-symbiotic' relationships between fermentative bacteria, obligate proton reducers, acetogenic proton reducers and methanogens (see Zehnder *et al.*, 1982; Mah, 1983). In some steps a species can act alone, in other cases species act in very close partnership (i.e. as a couplet). A typical example of such a combination is that of *Methanobacterium bryantii* and the 'S-organism' (this combination was originally thought to be a single species *Methanobacterium omelianskii*) which converts ethanol to acetate and methane.

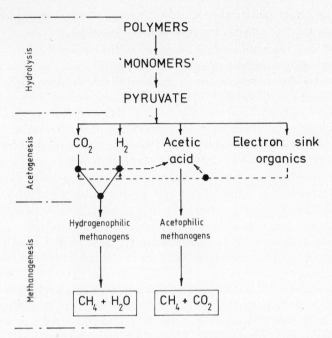

Fig. 1.18. A simplified outline of the processes taking place in anaerobic digestion.

The second part of this sequence is critical since hydrogen inhibits the growth of the 'S-organism'. In fact that partial pressure of hydrogen can be thought of as a regulator both of intermediate fatty acid catabolism and of methane formation. As such it is essential that the methanogens maintain the hydrogen concentration at a low level.

$$2\,CH_3CH_2OH + 2H_2O$$

$$\downarrow$$

$$2\,CH_3COOH + 4H_2$$

$$\vdash\!\!-\!\!-\!\!-\ CO_2$$

$$\downarrow$$

$$CH_4 + 2H_2O$$

Hydrogen is also involved in the inhibition of methane production by the presence of high concentrations of sulphate ions. These are converted to sulphide by the sulphate-reducing bacteria (e.g. *Desulphovibrio* spp.). These species compete for the methane precursors acetate and hydrogen and in fact utilise them more effectively than the methanogens. The production of methane is therefore reduced. A secondary inhibition of methanogenesis can occur if the soluble sulphide ion concentration exceeds 200 mg l^{-1}.

These discussions demonstrate the importance of having a full appreciation of the biology and the interactions which occur in wastewater treatment systems. Obviously not every combination has been fully covered nor has the effect of every type of substrate. However, specialist books and research papers are usually available to provide any supplementary data that may be needed.

2   Water pollution and its control

2.1   Defining pollution

The daily consumption of water in England and Wales is some
16×10^6 m³. This includes both domestic and industrial use. The
majority of this is eventually discharged to inland rivers and streams,
the total length of which is some 24000 miles (say 10^4–10^5 Ml). In
addition, about 20×10^6 m³ are abstracted directly from these rivers by
industry, used and then returned. Some of these waters will have
become contaminated during their use and it is therefore necessary for
them to undergo treatment before they can be discharged. Failure to do
this could result in serious changes in the chemical composition of the
river water, causing deleterious changes in the river ecology, possibly
coupled with a significant degree of oxygen depletion. At worst, toxic
contaminants could cause the total eradication of life within the river.
One can therefore consider pollutants as being oxygen-depleting or
directly toxic to the river fauna. Discharges of these types certainly
cause the more spectacular effects on river systems. However, there are
other types of pollutant which have more insidious effects. Pollution
can result from the addition of water whose temperature is greater than
that of the river itself. If the volume of water added or the temperature
differential is sufficient to cause an increase in the river temperature, for
even a short stretch, the biological activity and productivity within the
river will be increased. Furthermore, the capacity of the water to retain
oxygen will be lowered. Again a change in the ecological balance will
result. Similarly, if the pH of the river water is changed to any marked
degree, the balance within the biological food webs will be altered.

Pollution can also be caused by the addition of settleable inert solids.
These can produce a blanket of fine silt on the river bed. If this were
originally sand or gravel, the result would be a change in the biological
communities inhabiting the bed and, therefore, a change or at least an
imbalance in the food chains within that stretch of river. Pollution,
therefore, can be thought of as any discharge to a watercourse which is
capable of causing changes to the stream communities either on a
long- or short-term basis. Rivers within the UK have to accept a
significant load of oxygen-demanding pollutants. However, as long as
the load on any particular stretch is not excessive, the river can

Table 2.1. *Sources and sinks for dissolved oxygen and BOD within a river system*

Parameter	Source	Sink
DO	Photosynthesis	Bottom mud respiration Plant respiration at night
BOD	Surface run-off Bottom deposits, both soluble and particulate	Particulate settlement

assimilate it. Discharges of this type which have occurred on a regular, continuous basis for some time are likely to have caused a change in the down-stream ecology (relative to the time before the discharge). As long as the load is not increased, this 'new' down-stream ecology will be stable and, in a lot of cases, will be acceptable. Pollution control measures must therefore be aimed at:

(a) reducing the polluting load where the down-stream ecology is unacceptable
(b) ensuring that existing loads are not increased to a level where the ecology becomes unstable or unacceptable
(c) ensuring that discharges containing material which is toxic, rather than oxygen-demanding, do not take place.

Although the ecology is the aspect which must be protected, in practice the control of pollution is exercised in terms of chemical determinands. The most usual way of judging the effect that a single point discharge has on a river is by monitoring the concentrations of the biochemical oxygen demand (BOD) and dissolved oxygen (DO) down-stream of that discharge. Alternatively these can be predicted by using the Streeter–Phelps equation:

$$D_t = \frac{k_1 L_a}{k_2 - k_1}[10^{-k_1 t} - 10^{-k_2 t}] + D_a 10^{-k_2 t}$$

where D_t = DO deficit at time = t, D_a = DO deficit at time = 0, L_a = ultimate BOD of water immediately below discharge, k_1 = BOD decay constant, k_2 = re-aeration constant.

Although the derivation of this expression is based on a number of assumptions (e.g. BOD is removed *only* by biological oxidation; DO replenishment occurs only by re-aeration from the atmosphere), it is widely used and usually gives an acceptable analysis (Tebbutt, 1979). The BOD decay constant (k_1) will depend on the nature of the discharge, but a typical value for domestic sewage is 0.17–0.36 d^{-1}. The re-aeration constant (k_2) can either be measured or calculated from the depth and flow-rate of the river (Owens, Edwards & Gibbs, 1964). However, in many models it is taken as being 1.0 d^{-1}. Although this technique will give a relatively accurate model of the DO sag, it must be remembered that there will be several other sources and sinks of oxygen within a normal river situation. Also, BOD inputs and removals will occur through natural processes unrelated to biological oxidation (see Table 2.1 and Downing, 1971).

The actual concentration of organic pollutants at any point down-stream of a discharge can be calculated, in terms of the ultimate oxygen demand (UOD), from:

$$L_t = L_a 10^{-k_1 t}$$

The interconversions of BOD and UOD are made by:

$$B = L(1 - 10^{-5k_1})$$

where L_t = the UOD at time = t, B = the BOD at any time, L = the UOD at any time. The way in which these expressions are used can be demonstrated by the following simple example. In a more complex situation, where the calculations become repetitive, a computer would probably be used (Tebbutt, 1982).

A sewage works discharges an effluent with the following *average* characteristics: flow = $1 \text{ m}^3 \text{ s}^{-1}$, BOD = 25 mg l^{-1}, DO = 6.25 mg l^{-1}. The average flow in the river is $2.75 \text{ m}^3 \text{ s}^{-1}$ with a velocity of 0.14 m s^{-1}. If the BOD and DO of the river immediately upstream of the discharge were 6.1 mg l^{-1} and 10 mg l^{-1} respectively, calculate the point of maximum oxygen deficit in the river and the BOD at a point 10 km downstream. Assume that $k_1 = 0.17$, $k_2 = 0.4$ and the saturation DO concentration is 11 mg l^{-1}.

(i) Calculate time of travel

$$t = \frac{10 \times 10^3}{0.14 \times 60 \times 60 \times 24} = 0.83 \text{ days}$$

(ii) Determine BOD below discharge by mass balance

$$(2.75 \times 6.1) + (1 \times 25) = 3.75 \times B$$
$$B = 11.14 \text{ mg l}^{-1}$$

(iii) Convert BOD to UOD

$$L(1 - 10^{-0.17 \times 5}) = B = 11.14$$
$$L = 12.97 \text{ mg l}^{-1}$$

(iv) Calculate UOD 10 km down-stream

$$L_t = 12.97 \times 10^{-0.17 \times 0.83}$$
$$= 9.38 \text{ mg l}^{-1}$$

(v) Convert UOD to BOD

$$B = 9.38 (1 - 10^{-0.17 \times 5})$$
$$= 8.06 \text{ mg l}^{-1}$$

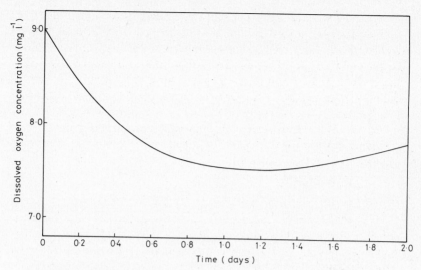

Fig. 2.1. Oxygen sag curve.

(vi) Determine DO below discharge by mass balance

$$(2.75 \times 10) + (1 \times 6.25) = 3.75 \times d$$
$$d = 9 \text{ mg l}^{-1}$$
$$D_a = 11 - d = 2$$

(vii) Apply Streeter–Phelps

Let $t = 0.05$

$$D_t = \left(\frac{12.97 \times 0.17}{0.4 - 0.17}\right)(10^{-0.17 \times 0.05} - 10^{-0.4 \times 0.05})$$
$$+ (2 \times 10^{-0.4 \times 0.05})$$
$$= 9.587 \, (0.9806 - 0.9550) + (2 \times 0.9550)$$
$$= (9.587 \times 0.0256) + 1.91$$
$$= 0.245 + 1.91$$
$$= 2.155$$

$$\therefore \text{DO} = 11 - 2.155 = 8.845$$

t	0.05	0.1	0.4	0.8	1.0	1.2	1.4
D_t	2.16	2.30	2.95	3.38	3.46	3.48	3.45
DO	8.84	8.70	8.05	7.62	7.54	7.52	7.55

From Fig. 2.1, the maximum oxygen sag occurs after a period of 1.15 days.

2.2 Measurement of pollution

The precise experimental details of the tests involved in the measurement of pollution may be found in any recognised text of

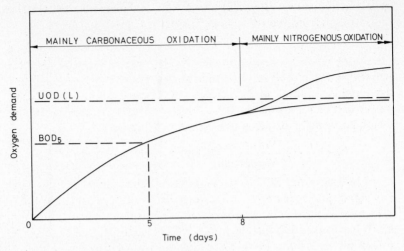

Fig. 2.2. Typical oxygen demand curve.

standard analytical methods (e.g. Department of the Environment, 1972).

2.2.1   *Biochemical oxygen demand*

The most usual method for measuring organic pollution is the biochemical oxygen demand (BOD). This test depends on the fact that when organic matter is mixed with bacteria and oxygen, the organic matter is oxidised and the concentration of the dissolved oxygen is reduced. If the sample volume is fixed and the amount of available oxygen is both restricted and known then the amount of oxygen used, after an incubation period of 120 ± 1 h (5 days) at a temperature of 20 °C in the dark, is a measure of the amount of organic matter. These restrictions are achieved by using

(a) a stoppered bottle
(b) a fully aerated sample.

To ensure that the oxygen is not totally depleted, in which case it would be impossible to calculate a BOD value, the sample should be diluted. It is usually advisable to test a series of dilutions, the ideal dilution being one which uses 50 per cent of the oxygen initially available. Another important feature, when industrial effluents are being tested, is to ensure that the microbial flora being used to perform the oxidation is fully acclimatised to the waste under investigation. If these details are not followed, then significant errors will result (Davies, 1971).

If the normal oxygen demand curve is followed for an extended period it can be seen (Fig. 2.2) that there is a departure after a period of 8–10 days from the theoretical first order curve given by:

$$\frac{\mathrm{d}c}{\mathrm{d}t} = -Kc$$

where c = concentration of organic matter, K = rate constant. This deviation is the result of the nitrification demand being superimposed on the carbonaceous demand. Nitrification is a two-stage process in which ammonia is oxidised to nitrate (see Chapter 3):

$$NH_4^+ + 2O_2 \xrightarrow[\textit{Nitrobacter}]{\textit{Nitrosomonas}} NO_3^- + 2H^+ + H_2O$$

In the laboratory BOD test therefore this effect is not normally of any significance. However, when treated effluents are being tested there may be a sufficiently large number of nitrifying bacteria present for this secondary demand to have a considerable effect. If this is the case and it is of benefit only to know the carbonaceous demand then it is usual to suppress nitrification by adding an inhibitor, allyl thiourea (ATU). The BOD test with all its potential errors is one which is well established, having been used since the early part of this century. Because of this, it has considerable value, and most workers would claim to understand both what the test itself means and what the significance of a particular BOD value is in any particular context. However, a major problem with the test is the length of time necessary to obtain a result. Because of this, tests have been developed which are much more rapid. These are based on the chemical oxidation of organic matter.

2.2.2 Chemical oxygen demand (COD)

The most commonly used chemical oxidant is acidic potassium dichromate. When a known excess of this reagent is refluxed with an aqueous sample containing organic matter, a very high degree of oxidation of most of the organics is achieved. It is therefore possible, by measuring the amount of unreacted dichromate (a simple titration with ferrous ammonium sulphate), to determine the amount of organic matter in the original sample. As with the BOD test it is essential for there to be an adequate residue of the oxidant at the end of the reflux period (2 hours) and therefore it is quite common to use diluted samples. Although this test has the potential for providing a rapid assessment of the degree of pollution, it is not without shortcomings. Probably the most significant of these is that it gives no indication as to whether the organic matter can be degraded biologically and, if so, at what rate. Also, not all molecules are oxidised by this type of treatment. However, it is a test which is widely used, particularly in

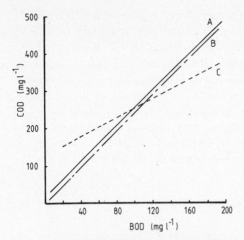

Fig. 2.3. Regression lines for COD/BOD relationships. A: Thames Water Authority (personal communication) – $y = 2.37x + 16.64$; B: Aziz & Tebbutt, 1980 – $y = 2.42x - 2.95$; C: North West Water Authority (personal communication) – $y = 1.27x + 125.07$.

trade effluent control (see Chapter 11), and as the reaction conditions are so intense the degree of error is much less than that resulting from the other oxidants which have been used from time to time by the Water Industry. Also, for a given effluent, it is possible to develop statistical relationships between COD and BOD values (see Fig. 2.3). As a first approximation, therefore, the COD value can be used to calculate the BOD of a sample. The uses of this approach for quality control purposes are obvious.

2.2.3   *Total organic carbon (TOC)*

This is an instrumental method for determining the amount of organic matter in an aqueous sample. With a fully calibrated system, a single determination could take as little as ten minutes. There are a variety of instruments available and in the main they rely on converting the carbonaceous organic matter into a detectable gas using an elevated temperature in conjunction with a catalyst. In most of the cases, the gas is carbon dioxide which is detected by an infra-red analyser. The inorganic carbon (carbonates and bicarbonates) is either determined by a separate analysis (again as carbon dioxide) or is removed, by acidification, stripping and absorption, before the main analysis. The output from the detection devices is usually fed to a chart recorder and the peak height taken to be equivalent to the carbon concentration. This is acceptable as long as the instrument is adjusted to give a sharp peak since under these circumstances peak area (the true measure of carbon concentration) and peak height approximate to the same answer. In some cases, this will depend upon the way in which the sample is introduced and certainly with one instrument, this will depend upon the technique of the operator. However, this is usually a question of training and good instrument maintenance. Given this, the method provides reliable and repeatable data which, as with COD values, can be related to the BOD of the sample.

In addition, because of its speed it enables a large number of replicate measurements to be made, thus improving the accuracy if necessary. However, any TOC:BOD (or TOC:COD) relationships should only be used as guidelines; there is no theoretical basis for any of the relationships.

2.2.4 Ultimate oxygen demand (UOD).

The BOD test as it is normally carried out (5 days at 20 °C) was designed to simulate the conditions prevailing when an element of organic matter was introduced into a typical river in the UK. However, as can be seen from Fig. 2.2, after the 5-day test period a significant amount of the organic matter still remains to exert an oxygen demand. It is therefore necessary, on occasions, either to measure a long-term BOD (quite often after 20 days) or to calculate a theoretical ultimate oxygen demand (L). This can be done from a knowledge of the 5-day BOD (B) and the BOD rate constant (k_1):

$$B = L(1 - 10^{-k_1 \times 5})$$

The UOD is used in river-modelling calculations and either the 20-day BOD or the UOD may be of use in assessing the effect that suspended organic matter could have on a river system if it were to become deposited on the river bed.

2.2.5 Other determinands

Although oxygen demands are probably the most commonly used parameters for defining pollution, other determinands are also important. For domestic sewage and simple organic trade effluents, the concentrations of suspended solid matter and of ammoniacal nitrogen are significant parameters. The former gives a measure of the material which could be deposited within the river system either to exert a long-term oxygen demand or to blanket the river bed and thus alter the ecology of that part of the river. Ammoniacal nitrogen must be considered as an important pollutant for three main reasons:

(a) It will exert an oxygen demand
(b) It can be toxic to fish
(c) It will increase the chlorine demand of the water if it is to be abstracted, treated and chlorinated at a point down-stream of the discharge.

Table 2.2. *Concentrations of total ammonia which contain an un-ionised ammonia concentration of 0.025 mg l^{-1}*

Temperature (°C)	pH			
	7.0	7.5	8.0	8.5
5	19.6	6.3	2.0	0.65
10	13.4	4.3	1.37	0.45
15	9.1	2.9	0.93	0.31
20	6.3	2.0	0.65	0.22

From European Inland Fisheries Advisory Commission, 1970.

The oxygen demand is the result of the bacterial conversion of ammonia to nitrate. On the basis of the stoichiometric equation, each unit mass of nitrogen, in the form of ammonia, will require 4.57 units of oxygen. This can mean that, in the event of a discharge containing appreciable quantities of ammoniacal nitrogen, the oxygen demand due to nitrification can have a greater potential for de-oxygenation than that of the carbonaceous BOD. The toxicity to fish is caused by the un-ionised form of ammonia, NH_3. The level of ammoniacal nitrogen that can be tolerated in waters that are to be used as fisheries will therefore depend on those factors which affect the pH of the water and hence the concentration of the non-ionised form. These have been discussed in detail by the European Inland Fisheries Advisory Committee (EIFAC, 1970). The main suggestion made by this committee about ammonia toxicity was that the maximum concentration of un-ionised ammonia that could be tolerated by fish or fry over an extended period ought to be taken as 0.025 mg l^{-1}. The concentrations of total ammonia which will contain this value can be assessed from the temperature and the pH of the water (see Table 2.2). The toxicity of free ammonia (and, for that matter, of other potentially noxious chemicals) is often assessed on the basis of the LC_{50} (48 hours) value. This is the concentration of toxin which is lethal to 50 per cent of the test fish after an exposure time of 48 hours. For most freshwater fish species this value is around 0.5 mg free ammonia l^{-1}. Work by the Water Pollution Research Laboratory (Ministry of Technology, 1967) has shown that free ammonia concentrations of one-tenth of this value ought to be harmless to most fish. This figure is comparable with the level of 0.025 mg l^{-1} suggested by EIFAC.

The flora and fauna of inland streams also need to be protected from toxic pollutants. Typical of these are phenols, heavy metals and cyanides. In those cases where such materials are known to be present, their concentration in the final discharge will need to be restricted. In

Table 2.3. *EIFAC limits for toxic materials (mg l⁻¹)*

Toxin/Fish	Salmonid	Cyprinid
phenols	1.0 ⎫	2.0 ⎫
cresols	1.0 ⎬ a	2.0 ⎬ a
xylenols	1.0 ⎭	2.0 ⎭
2,5-xylenol	0.5	—
zinc	0.03[b]	0.3[b]
	0.3[c]	1.0[c]
copper	5.0[b]	—
	40.0[c]	—

[a] either singly or in total.
[b] 95 percentile value for water hardness = 10 mg CaCO$_3$ l⁻¹.
[c] 95 percentile value for water hardness = 100 mg CaCo$_3$ l⁻¹.

general, the level of restriction will depend on the type of fish which
dominate the receiving stream, that is to say salmonid or cyprinid
(game or coarse fish). The former are usually more sensitive to the
action of poisons. EIFAC recommendations have been made for the
more commonly occurring toxic agents (see Table 2.3). However, these
figures refer to individual toxins acting in isolation, a situation unlikely
to occur very often in practice. What is more important is to be able to
assess their cumulative effect.

Attempts have been made to do this by determining a proportional
toxicity factor (PT) for each toxin present, where:

$$PT = \frac{\text{concentration of toxin}}{LC_{50} \text{ (48 hour)}}.$$

The total toxicity factor is then found from the summation of the
individual PT values (Brown, 1968). However, although it has been
shown that the value of the total toxicity factor can be related to the
presence or absence of fish (Solbe, 1973), the errors inherent in
calculating the PT values are such that the total toxicity factor is an
inadequate method for assessing water quality with the accuracy that
would be required for the setting of statutory or quasi-legal standards.

2.3   The classification of surface water

Water quality is almost invariably defined, in the first instance, in terms
of the chemical characteristics of the water. Within the UK, the
chemical classification currently in use is that recommended by the
National Water Council (1977) (see Table 2.4). This method defines
four general qualities of water (good; fair; poor; bad) in terms of five

Table 2.4. *Suggested classification of river quality*

River Class	Quality criteria	Remarks	Current potential uses
1A	**Class limiting criteria** (95 percentile) (i) Dissolved oxygen saturation greater than 80% (ii) Biochemical oxygen demand not greater than 3 mg l^{-1} (iii) Ammonia not greater than 0.4 mg l^{-1} (iv) Where the water is abstracted for drinking water, it complies with requirements for A2 water (v) Non-toxic to fish in EIFAC terms (or best estimates if EIFAC figures not available)	(i) Average BOD probably not greater than 1.5 mg l^{-1} (ii) Visible evidence of pollution should be absent	(i) Water of high quality suitable for potable supply abstractions and for all other abstractions (ii) Game or other high class fisheries (iii) High amenity value
1B	(i) DO greater than 60% saturation (ii) BOD not greater than 5 mg l^{-1} (iii) Ammonia not greater than 0.9 mg l^{-1} (iv) Where water is abstracted for drinking water, it complies with the requirements for A2^a water (v) Non-toxic to fish in EIFAC terms (or best estimates if EIFAC figures not available)	(i) Average BOD probably not greater than 2 mg l^{-1} (ii) Average ammonia probably not greater than 0.5 mg l^{-1} (iii) Visible evidence of pollution should be absent (iv) Waters of high quality which cannot be placed in Class 1A because of high proportion of high quality effluent present or because of the effect of physical factors such as canalisation, low gradient or eutrophication (v) Class 1A and Class 1B together are essentially the Class 1 of the River Pollution Survey	Water of less high quality than Class 1A but usable for substantially the same purposes

2	(i) DO greater than 40% saturation (ii) BOD not greater than 9 mg l⁻¹ (iii) Where water is abstracted for drinking water, it complies with the requirements for A3[a] water (iv) Non-toxic to fish in EIFAC terms (or best estimates if EIFAC figures not available)	(i) Average BOD probably not greater than 5 mg l⁻¹ (ii) Similar to Class 2 of RPS (iii) Water not showing physical signs of pollution other than humic (or colouration and a little foaming below weirs	(i) Waters suitable for potable supply after advanced treatment. (ii) Supporting reasonably good coarse fisheries (iii) Moderate amenity value
3	(i) DO greater than 10% saturation (ii) Not likely to be anaerobic (iii) BOD not greater than 17 mg l⁻¹[b]	Similar to Class 3 of RPS	Waters which are polluted to an extent that fish are absent or only sporadically present. May be used for low grade industrial abstraction purposes. Considerable potential for further use if cleaned up.
4	Waters which are inferior to Class 3 in terms of dissolved oxygen and likely to be anaerobic at times	Similar to Class 4 of RPS	Waters which are grossly polluted and are likely to cause nuisance
X	DO greater than 10% saturation		Insignificant watercourses and ditches not usable, where objective is simply to prevent nuisance developing

(a) Under extreme weather conditions (e.g. flood, drought, freeze-up), or when dominated by plant growth, or by aquatic plant decay, rivers usually in Classes 1, 2 and 3 may have BODs and dissolved oxygen levels, or ammonia content outside the stated levels for those Classes. When this occurs the cause should be stated along with analytical results

(b) The BOD determinations refer to 5 day carbonaceous BOD (ATU). Ammonia figures are expressed as NH_4

(c) In most instances the chemical classification given above will be suitable. However, the basis of the classification is restricted to a finite number of chemical determinands and there may be a few cases where the presence of a chemical substance other than those used in the classification markedly reduces the quality of the water. In such cases, the quality classification of the water should be downgraded on the basis of the biota actually present, and the reasons stated

(d) EIFAC (European Inland Fisheries Advisory Commission) limits should be expressed as 95% percentile limits

[a] EEC category A2 and A3 requirements are those specified in the EEC Council Directive of 16 June 1975 concerning the Quality of Surface Water intended for Abstraction of Drinking Water in the Member States.
[b] This may not apply if there is a high degree of re-aeration.
From National Water Council, 1977.

Table 2.5. *River water quality in England and Wales*

Class	Description	Current potential use	Length[a] (km)
1A	Good quality	Water of high quality suitable for potable supply abstractions; game or other high class fisheries; high amenity value	14450
1B	Good quality	Water of less high quality than Class 1A but usable for substantially the same purposes	13190
2	Fair quality	Waters suitable for potable supply after advanced treatment; supporting reasonably good coarse fisheries; moderate amenity value	8610
3	Poor quality	Waters which are polluted to an extent that fish are absent or only sporadically present; may be used for low grade industrial abstraction purposes; considerable potential for further use if cleaned up	3010
4	Bad quality	Waters which are grossly polluted and are likely to cause nuisance	610
		Total in survey	39880

[a] Lengths are rounded independently to nearest 10 km and may not sum to the total.
From National Water Council, 1981.

specific classes of river water. These classes are defined on the basis of the dissolved oxygen, the allyl thiourea suppressed BOD and the ammoniacal nitrogen concentrations together with, in certain cases, the EIFAC specifications for conditions which are non-toxic to fish. These classifications have been used in the most recent survey into the quality of rivers in England and Wales (National Water Council, 1981), a summary of which is given in Table 2.5. This shows that almost 70 per cent of the total length of the non-tidal rivers and canals surveyed were classified as being of good quality (i.e. 1A or 1B). The main feature of the NWC classification is that it uses the 95 percentile values of the chemical determinands. In the most simplistic terms this means the value which is exceeded by only 5 out of every 100 measurements. More correctly the 95 percentile value is calculated from a plot of determinand concentration against the percentage probability (P).

However, the problem is to decide which probability plot to use (e.g. normal, log-normal or extreme-value) and which technique to use to calculate the values of P.

Several techniques are used (see Cluckie & Forster, 1982; Ellis & Lacey, 1980). The simplest method is to assume the distribution which is to be used (usually normal or log-normal) and to calculate P from

$$P = {}^{(i-\alpha)}/(N+1-2\alpha)$$

where i = rank, N = sample size, α = 0, 0.375 or 0.44.

An alternative is to use distribution fitting techniques. With this method, no assumption is made as to the type of distribution used. The distribution of the actual data is compared with the theoretical distributions being considered. In each case an equal probability of occurrence is assumed. The fit is then examined statistically by a single-tailed Kolmogorov–Smirnov test. The actual array of data is assumed to fit the theoretical distribution being tested if the maximum difference between the theoretical and actual distribution probability is less than the expected difference. Once the most appropriate distribution has been found, any percentile value for that distribution can be calculated by a simple parametric formula. For example, the 95 percentile value (P95) of a normal distribution is given by:

$$P95 = \bar{x} + 1.645\sigma$$

where $\bar{x}$ = data mean, σ = data standard deviation. For the type of data being examined in river quality work, this technique is more likely to give a statistically correct value than any other. In addition, it provides a complete description of the distribution for use in subsequent analyses (e.g. the 'Monte Carlo' simulation method for determining consent conditions).

Despite the widespread use of chemically-based classification methods, there is also a role for biologically-based methods. The biological quantification of water quality depends on assessing the river biota in relation to the biota that would be expected for that stretch of river if it were totally unpolluted (see Chapter 1). Not all the changes in stream biota will affect water quality in an adverse way (for example, limited aquatic vegetation can encourage fish production). Nevertheless ALL changes are useful in assessing the degree of pollution and it must be remembered that (a) any use of water by Man will alter the water quality to some degree and (b) this will bring about an alteration in the natural stream biota, to a greater or lesser degree.

The biological assessment of water quality tries to quantify the degree of change in the biota. Biological assessment is of particular benefit when the polluting discharge is intermittent (or is timed to occur at 2 a.m!).

A number of lists have been published which classify aquatic

Table 2.6. *Trent biotic index*

Part 1 Classification of biological samples

Key indicator groups	Diversity of fauna	Total number of groups (see Part 2) present					Line No.:
		0–1	2–5	6–10	11–15	16+	
Column No.: 1	2	3	4	5	6	7	
		Biotic index					
Plecoptera nymphs present	More than one species	—	VII	VIII	IX	X	1
	One species only	—	VI	VII	VII	IX	2
Ephemeroptera nymphs present	More than one species[a]	—	VI	VII	VIII	IX	3
	One species only[a]	—	V	VI	VII	VIII	4
Trichoptera larvae present	More than one species[b]	—	V	VI	VII	VIII	5
	One species only[b]	IV	IV	V	VI	VII	6
Gammarus present	All above species absent	III	IV	V	VI	VII	7
Asellus present	All above species absent	II	III	IV	V	VI	8
Tubificid worms and/or Red Chironomid larvae present	All above species absent	I	II	III	IV	—	9
All above types absent	Some organisms such as *Eristalis tenax* not requiring dissolved oxygen may be present	0	I	II	—	—	10

organisms according to the degree of organic pollution with which they have been associated, but these must be treated with care. The presence or absence of individual organisms should not be taken as the real indication of the degree of pollution; it is the relative abundance in relation to other organisms in the community and in relation to the nature of the habitat which is significant. Thus the finding of *Asellus* (a mild pollutional type) or even a few *Chironimus* (gross pollutional indicators) in sluggish stretches of a river would not necessarily indicate pollution; HOWEVER if these species were found to dominate the community in stony rapids one could safely accept that there was organic pollution. One of the big problems with using biological

Table 2.6. (*cont.*)

Part 2 Groups
The term 'Group' here denotes the limit of identification which can be reached without resorting to lengthy techniques. Groups are as follows:

1 Each species of Platyhelminthes (flatworms)
2 Annelida (worms) excluding *Nais*
3 *Nais* (worms)
4 Each species of Hirudinea (leeches)
5 Each species of Mollusca (snails)
6 Each species of Crustacea (log-louse, shrimps)
7 Each species of Plecoptera (stone-fly)
8 Each genus of Ephemeroptera (mayfly) excluding *Baetis rhodani*
9 *Baetis rhodani* (mayfly)
10 Each family of Trichoptera (caddis-fly)
11 Each species of Neuroptera larvae (alder-fly)
12 Family Chironomidae (midge larvae) except *Chironomus thummi* (= *riparious*)
13 *Chironomus thummi* (blood worms)
14 Family Simulidae (black-fly larvae)
15 Each species of other fly larvae
16 Each species of Coleoptera (beetles and beetle larvae)
17 Each species of Hydracarina (water mites)

---

[a] *Baetis rhodani* excluded.
[b] *Baetis rhodani* (Ephem.) is counted in this section for the purpose of classification.
From Woodiwiss, 1964.

methods is that whilst the results are meaningful to the biologist, their significance is often difficult for chemists and engineers to appreciate. In an attempt to overcome this problem the concept of the *Biotic Index* has been devised. This attempts to give a number to the results of biological sampling. Two indices are worth considering: the Trent Index and the Chandler Index.

The Trent Index (Woodiwiss, 1964) is determined from a matrix (Table 2.6) of ten lines (based on key organisms) and five columns (based on the number of identifiable species that are present). The actual value of the index, ranging from 0 to 10, is obtained by:

(a) measuring the total number of groups present; this determines which column is to be used
(b) determining which of the key organisms are present. The organism which is least tolerant to pollution, and the number of species, defines the line that is to be used.

The value of the Index is then obtained from the intersection of the selected line and the selected column. This method is based on two assumptions; that pollution tends to restrict the number of organisms and that the key organisms tend to disappear in the order given in Table 2.6 as the degree of pollution increases.

However, the Trent Index does not really take into account the

Table 2.7. *Biotic score*

	Abundance in standard sample				
Groups present in sample	Present 1–2 Points scored	Few 3–10	Common 11–50	Abundant 51–100	Very abundant 100+
Planaria alpina Each species of Taenopterygidae, Perlidae, Perlodidae, Isoperlidae, Chloroperlidae	90	94	98	99	100
Each species of Leuctridae, Capniidae, Nemouridae (excluding *Amphinemura*)	84	89	94	97	98
Each species of Ephemeroptera (excluding *Baetis*)	79	84	90	94	97
Each species of Cased caddis, Megaloptera	75	80	86	91	94
Each species of *Ancylus*	70	75	82	87	91
Each species of *Rhyacophila* (Trichoptera)	65	70	77	83	88
Genera *Dicranota*, *Limnophora*	60	65	72	78	84
Genus *Simulium*	56	61	67	73	75
Genera of Coleoptera, Nematoda	51	55	61	66	72
Genera of *Amphinemura* (Plecoptera)	47	50	54	58	63
Genera of *Baetis* (Ephemeroptera)	44	46	48	50	52
Genera of *Gammarus*	40	40	40	40	40
Each species of Uncased caddis (excl. *Rhyacophila*)	38	36	35	33	31
Each species of Tricladida (excluding *P. alpina*)	35	33	31	29	25
Genera of Hydracarina	32	30	28	25	21
Each species of Mollusca (excluding *Ancylus*)	30	28	25	22	18
Each species of Chironomids (excl. *C. riparius*)	28	25	21	18	15
Each species of *Glossiphonia*	26	23	20	16	13
Each species of *Asellus*	25	22	18	14	10
Each species of Leech (excl. *Glossiphonia*, *Haemopsis*	24	20	16	12	8
Each species of *Haemopsis*	23	19	15	10	7
Each species of *Tubifex* sp.	22	18	13	12	9

Table 2.7. (*cont.*)

	Abundance in standard sample				
	Present 1–2	Few 3–10	Common 11–50	Abundant 51–100	Very abundant 100+
Groups present in sample	Points scored				
Each species of *Chironomus riparius*	21	17	12	7	4
Each species of *Nais*	20	16	10	6	2
Each species of air breathing species	19	15	9	5	1
No animal life			0		

From Chandler, 1970.

relative abundance of the organisms in a community. The two categories, 'one species only' and 'more than one species' is insufficient. To overcome this, there is a need to use something comparable to the Chandler Index which defines 5 levels of abundance based on the numbers collected in a five minute sampling with a hand net (Chandler, 1970; Hellawell, 1978):

Level of abundance	No./standard sample
Present	1–2
Few	3–10
Common	11–50
Abundant	51–100
Very abundant	> 100

The Chandler Index is based on a matrix with 26 lines and 5 columns (Table 2.7). The columns indicate the abundance and the lines the key organisms. Each intolerant species attracts a high score, each tolerant species a low score. The index is the sum of the scores for each species. There is no upper limit in theory but it would rarely reach 2000.

The shortcomings of both systems are that:

(a) not all the macro-invertebrates are included (largely because their pollution tolerance has not been properly established).

(b) not all biologists would agree to the relative positions of the species jn the Chandler table.

Nevertheless the Chandler Index does meet the requirements for a good pollution index in that:

(a) it makes a reasonable assessment of the diversity of the community

(b) it makes a reasonable assessment of the relative abundance

Table 2.8. *A comparison of the chemical classifications of river water and the average biological score for major rivers in England and Wales*

Chemical class	Biological score
1A	95
1B	93
2	50
3	23
4	12

From National Water Council, 1981.

   (c) it measures the overall trend of the community to environmental stress

   (d) it provides a weighting to the individual response to environmental stress

Despite the detail of these classifications and their potential for detecting intermittent pollution, biotic indices have not been used over-widely to define water quality. However, the 1980 river quality survey for England and Wales (National Water Council, 1981) includes an assessment of the rivers in terms of a biological score system which is not dissimilar from the Chandler Index in that the individual scores attributed to key species are added to give the final value. Because this system has only recently been introduced, little work has been done to assess its effectiveness. Individual data sets from the 1980 survey however, show that, on average, the biological score system and the chemical classification give similar gradations in water quality (Table 2.8).

An alternative approach is the use of water quality indices. These are systems which have yet to be fully developed. They are based on a series of determinands (e.g. BOD; pH; Amm. N; DO), each of which carries a weighting factor selected according to the relative importance of each parameter in determining water quality. The quality index can then be calculated in a number of ways (Scottish Development Department, 1976). Two of the more popular are:

   (a) An arithmetic type; $\sum\limits_{i=1}^{n} q_i w_i$

   (b) A geometric type; $\prod\limits_{i=1}^{n} q_i^{w_i}$

where n = number of parameters, q_i = value of ith parameter, w_i = weighting for ith parameter.

However, to date it is considered that water quality indices will have a greater role for monitoring trends within a catchment system than for use in predictive models. This means that really the only way of defining quality, for the purposes of calculating discharge control limits, is to rely on simple chemical limits as used in the NWC classifications.

2.4   Control of pollution

There is little point in knowing what pollutants are present, either in an effluent discharge or in the river water itself, or knowing what effect those pollutants may have on the stream biota, if their addition to natural waters cannot be controlled. Controlled, that is, in such a way as to reduce their impact to an acceptable level. There are several ways in which this can be achieved and, in the main, they rely on limitations being placed upon the concentrations of pollutants. These limitations can be applied in one of three ways: as zero discharge standards, as uniform emission standards or as local discharge standards. Zero standards do not in fact mean the complete elimination of specific pollutants, rather they mean that as complete a removal as is currently technically possible should be achieved. This method has the advantage that the protection of the environment is maximised and that where new techniques become established, water quality can be improved rapidly. However, it is a method which takes no account of the capacity of the river to absorb or to oxidise pollutants. This means that there is the potential for over-treatment and therefore for an over-expenditure in treatment capacity. The other major disadvantage of applying zero discharge standards is defining in precise legal terms what constitutes the 'best available technology'.

Uniform standards require that the control concentration for any pollutant be the same within the jurisdiction of the pollution control authority irrespective of the location of the discharge. The control levels tend to be based either on the average polluting effect of the effluents or on the average performance of existing treatment processes. As a system, it is both easy to administer and to control. In addition, it unifies the treatment costs imposed upon similar industries within that area. Despite these apparent advantages, this approach has no consideration for the relative volumes of the discharge and the receiving water and as such tends to produce areas of over-protection and under-protection, neither of which is either sensible or desirable.

Local standards, on the other hand, take account of not only these relative volumes but also the capacity for self-purification within the river, the quality requirements of the river down-stream of any discharge and the frequency with which discharges are accepted into the river. The result is a system which is very flexible and which does not cause any unnecessary expenditure on treatment processes. However, it is a system which requires greater skill and attention over the setting of the control levels and it is a system which could be applied only with difficulty to large international rivers.

Within the United Kingdom, the discharge of wastewaters is controlled by imposing consent conditions on discharges which are determined by local conditions. The logical way of achieving the correct limits is to:

(a) Determine the Environmental Quality Objectives (both present and future) for the stretch of river being considered. For example, to maintain a healthy population of game fish.

(b) Determine the Environmental Quality Standards necessary to achieve the objectives. For example, the maximum concentration of ammoniacal nitrogen that is compatible with game fish.

(c) Calculate the discharge control limits bearing in mind the up-stream river quality and the possible need to accommodate discharges in the future.

The first step that needs to be taken in setting the objectives is one of consultation with local industry, with planning authorities (both locally and nationally) and with local government; in this way a comprehensive assessment of the demands on the river system can be obtained. In addition, the conditions which affect the natural quality of the river need to be considered when the objectives are being determined. For example, a catchment which is based on permeable rock and does not, as a general rule, allow much direct surface run-off will produce a better natural quality of river water than a catchment which produces heavy surface run-off. Similarly, watercourses which have very low gradients and are dominated by plant growth for a large part of the year (such as occur in the Somerset levels) cannot be expected to attain as high a quality as, for example, a chalk stream.

The determination of the quality standards that will be placed on any stretch of river must take into account not only the criteria listed in Table 2.4 but also the increasing number of standards resulting from EEC directives. Once the objectives and standards have been assigned to a stretch of river, consent limits can be calculated for any discharges to that part of the river.

The currently accepted way of calculating consents for a discharge relies on using the class limiting criteria which are given in Table 2.4. These in turn are governed by the river quality objectives agreed for the water down-stream of the discharge. The simplest way of converting the class limiting criteria into consent conditions is to perform a mass balance across the discharge (see Fig. 2.4) using 95 percentile high and

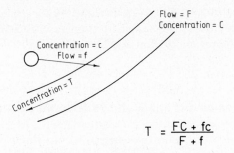

$$T = \frac{FC + fc}{F + f}$$

Fig. 2.4. The mass balance equation.

Table 2.9. *A comparison of the 95 percentile values for down-stream river quality (mg l^{-1})*

	BOD	Amm. N.
'Monte Carlo'	5.87	1.10
Mass balance	9.58	3.00

From Cluckie & Forster, 1982.

low values for the up-stream concentration and flow respectively. However, in statistical terms the consent conditions calculated in this way will not produce a valid result, even if the 95 percentile values have been calculated correctly (Warn & Brew, 1980; Cluckie & Forster, 1982). This is because the distribution of the down-stream water quality depends upon interactions between the up-stream flow and quality and these are not modelled by the mass balance equation.

A more sophisticated and more correct alternative is to employ the 'Monte Carlo' analysis (Warn & Brew, 1980). This approach requires that sufficient data be available to define the distributions for each known determinand. Values are then drawn randomly from each of the theoretical distributions and used in the mass balance equation to calculate a value for the unknown or the required determinand. This is usually either T or c. The process is then repeated many times until sufficient values have been generated to define the distribution for this parameter. Once this has been obtained any percentile of it may be calculated. Assessments for the number of times that the process of random selection and mass balance must be performed vary from 3000 (Warn & Brew, 1980) to between 200 and 400 (Cluckie & Forster, 1982). Obviously the greater the number the greater is the accuracy. It is equally obvious that the technique requires the use of a computer. The actual number used therefore will depend on the speed of the computer and what is considered to be an economic expenditure of computer time. A comparison of the results obtained by this simulation method with those determined by the simple mass balance calculation (Table 2.9) shows the differences that can occur.

2.5   Conclusions

The objectives of pollution control are to protect existing water quality and, in due course and where necessary, to improve water quality. To achieve these objectives it is necessary to define, to quantify and to control pollution. This, in turn, means that quality must be defined in a quantifiable way and that quality objectives for the various stretches of any river must be established. The final stage of any pollution control program is to ensure that the discharges from treatment works comply with the pre-determined standards necessary to produce the desired quality.

Pollution control should therefore not just be thought of as applying to a single discharge or even to a series of discharges. Rather it is the management of the entire river basin. The use of mathematical models may well assist this process. However, although models have been developed which vary considerably in their complexity (US Environmental Protection Agency, 1981; Casapieri et al., 1978; Holmes, 1982), their use, at least in the United Kingdom, is very limited.

3   Reactor types

3.1   General objectives

The specific objectives of any one effluent treatment plant will be
dependent on the nature of the receiving watercourse. Thus, a coastal
plant discharging to the sea may be designed to achieve a very different
standard of treatment from the works which discharges to an upland
stream. In other words, the function of the treatment works is to ensure
that there is little or no ecological impact on the receiving water.
Nevertheless, the general principles are that a treatment plant should
reduce: suspended matter; organic matter; and inorganic plant
nutriments (when required). This should be achieved on a regular and
reliable basis and to a degree determined by the consent conditions. To
do this an effluent treatment plant is assembled from combinations of
the following processes (Fig. 3.1):
preliminary treatment
primary treatment
bio-oxidation (secondary treatment)
tertiary treatment
sludge treatment.

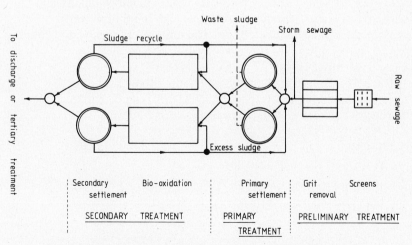

Fig. 3.1. Schematic representation of a typical sewage treatment works.

61

The design of a treatment works can be thought of as taking place in two stages: the initial 'broad-brush' design and the final detailed design. However, before any form of design is started, it is essential to determine (as far as possible) the quantity and composition of the wastewater to be treated and the standard of treatment required. The latter will be controlled by the discharge consent conditions (see Chapter 2). The amount of information that can be obtained about the former will depend on whether extensions or a new works are being planned. If the design is for the extension of an existing works it will be possible to measure the quantity and quality of the effluent. For a new works, assumptions will have to be made.

Except in unusual circumstances, the flow to the works would be taken as (Ministry of Housing and Local Government, 1970):

$$0.001PG + I + 3E + 1.364P \text{ m}^3 \text{ d}^{-1}$$

and full treatment would be given to:

$$0.003PG + I + 3E \text{ m}^3 \text{ d}^{-1}$$

where P = population served, I = infiltration (m³ d⁻¹), E = trade waste (m³ d⁻¹), G = water consumption (l *capita*⁻¹ d⁻¹)

The rates for the maximum flow and the flow to full treatment are still referred to as six times and three times the dry weather flow (6 DWF and 3 DWF) respectively, despite the fact that they ought to have been superseded by the Ministry of Housing and Local Government formulae.

The major problem is assessing the amount of infiltration. This will depend on the age and condition of existing sewers and on the type of soil through which the sewers run. For example, if an old sewer passed through a shallow gravel layer which was situated on top of impervious strata (e.g. clay), the level of the water table would rise rapidly and fall only slowly. Such a situation would give high infiltration which continued for some time after rain. There is, unfortunately, no formula for assessing infiltration. It must be based on experience, local knowledge and a prayer.

The concentration of the main pollutants (BOD, ammoniacal nitrogen (Amm. N) and suspended solids (SS)) can be estimated from typical *per capita* production figures (kg *capita*⁻¹ d⁻¹):

BOD   = 0.05–0.06
SS   = 0.06–0.09
Amm. N = 0.0032–0.0077

It is therefore possible to obtain realistic estimates, both for the flow and the polluting load, upon which the design can be based.

3.2   **Preliminary treatment**

This consists of the removal of coarse solids, the removal of grit and the separation of storm water.

All the channels associated with these inlet works should be designed to be self-cleaning at the *average daily flow* (often taken as 1.3 × dry weather flow) which is to say there should be a velocity of ⩾ 0.76 m s⁻¹.

Coarse solids are most frequently removed by screens – either coarse, conventional or fine. Coarse screens are in fact very coarse, with spaces of greater than 50 mm, and are used mainly at larger works as protection against quite large debris. Fine screens are usually constructed of mesh and as such many designers would require that they should be installed after grit removal. As the name would suggest, conventional screens (with spaces of 15–25 mm) are the most commonly used. They are raked either manually, in which case they are angled at 60° to the flow to facilitate this, or mechanically. The latter is preferred when flows exceed 1000 m³ d⁻¹. The mechanism is activated either on a time basis or when the flow level reaches a predetermined point. It is important to remember that with automatic screens duplicate units ought to be installed or at least there should be a bypass manual screen.

It is also important to ensure that the velocity of flow through a screen does not drop below 0.3 m s⁻¹ (in which case, grit could be deposited in the screen chamber) and that it does not exceed 0.9 m s⁻¹ (in which case material trapped on the screen could become dislodged). The width (W) of a screening chamber would normally be calculated from:

$$W = \frac{B+S}{S} \cdot \frac{Q}{VH} \text{ metres}$$

where B = width of bars, in mm, S = width of spaces, in mm, Q = maximum flow-rate, in m³ s⁻¹, V = maximum velocity, in m s⁻¹, H = depth of flow at maximum rate, in m.

Screenings are messy to handle and their disposal is awkward. The options available are burning, burying or tipping. A possible alternative is to macerate them and return them to the main flow through the works. Indeed, in some cases it is even thought preferable to macerate the full flow. Macerators or comminutors, however, need the protection of a coarse screen and grit removal. In addition, a manual bypass should be provided for use during servicing.

Macerated rags tend to attach themselves to the slightest protrusion, forming large unsightly balls. Because of this, most operators would consider that, once screenings had been removed, they should be kept separate. The handling of screenings has been greatly facilitated by a relatively recent development which macerates, washes and presses the screenings into a board-like cake. This has none of the more objectionable characteristics of untreated screenings (e.g. in terms of aesthetics and smell).

The removal of grit is necessary to prevent pump damage and to minimise silting problems. It is achieved by creating a settlement zone in which conditions are such that grit will settle whereas the majority of the suspended organic matter will not. These conditions can be brought about by maintaining a constant velocity of 0.3 m s^{-1}. Unless some proprietary system is used, constant velocity grit channels are practically universal. These are usually trapezoidal in section as this is easier to construct than the parabolic section which is theoretically correct. The flow is controlled by a standing wave flume and the channel width (W) is given by:

$$W = \frac{4.9Q}{H} \text{ metres}$$

where Q = flow, in m^3 s^{-1}, H = depth of flow, in m.

Since grit falls vertically at about 0.03 m s^{-1}, when the flow velocity is 0.3 m s^{-1} the theoretical length required is

$$L \text{ (m)} = \frac{\text{depth of flow} \times \text{velocity}}{0.03}$$
$$= 10 \times \text{maximum flow depth}$$

This is normally doubled to allow for turbulent effects. Although constant velocity channels are the most common means of removing grit, other techniques are used; for example, detritors or Pista grit traps (Institute of Water Pollution Control, 1972). Whichever system is used the grit is removed by pumps, dredgers or, at smaller works, manually, and after washing is dumped, usually on site.

As has already been explained only a proportion of the flow arriving at the works will receive full treatment. For a combined or partially separate sewerage system, the residue is given by $0.001P$ $(1364 - 2G)$ and will require 'storm treatment' (Ministry of Housing and Local Government, 1970); that is to say it should have some degree of settlement prior to discharge. The separation of flow is achieved by weirs set at the appropriate height. The storm tanks in which settlement is carried out are often designed on the somewhat arbitrary basis of 68 litres per head of population served and wherever possible facilities should be incorporated to enable storm sewage to be returned to full treatment when reduced flows occur.

3.3   **Primary treatment**

Primary settlement of sewage is used at the majority of works. This is
the stage whereby up to 70 per cent of suspended matter and 40 per
cent of the BOD is removed by the combined processes of flocculation,
adsorption and sedimentation. For anything other than the small rural
works it is unusual and dangerous to have a single primary tank. It is
therefore necessary to divide the flow (and the load) equally between a
number of primary tanks. This is best achieved by (a) flow splitting,
and (b) a distribution chamber. With flow splitting devices it is essential
that never more than two splits are made at any one time. Also, if it is
possible, there should be some fine control of each flow by a penstock
and measuring flume. With a distribution chamber, the situation where
the feed channel could impart a velocity vector into the chamber such
that some outlet pipes obtained a preferential flow should be avoided.
Also if the feed pipes to the tanks were, of necessity, of different
lengths, partitions and weirs, or preferably weir penstocks, should be
used (Institute of Water Pollution Control, 1973).

The theory of sedimentation in general, as practised by the water
industry, is based on the work of Hazen done at the turn of the
century. The key finding of this work was that the proportion of solids
removed was independent of the depth of the settlement tank. The main
problem in applying this to the settlement of sewage solids is that the
solids are flocculent in character and thus tend to increase in size during
settlement.

There are basically three types of settlement tank (Institute of Water
Pollution Control, 1973): upward flow; horizontal flow; and radial
flow.

3.3.1   *Upflow tanks*

These are fairly common on small works and may be conical (45° slope)
or pyramidal (60° slope) (Fig. 3.2). Sludge is collected in the deep
hopper (lower $\frac{2}{3}$) and removed by hydrostatic pressure. In size, it is
generally recommended that they are 5–9 m square; if less than this, the
weir loadings are too low and if greater, construction costs are
excessive. Because of their depth, they can be difficult to construct in
poor or waterlogged ground. The usual design criteria are:

Retention period	2 hours at 3 DWF
Upflow velocity	$\not> 1.5$ m h^{-1}

The weir loading rates need to be watched; if these are too low and
therefore the weir not self-cleaning it may be necessary to use V-notch
or castellated weirs.

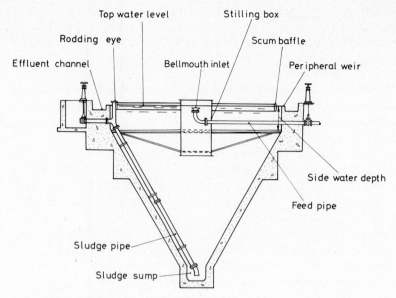

Top water level
Stilling box
Rodding eye
Scum baffle
Effluent channel
Bellmouth inlet
Peripheral weir
Side water depth
Feed pipe
Sludge pipe
Sludge sump

Fig. 3.2. Upflow settlement tank.

3.3.2   *Horizontal tanks*

Length:width	3:1 or 4:1
Depth	2 m minimum
Floor slope	1 in 40 manual desludging
	1 in 100 automatic
Retention time	2 hours at 3 DWF
Surface loading	$30 \text{ m}^3 \text{ m}^{-2} \text{ d}^{-1}$ at maximum design flow
Weir loading	$300 \text{ m}^3 \text{ m}^{-1} \text{ d}^{-1}$ at maximum design flow

Some attention needs to be paid to the design of the tank inlet as this determines the distribution to the tank – whether or not there is short-circuiting – and the tank efficiency. There are a variety of designs that have 'worked' and these are well documented. Perhaps the only best advice is – keep it simple. The outlet weir is usually of full width and should have the protection of a scum baffle. For the most accurate levelling it is best to use an adjustable weir plate of co-plastic or aluminium. If the tanks are thinner rather than fatter and large flows are being handled it may be necessary to use double or even triple weirs to get the proper loading rates.

Wherever possible automatic desludging is preferable to manual desludging as this entails emptying a tank and putting a man into it, but on small works the manual method usually has to be employed. Of the automatic techniques, the travelling bridge scraper is best as the equipment can in the main be serviced without taking the tank out of operation. Flight scrapers which operate on an endless chain with some of the pulleys on the bottom of the tank are not as good because of maintenance problems.

3.3.3 *Radial flow*

These are circular in plan ranging in diameter from 5 to 50 m with a centre feed (Fig. 3.3). The floor slopes to a central sump and sludge is gathered by scrapers to this sump.

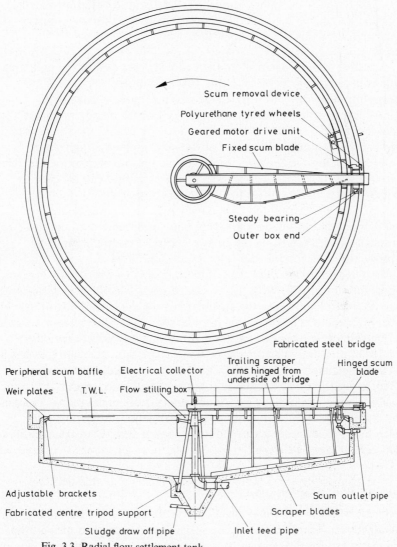

Fig. 3.3. Radial flow settlement tank.

Retention time   2 hours at 3 DWF
Upflow velocity = $\not> 1.5$ m h^{-1}
Side-wall depth = 2 m minimum
Weir loading $\not> 300$ m^3 m^{-1} d^{-1}
                  $\not< 100$ m^3 m^{-1} d^{-1}
Floor slope $7\frac{1}{2}°-10°$
Sludge hopper   This should provide for 18 hours storage at
                 large works and 24 hours at small works
                 on the basis of 0.09 kg sludge
                 capita^{-1} day^{-1}. Thus, if withdrawn at 2%
                 TSS, a capacity of 4.5 l *capita*$^{-1}$ must be
                 provided.

The inlet diffuser drum should not exceed 5 per cent of the tank area and is usually half the mean depth. It should extend about 0.15 m above top water level (TWL). Large tanks can give satisfactory performance without a diffuser box. This is worth considering when the tank diameter is > 30 m. Scrapers are used to 'sweep' the sludge into the collection hopper. These are rubber-edged blades hung from a rotating bridge with the arms hinged at the bottom and/or the top. The latter is not recommended by some designers as they can lift over solids – particularly raw sludge. It is essential that the bridge/arm/blade assembly is relatively rigid so that solids are not left on the tank bottom. Side-wall scrapers are sometimes used but must be justified rather than being put in as a matter of course. Peripheral speeds are 1.8–2.5 m min^{-1}.

Sludge withdrawal from the central hopper is by hydrostatic head or sometimes by air-lift. With flat-bottomed tanks which are sometimes used for secondary tanks the air-lift system or the hydrostatic or a suction take-off is incorporated into the rotating bridge/scraper system.

On primary tanks and sometimes on secondary tanks (where there has been no primary settlement or where there are settlement problems) scum collection is incorporated with the rotating bridge or scraper. Once every rotation the scum that has been collected is swept into a scum trough. The outlet weirs can be single or multiple; plane, V-notch or castellated. They should be protected by baffles. Adjustable weir plates may ease levelling and should be used if there is any danger of differential tank settlement.

3.4   Biological filtrations

3.4.1   *Basic considerations*

Biological filtration as a process was developed at the end of the nineteenth century. However, it is not a filtration process in that its function is not one of straining. Rather it is a biological fixed-film reactor in which a carefully balanced eco-system is used to absorb and metabolise the pollutants in settled sewage. The reactor configuration is that of a packed bed in which there is a counter-current flow of liquid (settled sewage) and air. These beds can be either circular or rectangular and the packing can be stone, plastic or, in some cases, wood. These packings provide the habitat for the biological film which will oxidise the applied load of pollutants. Filters can be considered in two very broad categories: conventionally loaded and high-rate systems.

3.4.2. *Conventionally loaded filters*

In general, the filter depth should not be less than 1.5 m and should not exceed 2.5 m. With deeper beds a larger diameter media will be required. The choice between rectangular and circular filters will depend on the nature of the site, but usually the circular design is preferable. If rectangular filters must be built, their lengths should not be greater than 75 m, unless they are divided into bays, nor their width greater than 45 m. Circular filters should not exceed 40 m diameter (Fig. 3.4).

Filter beds are usually constructed on a concrete floor (100–150 mm thick) which is then covered with drainage tiles. In addition, under-drains must be provided. The layout of these will depend on the fall of the land and can either be a radial pattern (with some

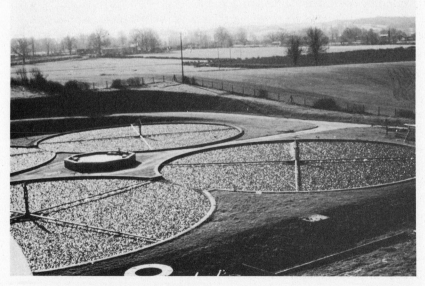

Fig. 3.4. Circular trickling filters.

Table 3.1. *Properties of mineral media*

Material	Nominal size (mm)	Voids (%)	Specific surface (m² m⁻³)
Slag	50	45–55	100–118
Slag	100–150	45–55	50
Clinker	62	45–55	120
Rounded gravel	62	45–55	67–77

herring-boning on larger filters) or a cross flow pattern. In rectangular filters the treated effluent is discharged by under-drains or drainage tiles into culverts, which are usually constructed beneath the feed channels and which are large enough to give a good air-flow for aeration.

Aeration is of paramount importance to the operation of a biological filter and the media must therefore be packed to ensure an even distribution of air. In addition, the outlet channels should not drown the air vents. Air bricks in the side-walls have been used to provide additional ventilation as have dry retaining walls built of large pieces of filter medium. Their effect on the degree of ventilation has not been quantified but both systems provide additional breeding grounds and exit routes for flies and their use is therefore not recommended.

Filter wall can be built from bricks or reinforced concrete. In addition, proprietary prefabricated dry concrete blocks have been used but the structural integrity has yet to be fully proved. Buried beds should be considered whenever possible. This allows for thermal insulation by the surrounding earth and also enables cheaper constructions materials (e.g. breeze blocks) to be used for the filter walls.

The distributors can be driven by the water reaction, by water wheels or, in specialised cases, by electricity. Whichever system is used, dosing chambers must be provided to give reasonable head of liquid under low flow conditions. Rectangular filters should have travelling distributors preferably driven directly by water wheels or by cables. Supply channels must be provided either down the longitudinal centre or along the side of the filter so that the distributors can be fed through moving cycles. The distributors will have guide-wheels which run along the top of the filter walls. Where the side-walls are used, these must be provided with a track or rails for the guide-wheels. It would probably be best to arrange the distributors in pairs, moving in opposite directions to balance wind effects.

The media for conventional biological filters must comply with the specifications laid down in BS1438/1971 and may be any durable angular aggregate such as clinker, granite, basalt or slag. The lowest

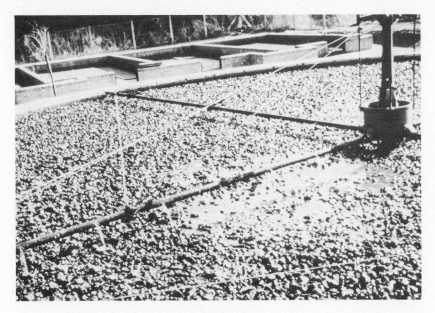

Fig. 3.5. 'Ponding' on an over-loaded filter.

0.3 m of the bed should be filled with 100–150 mm aggregate and the remainder of the bed with 40–50 mm aggregate. In two-stage filtration, the primary filter should be packed entirely with 100–150 mm aggregate.

Dosing periodicity. With biofiltration, the condition to be avoided is an accumulation of solids at the surface such that voids become blocked and the filter 'ponds' (Fig. 3.5). During winter months, low temperatures suppress the activity of grazing organisms and there is an increase in film growth. With an old or overloaded filter system this can lead to ponding with the concomitant deterioration in effluent quality. One way of limiting film growth at the top surface of the filter is to reduce the dosing frequency from every 0.25–2 minutes to once every 5–12 minutes. This produces a better distribution of nutriments deeper into the filter bed. It also increases the time of quiescence, during which diffusion of nutriments from liquid to biofilm occurs, to such an extent that the growth of the film can be limited by lack of nutriments. However, unless the periodicity can be varied, effluent quality can deteriorate during summer months. In other words, dosing should only be slowed to an extent which controls film growth.

It must be recognised, however, that control measures of this type are not always possible and that therefore film will accumulate during the colder months and that equally well, this excess film will be sloughed off in the spring. When this occurs, humus tanks tend to become overloaded and consent conditions exceeded.

The most usual way of sizing a biological filter is by using the organic loading rate based on settled sewage. Recommended values for these rates are given below:

Process	Organic loading rates (kg BOD m^{-3} d^{-1})
Single	0.06–0.12
Re-circulation	0.09–0.15
Alternating double filtration (ADF)	0.15–0.26
2-stage filtration; primary	1.56–2.29
secondary	0.04–0.12

Thus, from a knowledge of the daily flow (Q) and the BOD (L_i) in that flow, the applied load QL_i (kg BOD d^{-1}) can be calculated. The volume (V) of filtration medium that is required is then obtained from QL_i/R, where R is the organic loading rate.

An alternative method of estimating the volume of media required, for example at a new works where the precise strength of the sewage is not known, is to base the volume on population served using a figure of 0.41 m^3 per head of population equivalent for single filtration.

If the sewage is particularly strong or contains a high proportion of strong trade waste (e.g. from dairies or meat processing), a more complete treatment will be achieved if either re-circulation or ADF is used. The re-circulation involves the dilution of the feed with settled final effluent. The ratio of effluent to feed is usually in the range 1:1 to 2:1. There are three ways of applying the re-circulation:

(a) by varying the rate of re-circulation directly with the sewage flow, thus maintaining a constant re-circulation ratio
(b) by varying the rate of re-circulation inversely with the sewage flow, thus maintaining a constant total flow to the biological filter
(c) by maintaining a constant rate of re-circulation.

Of the three methods, the third is the simplest and most economic but (a) is the ideal. The effect of re-circulation is to increase the effective hydraulic loading (m^3 m^{-2} d^{-1}) on the filter causing greater scouring within the bed. The strength of the applied feed is reduced correspondingly which has the effect of suppressing fungal growth near the surface of the filter. However, since the removal kinetics are first order a reduction in removal efficiency might be expected. This in fact does not occur at low rates of re-circulation and this is thought to be

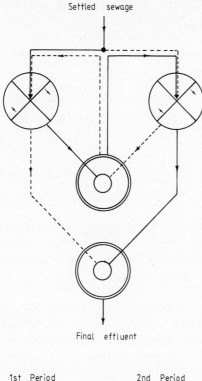

Settled sewage

Final effluent

1st Period   2nd Period

Fig. 3.6. Sequence of operation for alternating double filtration (ADF).

due to a greater wetting of media surfaces resulting in a more efficient use of the film on those surfaces.

In alternating double filtration (ADF), there are two sets of similar filter beds and two humus tanks (Fig. 3.6). By installing some additional pumping and flow diversion valves, the working sequence of the filters can be changed, usually at intervals of 1–2 weeks. It should be noted that although the order of the filters is changed, that of the humus tanks is not. This means that two distribution chambers are required (one for the filters and one for the humus tanks) and that the secondary settlement tank will have to be of a larger size (6 hours at DWF) than the inter-stage tank (3 hours at DWF). ADF filters are often packed with a slightly larger medium (63–75 mm) than that used in single filtration.

The effect of ADF is therefore to alternate between nutriment-rich and nutriment-limiting conditions which in turn promote heavy film

Table 3.2. *Characteristics of filters used outside the UK*

Country	Filter depth (m)	Media size (mm)	Loading (m³ m⁻³ d⁻¹)	(Kg m⁻³ d⁻¹)
Belgium	2.5–3	60–100	0.27–0.32	0.07
W. Germany	2–5	—	—	0.3–0.4
Eire	1.8	25–50	0.3–0.5	0.09–1.2
Holland	1.5–3	40–80	—	0.5–0.8
Sweden	3	70–90	0.3	0.5–0.8
USA	1.5–3	—	—	0.1–0.4

From Pike, 1978.

growth and film reduction respectively. By judiciously selecting the frequency of alternation, high BOD loading rates can be achieved with ponding conditions just failing to be established. Thus, ADF is commonly used with high strength, readily degradable wastes (e.g. milk processing).

Although the most common approach for designing filters, in the UK, is to use the organic loading rate, other techniques are available and are used (Pike, 1978). These use mathematical expressions that have been derived either from first order reaction kinetics or on an empirical basis. The latter type is probably best typified by the formula derived by the National Research Council (1946):

$$\frac{L_i - L_e}{L_i} = \frac{1}{1 + 0.44\{W/(fV)\}^{0.5}}$$

where L_i = BOD of influent, L_e = BOD of final effluent, W = BOD load (kg d⁻¹), V = volume of filter media (m³). The term f is a re-circulation factor. Thus, for a straight-through system $f = 1$ and if re-circulation is used f is given by:

$$f = \frac{1 + \alpha}{(1 + 0.1\alpha)^2}$$

where α is the re-circulated flow:settled sewage flow ratio.

The basic first order equation is:

$$L_e = L_i \exp(-KS/Q)$$

where S = specific surface of medium (m² m⁻³), Q = hydraulic loading rate (m³ m⁻³ d⁻¹), K = first order rate coefficient. This expression has been expanded to incorporate the effect of temperature (Bruce & Merkens, 1973):

$$L_e = L_i \exp(-K\theta^{(T-15)}S/Q)$$

Table 3.3. *Calculated values for media volume and loading rates*

Method	Media volume (m³)	Organic loading rate (kg BOD m⁻³ d⁻¹)	Hydraulic loading rate (m³ m⁻³ d⁻¹)
Pike	356	0.485	2.43
Bruce & Merkens	1071	0.161	0.81
NRC	7627	0.023	0.11
UK practice	1728	0.100	0.50

More recently (Pike, 1978), further modifications have been made, based on multiple regression analysis of experimental data, to give:

$$L_e = L_i \exp\left(-K\theta^{(T-15)}S^m/Q^n\right)$$

where θ = temperature coefficient, m, n = constants. The coefficients m and n are thought to relate to the physical nature of the surface and efficiency with which it is wetted. The use of these coefficients is claimed to enable the expression to be used over a wider range of hydraulic loading rates, temperatures and types of media. However, its use as a design tool is limited to straight-through filtration since the values of K, m and n vary with the degree of treatment that the sewage has received.

It is interesting to examine how these various methods perform, using published values for the constants. Pike reports the values $K = 0.0204$, $\theta = 1.111$, $m = 1.407$ and $n = 1.249$. Wilson (1981), in demonstrating the use of the Bruce & Merkens formula, uses $K = 0.037$ and $\theta = 1.08$. If these values are used to calculate the filter volume required for the following conditions:

$$
\begin{aligned}
L_i &= 200 \text{ mg l}^{-1} \\
L_e &= 15 \text{ mg l}^{-1} \\
\text{flow-rate} &= 0.01 \text{ m}^3 \text{ s}^{-1} \\
T &= 10\ ^\circ\text{C} \\
S &= 100 \text{ m}^2 \text{ m}^{-3}
\end{aligned}
$$

and compared with the values obtained from the NRC method and the organic loading rate methods (assuming a value of 0.1 kg BOD m⁻³ d⁻¹), the results differ quite widely (Table 3.3). Also, if these volumes are then used to calculate the hydraulic and organic loading rates, it can be seen (Table 3.3) that really only the Bruce & Merkens method gives rates which are at all compatible with current UK practice (and thus the organic loading rate method). It is therefore suggested that formulae based on theoretical reasoning or empirical relationships need to be used with some considerable care and certainly checked against accepted yardsticks.

Table 3.4. *Properties of plastic media used in high-rate filtration*

	Type	Material	Weight (kg m^{-3})	Specific surface (m^2 m^{-3})	Voidage (%)
Flocor E	M	PVC	38	85	98
Flocor R	RP	PVC	40	240	95
Cloisonyle	M	PVC	75	220	94
Filterpak	RP	Polypropylene	64	118	93
Actifil 90	RP	Polypropylene	44	95	95

M = modular; RP = random pack.

3.4.3   High-rate filtration

As has already been explained, one of the problems with conventionally loaded rock filters is their tendency to 'pond' when conditions of overload promote a sufficiently heavy growth of biofilm to block the voids at the surface. One way of avoiding this is to use a medium with a voidage considerably greater than that of rock. Plastic media are such a material. They were originally introduced to treat high strength industrial wastes. The specifications for their design were that, when compared with conventional media, they would be capable of removing more BOD at greater loading rates and would have a sufficiently open structure to facilitate oxygen transfer and avoid blockages. In addition, they should be strong enough to support the wet weight of the biofilm, be inert to biological and chemical attack and yet be light enough to reduce civil engineering construction costs. One benefit that can be obtained from the low bulk density of plastic media is that filters packed with this material can be built as towers up to 8–10 m high. The properties of the principal packings available in the UK are shown in Table 3.4. There are basically two types, modular sheet packing which were the first to be developed, and random packing (Fig. 3.7).

Plastic media filters are widely used for treating industrial wastes. They have also been used to treat screened (to 10 mm) and de-gritted domestic sewage either when: (a) the BOD is stronger than average; (b) the existing plant is overloaded; (c) works liquors need to be treated separately; or (d) a standard less stringent than Royal Commission is required.

It is most likely that in the majority of cases where plastic media are to be installed, the design will be done by the company manufacturing the media. Designs done in this way usually depend on company knowledge about the treatability of the waste in question and the nature of the media being used.

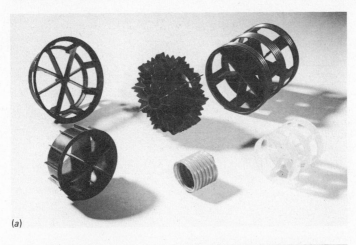

(a)

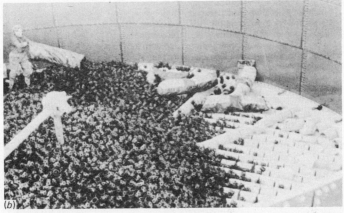

(b)

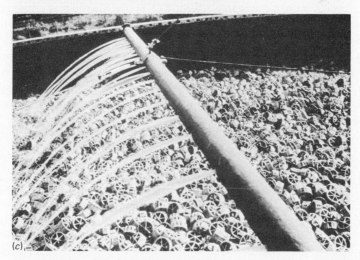

(c)

Fig. 3.7 *a*: Various types of random pack plastic media; *b*: packing of plastic media; *c*: plastic media in operation.

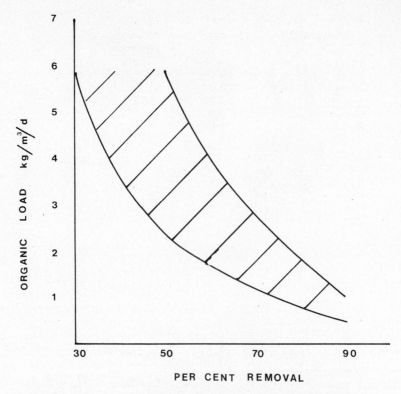

Fig. 3.8. Loading rate/efficiency envelope for plastic media filters.

In general, the volume of media to be used is calculated from the organic loading rate. This in turn is determined by the efficiency (in terms of the percentage removal of BOD) that the filter is expected to achieve. Although each manufacturer makes his own claims about efficiencies and loading rates, as a general rule they can be obtained from Fig. 3.8 which combines data from most of the manufacturers. The loading rate that is derived in this way is then multiplied by a treatability factor (Table 3.5). This gives the design loading rate which, together with the applied load, enables the volume of media to be calculated:

$$\text{Volume} = \frac{\text{applied load (kg d}^{-1})}{\text{design loading rate (kg m}^{-3}\,\text{d}^{-1})}$$

An alternative way of calculating the necessary volume of media is to use formulae of the type used for conventionally loaded filters. One, which has been suggested for high-rate filters (Hutchinson, 1975), is based on first order conditions within a plug-flow reactor;

$$L_e/L_i = \exp(kSH/F^x)$$

Table 3.5. *Treatability factors for various effluents*

Effluent	Inlet BOD < 400	Inlet BOD < 400
Domestic (at 20 °C)	1.0	1.0
(at 10 °C)	0.72	0.72
Dairy	1.2	1.0
Brewery	0.9–1.1	1.0–1.2
Distillery	0.8	1.1–1.3
Abattoir	0.7–0.9	0.7–1.0
Tanning	0.7–0.9	0.7–1.0
Dyestuffs	0.7	0.8–1.0
Paper	0.6–0.8	—
Pulp	0.7–0.9	0.8–1.0

where H = filter depth (m), F = flow rate (l s^{-1} m^{-2}), x = media factor (0.125–0.25). The removal rate constant (k) varies with temperature and may be calculated from

$$k = k_{20}(1.035)^{(T-20)}$$

However, this method is limited to influent BOD values of less than 500 mg l^{-1}. In other words formulae need to be used with caution and a precise reading of the 'small print'.

Having obtained a figure for the volume of media required the other dimensions (height and area) need to be calculated.

The height of the filter (and thus its cross-sectional area) is a more or less arbitrary choice. However, it has been shown that for a given volume of media the performance will be greater in a small diameter deep filter than in a large diameter shallow filter. This is thought to be due to improved wetting of the media surface and a greater residence time in the filter bed. In most cases plastic media is most effective when being used to achieve a BOD removal of 50–60 per cent. The other critical design parameter for plastic media filters is the irrigation rate. Effluent should be applied to filters so that the filter surface is continually wetted. In most cases the minimum irrigation rate is 1.5 m^3 m^{-2} h^{-1} although one manufacturer does claim a lower rate. If this minimum irrigation rate cannot be achieved by the normal flow of sewage then re-circulation must be introduced. Alternatively, a different height/area combination should be examined.

High-rate filters are quite frequently built as multi-stage units and the design of such systems is done in precisely the same way, with each filter being designed as a separate unit but obviously with a different influent BOD and removal efficiency.

The design and construction of the tower structure is relatively straightforward. Under normal operating conditions plastic media, particularly the modular type, does not exert a significant lateral thrust and there is therefore little requirement for the tower design to provide lateral support to the packing. However, wind resistance must be considered and it is normal to design in accordance with the British code of practice CP 3 (British Standards Institute, 1972). The towers are frequently made of a mild steel framework which must be capable of withstanding the weight of the cladding material used, the weight of the access facilities to the top of the filter and the weight of the loaded distribution system. Cladding material which is frequently used includes PVC sheet, acrylic plastic or steel.

Because of the high compressive strength of modular media it is possible to have packings up to depths of 4.2 m without any intermediate supports. The best type of support for a modular medium, such as Flocor, would be a grid system made up of narrow parallel beams (40 mm wide) spaced at 220 mm centres. For bed depths up to 4.2 m this grid could be constructed of impregnated redwood, but for deeper packings grids should be of epoxy or nylon coated steel.

The foundations for the tower should provide for reinforced concrete to support the main members of the filter shell. Unreinforced concrete can be used for the drainage pan beneath the packing supports. This should slope at 1:25 to allow the effluent to wash the voided solids from the filter.

The plastic media itself should be packed on support decking. This should be made from aluminium or steel and designed so as to allow the free passage of liquid and solids sloughed from the media. The decking should be capable of supporting weights equal to 240–370 kg m^{-3} per unit depth of packed bed.

The choice of distributor will depend on the configuration of the tower. Where a circular filter has been designed the simplest and cheapest distributor is the conventional rotary distributor made from galvanised mild steel and fitted with PVC bushed nozzles, steel spread plates and galvanised ropes. If a rectangular filter is to be used, then fixed spray units with splash plates would ensure full utilisation of the media. Proper safety facilities must be provided at the top of the tower. These should include walkways (particularly over random pack media) and access for rodding distributors.

3.4.4   *Rotary biological contactors*

One of the earliest reports of the treatment of sewage by a contact process involving partially submerged rotating plates was given in 1929 (by Doman). However, it was not until 1965 that a commercially available process became available. There are several different designs now available but in its simplest form a rotary biological contactor

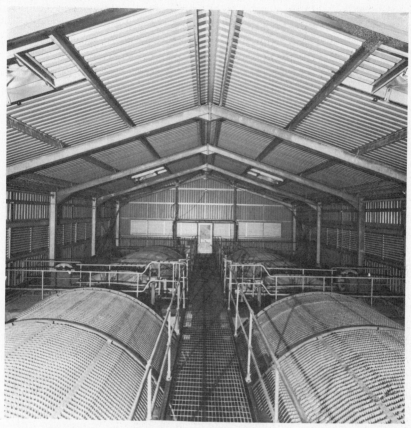

Fig. 3.9. Rotary biological contactors (by courtesy of Clearwater Systems Ltd).

(RBC) consists of a series of discs (2–3 m diameter) mounted on a shaft which is driven so that the discs rotate at right angles to the flow of settled sewage. The discs are usually made of plastic (polythene, PVC, expanded polystyrene) and are contained in a trough so that about 40 per cent of their area is immersed (Fig. 3.9). The discs are arranged in groups or packs with baffles between each group to minimise surging or short-circuiting. With small units the trough is covered and large units are often housed within buildings. This is to reduce the effect of weather on the active biofilm which becomes attached to the disc surfaces. As the discs rotate, this film alternately absorbs nutrients from the settled sewage and oxygen from the air. The speed of rotation is limited by shearing of the film at the periphery of the disc and is usually within the range of 0.5–10 revolutions per minute. Film that is sloughed off tends to remain in the reactor trough with a degree of

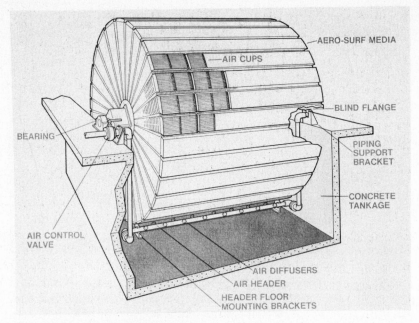

Fig. 3.10. The 'Aerosurf' system.

activity so that the process can, to a degree, be thought of as a hybrid; part fixed-film, part homogeneous in nature. After passage through the reactor trough, the liquors flow to a settlement tank to ensure that biological solids are removed before discharge to a watercourse.

As has already been stated, there are a number of variations to this basic concept. These have been described by Pike (1978) and therefore will not be discussed here. However, one variant is worth mentioning. This is the aerated RBC. With this process polythene cups are attached to the perimeter of the discs and a coarse bubble diffuser releases low pressure air into the cups causing rotation (Fig. 3.10). The concept has been used in two systems: as an alternative to electrically driven RBC's and as a means of uprating activated sludge processes. In this latter approach, the disc units are placed in existing aeration tanks, the effect being to increase the biomass concentration within the tanks quite significantly without requiring a corresponding increase in aeration capacity (Guarino *et al.*, 1980).

The design procedures for RBC systems vary according to the size (population equivalent) of the unit. However, the demarcation line between small and large units is ill-defined. In the absence of better information it is suggested that small means less than a population equivalent of 250. Plants of this type should be designed on the basis of a BOD loading rate per unit area of disc, both sides of the disc

Table 3.6. *A comparison between design methods for determining the surface area of RBC systems*

Example	Area (m²)		Error (%)
	Steels method	First order method	
Steels	7472	7218	−3.4
Wilson	15 500[a]	15 501	Negligible

[a] No correction for number of shafts.

contributing to this area. To achieve a Royal Commission (20:30) standard the loading rate should not exceed 6 g BOD $m^{-2} d^{-1}$ (Bruce & Merkens, 1975). In addition, the sizing of the reactor tank would need, in the UK, to be in accordance with CP 6297 (British Standards Institute, 1983) (formerly CP 302). For the design of larger systems, the technique described by Steels (1974) is recommended. This is based on the hydraulic loading rate per unit area of disc. The technique is involved and requires that a variety of factors are used according to the population being served and the number of stages being used. Readers are therefore recommended to refer either to Steels (1974) or to Wilson (1981). An alternative, but tentative, method is suggested by Pike (1978). This is based on first order kinetics and is similar to the formulae used for trickling filters. Thus:

$$\log e \frac{L_e}{L_i} = -K\theta^{(T-15)} (A/F)$$

Taking the examples quoted by Steels and by Wilson and comparing the values calculated for the required surface areas by the two methods, using $K = 0.2$ (Pike, 1978), $\theta = 1.05$ (Antonie, 1978) and $T = 10\ °C$, shows a good agreement between the methods (Table 3.6). A similar type of formula to that described by Pike, but based on soluble BOD, has been suggested by Wu & Smith (1982):

$$\frac{L_e}{L_i} = \frac{14.2\ (F/A)^{0.5579}}{T^{0.2477} L_i^{0.6837}} \exp(0.32N)$$

(note: F/A has the units gall d^{-1} ft^{-2}).

The various methods used in design have recently been reviewed by Lumbers (1983).

3.4.5 Fluidised beds

Fluidised and expanded bed reactors are one of the most recent developments in the field of fixed film reactors. In fact, their current

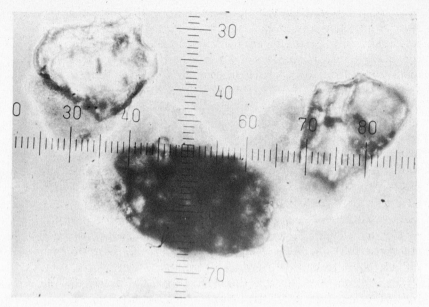

Fig. 3.11. Sand/biofilm from an oxygenic fluidised bed.

stage of development is such that no generally accepted design criteria have been established. Discussion of these reactors will therefore be limited to a description of their characteristics and modes of operation. For a more detailed appraisal, readers are referred to Cooper & Atkinson (1981).

Reactors of this type can be operated in three different ways: aerobically, anoxically or in an anaerobic mode. The principal advantages claimed for these systems are that they afford the means of operating at high biomass concentrations without recourse to solids recycle, that they can achieve the desired treatment in compact reactors thereby saving on land costs, and that the parameters governing performance are readily controllable. Irrespective of the mode of operation, the common feature of this family of reactors is that a solid support medium is expanded or fluidised by an upward flow of liquid. The support media that have been used include sand, anthracite and reticulated foam pads. However, sand (0.2–2 mm diameter) is the most common. The purpose of the media is to provide a surface which can be colonised by the microbial flora appropriate to the mode of operation (Fig. 3.11). Another common feature is the need to obtain an even distribution of the liquid into the support phase. This can be achieved by a downwards injection of the liquid into a conical base (Cooper & Wheeldon, 1982).

Anaerobic beds tend to be expanded rather than fluidised and, as will be shown in Chapter 8, are more suitable for the treatment of industrial wastewaters than for domestic sewage (Rockey & Forster, 1982). The main object of any anaerobic reactor treating liquid wastes is the conversion of carbonaceous pollutants to methane. As such therefore, anaerobic beds require an effective gas/liquid separation stage. Also, since most anaerobic processes are operated in the mesophilic range, heating/heat transfer facilities are required. This may involve using some of the methane generated by the process. Alternately, waste heat from the processes generating the wastewater can be used either in the form of low-grade steam, or hot process water which can be the wastewater itself or cooling water. At the present time, few full-scale plants are in operation. It is therefore not possible to judge whether the process is a serious competitor to the existing treatment technology.

Anoxic reactors are designed to remove nitrate and most of the developmental work has been associated with the need to reduce nitrate concentrations in surface waters that are required for the production of potable water (Gauntlett & Craft, 1979). However, the removal of nitrate from sewage can also be ecologically useful and anoxic fluidised beds have been used to treat sewages in which all the ammoniacal nitrogen has been oxidised to nitrate (Cooper & Wheeldon, 1980, 1982). Anoxic reactors have also been applied to the treatment of industrial wastes which are high in nitrate (Bosman & Hendricks, 1981). Denitrification requires the input of a carbon source. For the treatment of sewage, this is provided either by allowing a proportion of raw sewage to bypass the oxidation stage or by siting the anoxic bed before the oxidation unit and recycling a proportion of the nitrified effluent. In this way, the nitrate acts as an oxygen source for carbon in the raw sewage which reduces the requirement for oxygen in the aerobic stage. Other than this, anoxic fluidised beds have no special features.

Although air has been used for the aeration of fluidised beds, it has been suggested that this type of process has a limited value (Forster, 1980) and in fact most recent developments in this field are based on oxygenic systems. That is to say, systems using aeration with pure oxygen. The full-scale application of aerobic fluidised beds is basically restricted to two designs: the Oxitron system (Dorr–Oliver Co., Ltd,) and the Captor process (Simon–Harkley Ltd.). The Oxitron system (Fig. 3.12) consists of a fluidised bed of sand and an external, down-flow bubble oxygenator (see Chapter 5). In the plant described by Hoyland & Robinson (1983), sand with a size range of 250–550 μm was used and the average concentration of biomass on the sand was 10–14 kg m^{-3}. The Captor process not only uses a different support medium (plastic foam pads) but also uses a different aeration concept (diffused air directly into the main reactor). Thus fluidisation, or more precisely pseudo-fluidisation, is caused by the air/liquid mixture.

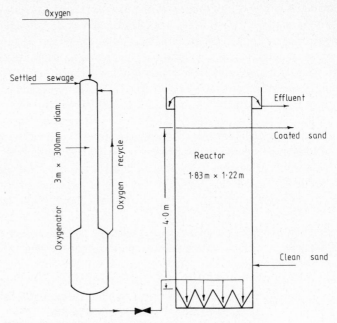

Fig. 3.12. Schematic representation of the 'Oxitron' system.

The other major difference between these two processes lies in the technology used to effect the separation of surplus biomass. This is an essential feature in maintaining optimal microbial activity. In the Oxitron process (and any other sand-based reactor, be it anaerobic, anoxic, or aerobic) the biomass is removed by shear. As operated in the UK, a portion of the bed is removed, partially de-watered and subjected to shear from a mechanical stirrer. The two solid phases, the cleaned sand and the biomass, are then separated by a vibrating screen (Cooper *et al.*, 1981). An alternative method is to effect the shear in a centrifugal pump and return the sheared mixture to the top of the fluidised bed to enable a hydraulic separation to occur; the sand then sinks back into the bed and the lighter biomass is carried out of the reactor with the treated effluent (Hoyland & Robinson, 1983). The vibrating screen method produces a highly concentrated sludge but is mechanically more complicated. However the hydraulic method requires the use of a sedimentation tank which adds to the cost of the treatment. A third method patented in America permits both the shear and the separation to take place within the bed itself and is initiated when the height of the bed reaches a predetermined point (Hickey & Owens, 1978). Since the excess sludge is removed with the treated liquors, this method also requires a settlement/thickening tank.

The Captor process, because of its unique support medium, can

Table 3.7. *Values of the constants E_m and
a in the expression* $E = E_m \left(1 - \dfrac{a}{t_r} \right)$

Type of waste	E_m	a
Shell-fish	85	0.153
Food processing	99	0.362
Fermentation liquors	95	0.052
Meat packing	100	0.044

remove excess sludge merely by passing the foam pads through a
compression roller unit. Concentrated sludge is obtained and there is no
need for it to be processed further.

3.4.6. *Submerged filters*

The final type of fixed film reactor to be discussed is the submerged or
upflow filter. This, in some ways, can be thought of as the precursor of
fluidised bed systems. It has been evaluated as an aerobic, anoxic and
anaerobic process (McHarness & McCarty, 1973; Bailey & Thomas,
1975; Anderson, Donnelly & McKeown, 1984). Various packings have
been used, ranging from stone to the random-pack plastic media.

The basic design of upflow filters is essentially the same irrespective
of the mode of operation. The major differences are similar to those
described for fluidised beds. Thus aerobic systems require an aeration
or oxygenation device; anoxic processes require that provision be made
for a carbon source to be added; and gas removal is needed for
anaerobic units. The major application of upflow filtration at the
present time is an anaerobic filter with plastic media being used
(Anderson *et al.*, 1984). The design of anaerobic filters is probably best
done on the basis of performance relationships using COD
reduction/organic loading rate curves. However, Young & McCarty
(1967) have also suggested a suitable empirical relationship:

$$E = E_m \left(1 - \frac{a}{t_r} \right)$$

where E = Organic removal (%), E_m = Maximum removal (%),
t_r = Hydraulic retention time, a = constant. The problem with using
this equation is that, unless accurate values for E_m and a are known,
pilot-plant evaluations are needed before a full-scale plant can be
designed. The range of values noted for these constants (Forster, 1984)
(Table 3.7) emphasises the need for having accurate figures.

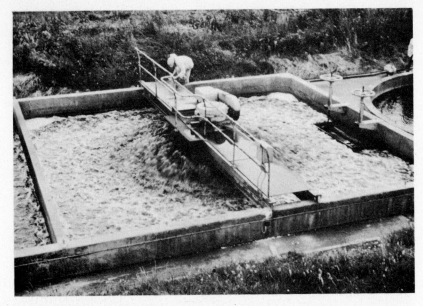

Fig. 3.13. An activated sludge aeration tank.

3.5   Homogeneous reactors

3.5.1   *Aerobic processes*

The activated sludge process is a purely aquatic system in which the sewage, which has usually been settled, is contacted with air and a flocculated mass of bacteria and protozoa (see Fig. 1.17). This is the activated sludge and the contents of the aeration tank are known as the mixed liquor solids (MLSS). After an appropriate contact time, usually upwards of 4 hours, the solids are concentrated by settlement and recycled. Air is supplied either by a compressor and diffuser system or by mechanical surface aeration (Fig. 3.13 and see Chapter 4).

An activated sludge system is therefore designed with two objectives: (a) to oxidise organic matter and (b) to produce a sludge with good settling properties. One of the key factors in achieving these objectives is adequate aeration/mixing and the aeration system must be sized so that it not only transfers sufficient oxygen to the mixed liquors but also transfers the oxygen at a rate which is greater than the maximum oxygen uptake rate of the microbial flora in the mixed liquor. Activated sludge systems can be considered in three categories: (a) Conventional aeration; (b) Extended aeration; and (c) High-rate aeration. Processes designed for conventional aeration will, in general, have liquid retention periods of between 4 and 8 hours at DWF, they will operate at an MLSS concentration of between 1500 and 4000 and the return sludge

Table 3.8. *Loading rates used for the design of activated sludge systems*

Process	Hydraulic loading rate (kg BOD m^{-3} day^{-1})	Sludge loading rate (kg BOD kg MLVSS^{-1})
Conventional aeration	0.56–0.80	0.25–0.45
Extended aeration	0.16–0.32	0.05–0.20
High rate process	2.40–4.00	0.5–5.0

pumps should be capable of pumping flows of up to 150 per cent DWF. A plant of this type should be capable of producing a final effluent of at least a 30:20 standard. Aeration would usually be either by surface aeration or by diffused air (see Chapter 4).

In terms of sizing, there are very few limitations to a diffused air plant; almost any width or length of tank may be selected. However, to achieve good plug-flow characteristics within the tank a length to breadth ratio in excess of 3:1 is preferable. The depth of the aeration tank should usually be about 4 m, although in exceptional circumstances either very shallow or very deep tanks may be used. It is essential that the returned activated sludge, the incoming sewage and the mixed liquor should be mixed as quickly as possible. One way of achieving this is to mix the sewage and returned sludge externally to the aeration tank and then to ensure a uniform distribution of this mixture across the full width of the aeration tank. The aeration compressors should be sized on the basis of 1 kg of oxygen per kg of carbonaceous BOD removed. This means a volume of 9–20 m^3 air m^{-3} of settled sewage depending on the presence or absence of trade wastes. The volume of the aeration tank will be determined by the loading factors given in Table 3.8. Usually the solids loading rate (food:mass) is used.

Diffused air systems are readily adapted to the *tapered aeration* approach. With this modification, aeration is intensified at the inlet end of the aeration tank, thus supplying additional oxygen at the point where the load and therefore the oxygen demand is greatest.

It is generally considered that mechanical surface aerators are more easy to maintain than air diffuser systems. A surface aeration plant should be designed so that the aeration tank is divided into pockets and so that there are between two and four pockets operating in series. This would constitute a single aeration stream. There is benefit in having more than one stream operating in parallel. Individual aeration pockets should reflect the characteristics of the aerator but in general terms they should be square in plan with the side-wall length not exceeding ten times the diameter of the aerator (this usually results in a length of between 6 and 15 m). The pockets should be flat-bottomed with a depth of between 2.5 and 5 m. An approximate guide to the depth can be obtained by using a ratio of 3:1 side-wall length:depth. The aeration cones should be driven by individual electric motors, the power requirements being of the order of 0.55 and 0.65 kWH per kg of BOD removed. A full discussion of aerators, their sizing and testing is given in Chapter 4.

Activated sludge plants having hydraulic retention times of greater than 15 hours should be considered as being in the extended aeration mode. In the main, this means oxidation ditches. These are continuous channels in which the aeration and the circulation of the ditch contents is achieved by mechanical aeration which in the majority of cases has a horizontal shaft and is placed across the ditch (see Barnes, Forster & Johnstone, 1983).

Oxidation ditches were developed in Holland and, as designed initially, operated on a fill and draw basis without a separate settlement tank. However, problems with retaining sludge during period of high rainfall soon led to the introduction of either internal or separate clarifiers. The earliest ditches were small and used horizontally mounted aerators of the 'Kessener brush' or 'TNO' type. Developments in technology have subsequently led to the construction of large ditches which adopt numerous configurations and use a variety of aeration devices. Many have lost the original character of being simple country ditches: indeed, ditches serving between 20 000 and 500 000 are common. The largest treats a mixture of industrial wastes and domestic sewage for BASF in Ludwigshafen, Germany, and has a population equivalent *c*. 6.5 million. However, the size of the original rotors and the depth of the ditches themselves limited the size of the population served to about 15 000. Thus, to enable the oxidation ditch configuration to be used for flows from population equivalents in excess of this, ditch systems using deeper and wider channels with larger mechanical aerators had to be developed. These can be operated either as extended aeration units or with more conventional retention times (i.e. 6–9 hours).

Generally, however, oxidation ditches can be considered as low-intensity activated sludge systems operating in the extended aeration range of sludge loading. Usually, they treat raw sewage and the use of primary sedimentation would be considered an unusual variation. Paramount among the attributes often mooted for oxidation ditches is their ability to produce high quality effluents in a simple, reliable manner with the production of a minimum quantity of 'stable' sludge. That this is so gives credit to Pasveer's original philosophy which was to provide simple systems that would treat sewage and aerobically digest sludge in one tank. Although important in their own right, the other capabilities of oxidation ditches, such as their ability to nitrify and denitrify in the one tank, must be considered to be secondary to the fundamental principle of simplicity.

In the UK, the design of extended aeration plants should conform to the specifications laid down in the Ministry of Housing and Local Government Technical Memorandum on activated sludge plants providing for a long period of aeration (1969). For oxidation ditches, the main criteria are:

> BOD load $\not> 210$ mg BOD l^{-1} of ditch capacity
> sludge loading of 0.05–0.15 kg BOD kg MLSS^{-1} d^{-1}
> aerators should give about 2 kg O$_2$ kg BOD^{-1}
> depth of ditch between 1.0 and 1.5 m
> aerators should give a flow of 0.3 m s^{-1}.

There are many possible arrangements and operating modes for oxidation ditches. The ditch itself can be arranged in almost any configuration as long as it forms a closed circuit. For smaller ditches the most common configuration is the single channel arranged in an oval shape. The development of larger ditches has led to a variety of layouts which provide a great deal of flexibility in design. The basic circuit can be formed in 'L'-shapes, horseshoes or other configurations to suit site conditions. Other systems use concentric arrangements of inter-connected multiple channels (Fig. 3.14 and 3.15).

In cross section, most ditches are either rectangular or trapezoidal, and liquid depths vary from about 1 to 4 m. With surface aerators, 4 m is about the limit of depth; above 4 m there is a possibility of sludge depositing on the tank floor.

Although a number of manufacturers market aeration devices for oxidation ditches they are all, in general, variations of standard surface aerators. By far the most common is the horizontally mounted (brush) aerator, although the vertical shaft aerator as used in the Carrousel system is gaining wide acceptance. Notable exceptions to these are the Orbal system, developed in South Africa, which uses an arrangement of discs mounted on a horizontal shaft (Fig. 3.15), and the Downdraft tube aerator which induces mixed liquor and entrapped air through a U-tube under a transverse barrier (see Chapter 4).

Aeration efficiency, reliability and cost are obviously paramount considerations in selecting an aerator for a particular system. However, as far as the operating mode is concerned, these criteria are of less importance than the distribution of aerators around the ditch, the velocity imparted to the liquor, and the change in aeration efficiency with rotor speed or depth of submergence.

Velocity imparted to the liquor is vitally important in keeping the solids in suspension throughout the whole length of ditch; the minimum

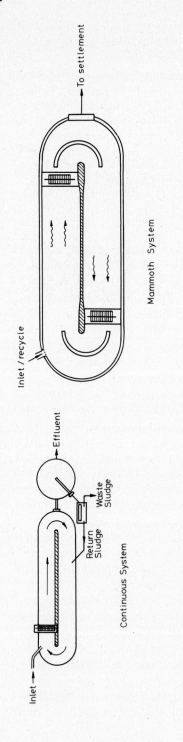
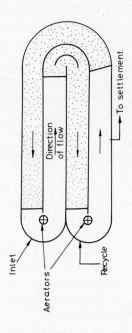

Fig. 3.14. Typical layouts for oxidation ditch systems.

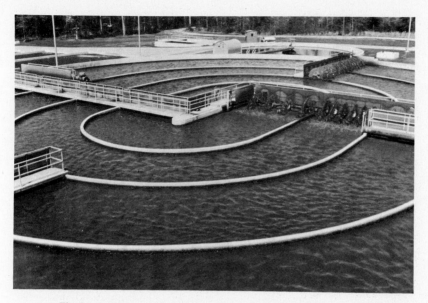

Fig. 3.15. 'Orbal' multi-channel oxidation ditch (by courtesy of Envirex Inc.).

velocity can be considered to be about 0.15 m s^{-1}. With vertically mounted aerators, which impart velocity by centrifugal force, the velocity (0.3–0.4 m s^{-1}) is usually far in excess of the minimum required, and the change in aeration efficiency with velocity is relatively small. However, with horizontal or brush aerators high velocity can affect aeration efficiency. If the velocity of liquor passing the aerator becomes too great, the differential speed between the rotor tip and the liquor becomes so low that aeration efficiency is impaired. In some cases it is necessary to introduce baffles to the ditch.

Distribution of aerators around the ditch can play a significant part in the process especially where nitrogen removal is required. Horizontally mounted aerators can be installed at any point along the length of the ditch. Generally they are mounted sufficiently far apart to allow a significant change in dissolved oxygen profile such that, if required, large enough anoxic zones will be present to permit denitrification. However, with some systems such as the Akvadan–Harvey Bio Denitro system, a different operational mode has been adopted to allow denitrification. In this system there are no separate final settling tanks, clarification being achieved by allowing settlement in the aeration tank. The problem arises in the resuspension of the settled solids with the horizontal aerators. Because of the restriction in velocity with this type of aerator it is not possible to successfully resuspend the solids throughout the whole ditch if the aerators are widely separated. Consequently, a larger number of smaller aerators are distributed over the whole ditch. While there are advantages in such a system (no settlement tank and no return sludge pumping) it means that the dissolved oxygen profile is not sufficient to permit the presence of anoxic zones large enough to allow denitrification. In this case, denitrification is achieved by reducing the speed of some of the aerators on a time cycle and allowing the whole ditch contents to become anoxic.

With vertical shaft aerators there is no option in the position of the aerators. They are located at one end of the channel in line with the centre dividing wall in an aeration section, the depth of which depends on the aerator diameter. To provide optimum aeration efficiency the depth of the aeration section must be at least equal to the diameter of the aerator. Thus some Carrousel systems have deeper aeration sections than channels. However, in all Carrousels the separation of the aerators is sufficient to allow the presence of anoxic zones for denitrification.

Most frequently, clarification of final effluent and thickening of return sludge is carried out in separate circular settlement tanks, although some have internal clarifiers which are accommodated in a central 'island' and some use a split ditch arrangement. In the latter option one leg of the circuit is divided into two channels equipped with control gates. The ditch is operated with one gate closed and one open, the closed leg becoming a horizontal flow settling zone. Less commonly, clarification is accomplished by using the whole volume of the ditch on an intermittent basis.

The design criteria for separate settlement tanks used with oxidation ditches are similar to those for other activated sludge systems. Average overflow rates between 16 and 20 $m^3 m^{-2} d^{-1}$ with peak rates of 40–45 $m^3 m^{-2} d^{-1}$ and a solids loading equivalent to 6 kg $m^{-2} d^{-1}$ are used in the USA where minimum side-wall depths are recommended to be between 3.7 and 4.3 m (12–14 ft). In Europe the practice has been to use similar overflow rates but there has been a tendency to use much lower side-wall depths (1.5 m) with relatively shallow floor slopes ($7\frac{1}{2}$ to 10°).

The simplest ditch system is probably that based on the small diameter, horizontal rotor. This can be used in a variety of ditch configurations, all of which are basically a continuous circuit having a trapezoidal cross section and a depth of 1.0–1.8 m. This channel can be formed into horseshoes or other configuration to fit the site, but in general an oval or circular configuration is used. The construction and in particular the lining of these ditches tends, in the UK, to vary with the size of the ditch. The linings can be reinforced concrete, concrete slabs, asphalt or butyl membrane. In some cases, most often small ditches, the ditch can even be unlined.

One of the major features of this type of ditch is its low capital cost in relation to other types of bio-oxidation – the feature specified by Paveer. It is thus very suitable for use in developing countries.

As well as oxidising carbonaceous pollutants most conventional and extended aeration plants will be required to nitrify. Nitrification is the microbial oxidation of ammoniacal nitrogen to nitrate and it is achieved in two steps by two specific species of chemolithotrophic bacteria.

$$NH_4^+ + 1.5O_2 \xrightarrow{\textit{Nitrosomonas} \text{ spp.}} NO_2^- + 2H^+ + H_2O$$

$$NO_2^- + 0.5O_2 \xrightarrow{\textit{Nitrobacter} \text{ spp.}} NO_3^-$$

Thus the complete oxidation of 1 kg of ammoniacal nitrogen, in theory, requires 4.57 kg O_2. However in practice, because of the release of oxygen during the assimilation of carbon dioxide, the amount of oxygen which must be supplied externally is slightly less, 4.3 kg. Nevertheless, whatever the absolute value, nitrification has a high oxygen demand relative to the requirements of carbonaceous oxidation. The main requirements for nitrification are therefore good and adequate aeration so that dissolved oxygen levels are at least 2–4 mg l^{-1} and a long (usually > 10 days) sludge age. This latter requirement ensures that the slower growing nitrifiers can maintain adequate colonisation of the sludge.

Sludge age is calculated from:

$$\text{Age (days)} = \frac{M \times V}{(S \times W) + (E \times Q)}$$

where M = MLSS concentration, in mg l^{-1}, V = Aeration tank volume, in m^3, S = Solids concentration of wasted sludge, in mg l^{-1}, W = Volume wasted, in m^3 d^{-1}, E = Effluent suspended solids, in mg l^{-1}, Q = Effluent flow-rate, in m^3 d^{-1}.

Activated sludge systems can also be operated as a high-rate process. This is a heavily loaded, short contact time process which is designed to give a final effluent of worse than 30:20. It finds application for coastal treatment or as a pretreatment of industrial effluents before discharge to sewer.

In addition to nitrifying, some activated sludge systems may be required to denitrify. This requirement may be necessary in order to meet discharge consent standards or to prevent spontaneous denitrification occurring in the final settlement tanks, so causing elements of the sludge blanket to rise to the surface with the nitrogen gas. Denitrification is the result of chemolithotrophic bacteria utilising nitrate as the terminal electron acceptor in their respiratory chain in the absence of molecular oxygen (anoxic conditions). The process also requires carbon as an energy source. It is therefore relatively easy to achieve denitrification in the activated sludge process by creating an anoxic zone within the main aeration tank. With conventional tank geometry there are two places where such a zone can be located: at the inlet where carbon is available as settled sewage and nitrate in association with the return sludge; or immediately prior to discharge to the final settlement tank. In this latter case a carbonaceous supplement is needed since the BOD at that point in the treatment cycle ought to be very low. The use of settled sewage would tend to increase the concentration of ammoniacal nitrogen in the final effluent and for this reason other carbon sources have been evaluated (see Jank & Bridle, 1983). Most conventional activated sludge plants that have anoxic zones for denitrification tend to have them located at the inlet end of the aeration tanks. Although denitrification rates are known, there seems to be little available data for the sizing of anoxic zones and those suggestions that have been made tend to be 'rule of thumb' guidelines (see Jank & Bridle, 1983; Barnes & Bliss, 1983).

Oxidation ditches have a greater potential for achieving and controlling denitrification since aeration is provided at fixed, well separated points within the aeration tank. Down-stream of these points there will be a gradual reduction in dissolved oxygen, due to aerobic respiration, until anoxic conditions are reached. For operational control purposes these are taken to be when the dissolved oxygen (DO) is less than 0.5 mg l^{-1} (Hanbury *et al.*, 1978). The size of the anoxic zone can be calculated from the time taken to achieve denitrification:

$$\tau = N/\gamma M$$

where $N =$ the concentration of nitrate, in mg l^{-1}, $M =$ the concentration of MLSS, in g l^{-1}, $\gamma =$ the denitrification rate, in mg g MLSS^{-1} h^{-1}. Taking a typical value for γ of 1 mg g^{-1} h^{-1} it has been shown that, for normal operating conditions, about 50 per cent of the ditch volume needs to be anoxic (Johnstone, Rachwal & Hanbury, 1983).

One advantage of operating any activated sludge system in a denitrifying mode is that some of the carbonaceous pollutants can be oxidised without the use of molecular oxygen which is expensive to transfer to the liquid phase. Indeed, it has been shown (Johnstone *et al.*, 1983) that the oxygen requirements of a ditch in which nitrification/denitrification is taking place can be calculated from:

$$R = B + 4.34 N_H - 2.85 N_T + 0.024 M V r_{20} \theta^{(T-20)}$$

where $R =$ oxygen usage, in kg d^{-1}, $B =$ BOD removal, in kg d^{-1}, $N_H =$ Amm. N removal, in kg d^{-1}, $N_T =$ Total nitrogen removal, in kg d^{-1}, $M =$ MLSS concentration, in kg m^{-3}, $V =$ aeration tank volume, in m³, r_{20} = basal respiration rate at 20 °C = 3.9 mg g MLSS⁻¹ h⁻¹, θ = temperature coefficient = 1.07.

This is less than the oxygen requirement of a ditch in which no denitrification is taking place by $2.85N_T$ kg d⁻¹. The control of the anoxic zones, and thus the denitrification, can best be achieved by controlling the DO automatically with oxygen electrodes (see Johnstone *et al.*, 1983). The control probe should be located between the point of aeration and the start of the anoxic zone. Upper and lower limits can then be set to ensure that:

(a) there is a DO concentration in the aerobic region which is adequate for nitrification (> 1.5 mg l⁻¹)
(b) the DO concentration at the start of the anoxic zone is $\leqslant 0.5$ mg l⁻¹ and
(c) these conditions are maintained even at the extremes of the loading rates.

The final point that needs to be considered when examining the design of activated sludge plants is the solids produced by the process. These originate in part from solid material in the incoming sewage and in part from biological growth. However, irrespective of their source the excess solids resulting from bio-oxidation will have to be processed and disposed of in one way or another. Three methods for calculating the mass of solids are worth discussing. The first is based on a solids balance within the aeration tank and gives the accumulation of solids (S_t) in terms of mass per unit time:

$$S_t = (cS_i + aL_r) - bS$$

where S_i = mass of solids in influent, c = fraction of non-biodegradable solids in influent, L_r = mass of BOD removed per unit time, a = mass of solids produced per unit mass of BOD removed (the yield coefficient), S = mass of solids being aerated, b = decay constant.

Most workers take the solids to be the volatile rather than the total solids. However, there are differences in opinion as to which BOD value should be used; for example, Tebbutt (1971) recommends the use of ultimate BOD whilst Eckenfelder & O'Connor (1961) use the normal five-day BOD. This latter point can be ignored as long as the value for the yield coefficient has been calculated or obtained from the literature on a compatible basis. The main problem with this method is using (or even finding) the current values for the yield coefficient and the decay constant and as a result this method is not widely used in practical design. An alternative and purely empirical approach (Wilson, 1981) is to calculate the sludge wastage rate (W) on the basis of:

$$W = QL(0.2 + SLR^{\frac{1}{2}}) \text{ in kg dry matter d}^{-1}$$

where SLR = sludge loading rate (kg BOD kg MLSS⁻¹ d⁻¹).

The third method is based on a partly theoretical and partly empirical derivation by Johnstone *et al.* (1983) for the sludge production in oxidation ditches:

$$\frac{S_T}{B} = 0.7 - \left[\frac{0.034 \times 1.07^{(T-20)}}{SLR}\right] + Kc$$

where S_T = total sludge produced, in kg d^{-1}, B = mass of BOD removed, in kg d^{-1}, K = influent total suspended solids:influent BOD.

This method is only valid for SLR values of 0.05 to 0.15. It can therefore be seen that there is no particular method which will enable the design engineer to calculate the mass of solids accurately other than perhaps for specialised cases.

3.5.2   *The Deep Shaft process*

This is a wastepaper treatment system, analogous to the activated sludge process, which was developed from fermentation technology with the objective of providing a high intensity treatment. The system is relatively simple, consisting of a single shaft either with a single central division or a central core or, more recently, a cruciform division. Thus the shaft is separated into a downflow section and an upflow zone (Fig. 3.16). The circulation of liquid within the shaft is brought about by air lift principles. Initially, air is injected into the riser at a relatively

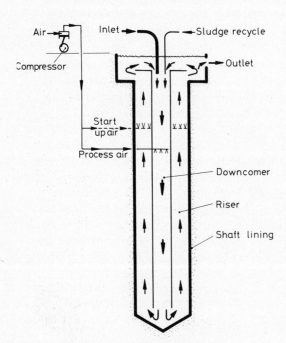

Fig. 3.16. The Deep Shaft process.

shallow depth. Air lift initiates the circulation and once this has started the majority of the aeration is transferred to the downcomer. The liquid velocity is of the order of 1–2 m s⁻¹, and at this velocity the downward flow of liquid has a greater speed than the rise rate of the air bubbles. Air is thus carried down the shaft.

The key feature of this circulation method is the gas voidage and the location of the air injection point. An examination of the voidage patterns shows that, within the aerated levels, the voidage in the downcomer is greater than that in the riser. This is because of the relative speeds of the gas and liquid: incipient contra-flow in the downcomer, giving a high bubble retention time, as opposed to co-current flow in the riser giving a short bubble retention time. However, because of the non-aerated section above the injection point, the downcomer has a *nett* lower voidage and therefore the greater weight of liquid. The result is circulation (Hemmings *et al.*, 1977; Hines *et al.*, 1975).

The dimensions of deep shafts vary with the organic load to be treated. Depths of between 50 and 150 m have been used in conjunction with diameters of 0.5 to 10 m (Hemmings *et al.*, 1977). Details of how the shafts are sunk are available in the literature (Collins & Elder, 1980; Cox *et al.*, 1980) and will not be discussed here.

The oxygen transfer is a key feature in the advantages claimed for this process. The high liquid velocities within the shaft give high Reynolds numbers. Bubble coalescence is therefore minimised and there is a high rate of surface renewal, both being factors which promote high levels of oxygen transfer (see Chapter 4). In addition, the driving force for the transfer of oxygen is significantly increased since the pressure at the bottom of a typical shaft can result in the solubility of oxygen in water being increased 5–10-fold. The net result is that transfer efficiencies of 3–4.5 kg O_2 kWh⁻¹ have been reported together with utilisations of better than 85 per cent (Hemmings *et al.*, 1977). The other major advantage claimed for the process is that high sludge loading rates can be supported by the high oxygen transfer efficiencies; a typical figure based on published data is 0.9 kg BOD kg MLSS⁻¹ d⁻¹.

One of the major problems with the Deep Shaft process has been gas disengagement. Micro-bubbles still exist in the mixed liquor when it is taken from the shaft. These prevent a settlement stage producing a final effluent of an acceptable quality. Various techniques have been tried to overcome this problem of turbidity. These have included vacuum de-gassing prior to settlement (Hemmings *et al.*, 1977; Collins & Elder, 1980), flotation (Bolton & Ousby, 1977) and bubble stripping (Cox *et al.*, 1980). None of these has proved to be totally satisfactory. The result is that current designs are based on the philosophy of a dual treatment (Fig. 3.17) in which a shaft, reduced in size, removes only a

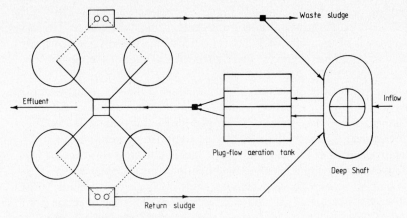

Fig. 3.17. Deep Shaft II.

proportion of load. The mixed liquor from the shaft is then passed to an aeration tank which affords the rest of the treatment necessary and de-gasses the liquors. These can then be settled in a conventional manner with the concentrated sludge being recycled to the shaft. It is claimed that the reduced size of both parts of this hybrid make it more cost beneficial than pure versions of either one of the components (Anon., 1983).

3.5.3   *Anaerobic reactors*

Homogeneous reactors can also be operated anaerobically and used to treat liquid wastes. Systems of this type are sometimes known as contact digesters, sometimes as anaerobic activated sludge and sometimes merely as conventional digesters. They may be operated either as batch or as continuous processes and may incorporate a recycle either of gas or of solids or both. Probably the simplest operational type is the continuously fed reactor without any form of recycle. Two tanks would be used; a primary tank which was heated and from which gas was collected, and a secondary tank which would preferably be open to the atmosphere and which separated liquid from solid. This type of digester is similar in design to that used for the treatment of sewage sludge and would best be used for treating wastes with a high solids content (e.g. farm slurries). Indeed, this approach has been used successfully by the Rowett Research Institute for the slurry from a 300 pig unit. The plant uses a retention time of 10 days and has a gas yield of 0.3 m³ gas kg total solids applied^{-1} (Hobson, 1984). When the treatment of liquors containing low solids concentrations is being considered, a similar type of design can be used although some form of solids recycle is necessary to prevent wash-out (Fig. 3.18). These plants

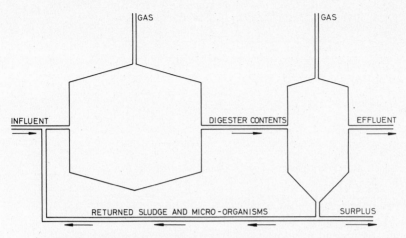

Fig. 3.18. Simple contact digester with solids recycle.

tend to be operated with relatively short hydraulic retention times (e.g. 0.5 to 5 days) and it is therefore essential that the settlement is efficient. Not only is this important in maintaining final effluent quality, but also in ensuring that the main digester carries as high a concentration of solids as is possible. In this way, the high solids retention time that is necessary for good treatment can be achieved.

One of the main problems that is encountered with the contact process is the poor settlement of solids, or to be more precise, an inability to settle due to an attachment of product gas to the solid particles. Several techniques have been employed to overcome this problem, vacuum de-gassing being one of the more common (Fullen, 1953). An alternative approach is that adopted by South African workers who modified a commercially available digester: the Dorr–Oliver 'Clarigester' (Cillie *et al.*, 1969; Stander, 1967). These modifications, which were made to improve solids retention, were:

(a) The installation of a conical section beneath the standard stilling box. This segregated any active solids from the quiescent zone and provided a region in which gas would separate, thus reducing the 'flotation risk' in the main clarifier.

(b) The use of a conical unit instead of the standard gas seal.

(c) The provision for external re-circulation of sludge (3.8 l s^{-1} for 10 minutes every half hour) to assist in flushing thickened sludge from the clarifier back to the digester zone.

This type of digester has been used to treat a variety of organic wastes and has achieved high removal rates of the polluting load (97 per cent based on COD for wine distillery residues). However, the maximum

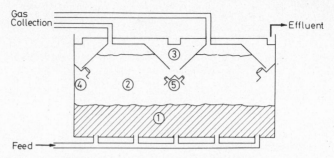

Fig. 3.19. Schematic diagram of an Upflow Sludge Blanket reactor.

loading rate that could be achieved without undue loss of solids was 3.2 kg COD m^{-3} d^{-1}.

In an attempt to improve on this relatively low loading rate, Dutch workers developed a system known as the Upflow Sludge Blanket (USB) reactor (Lettinga *et al.*, 1980). Although no support medium is specifically added to this type of digester (Fig. 3.19), the sludge produced is of such a granular nature that the process characteristics should perhaps be considered as a hybrid type. The underlying principles of the USB reactor are that a heavily flocculated sludge should be developed which can act almost as a separate fluidised bed (1) and withstand relatively high mixing forces. Having achieved this, wash-out of less stable particles can be reduced by having a quiescent zone (2) which enhances the potential for re-flocculation and hence settlement back into the sludge blanket by way of sludge collected in the settlement zone (3). The operation of the gas collection bowls, which should slope at an angle of 50° to promote the ready return of sludge from the settlement area, is made more effective by the use of vented gas traps (4) and gas seals (5). A full scale version (200 m³) of this type of digester has successfully treated sugar beet waste at a loading rate of 16 kg COD m^{-3} d^{-1} and a hydraulic retention time of 4 hours, achieving COD removals in excess of 90 per cent. Upflow sludge blanket reactors can also be used as a purely methanogenic process with the acidogenic phase being carried out in a separate reactor. It is claimed that by doing this each part of the overall biogas generation process can be optimised (see Morris & Burgess, 1984).

4　Aeration

4.1　Introduction

The very nature of any of the bio-oxidative processes (e.g. trickling filters; activated sludge) means that oxygen must be supplied to the microbial flora to maintain aerobic conditions. However, it must be remembered that this oxygen must be supplied at a rate sufficient to at least balance the rate of removal by the active biomass. In the case of trickling filters, the oxygen is supplied from the air which passes up through the filters. This can be thought of as natural aeration. In the activated sludge system, aeration is a positive process with specific equipment being used to ensure the transfer of oxygen into the mixed liquors. Although oxygen transfer is an essential part both of the activated sludge process and the operation of trickling filters, aeration as a technology is really confined to activated sludge systems. Activated sludge will contain many different bacterial species, each having differing responses to oxygen; some will be genuinely aerobic, some will be facultative anaerobes, whilst some may be micro-aerophilic. This means that not only will the removal rate vary with temperature (as would any chemical reaction) but also with the nature of the feed-stock (which will determine which species become dominant) and the rate of aeration itself. The balance between the transfer rate and the removal rate is of paramount importance. If transfer exceeds removal, the process becomes wasteful in energy; if the opposite occurs there will be an inadequate removal of pollutants.

4.2　Theory of oxygen transfer
4.2.1　Development of basic theory

To understand how oxygen is transferred into a fluid it is usual to consider the transfer from a bubble into water. The process needs also to be considered in terms of the equilibrium conditions which determine the solubility of the gas and therefore its ultimate concentration at the prevailing temperature and pressure. Thus for a given gas pressure and temperature there will be equilibrium concentration (C^*) in the liquid and, conversely, for a given concentration and temperature in the liquid there will be an equilibrium gas pressure (p^*) in the gas phase.

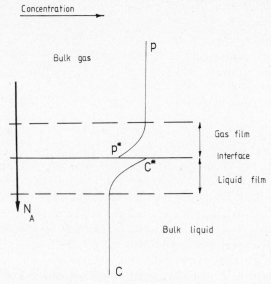

Fig. 4.1. Schematic representation of a bubble/water interface showing the oxygen pressure and concentration variation.

The transfer of oxygen from the bulk gas phase to the bulk liquid phase takes place in a series of stages:

(a) Diffusion from the bulk gas to the gas/liquid interface. This process is quick and establishes a saturation concentration at the interface.
(b) Passage across the interface.
(c) Diffusion from the liquid side of the interface into the bulk liquid phase.

The interface of a bubble is composed of three regions: the interface itself, a static gas film and a static liquid film (Fig. 4.1). The resistance to the transfer of oxygen resides in these films. This is because the molecules in the films have (a) a high velocity; (b) a short mean free path and therefore (c) a large number of collisions. The net passage of gas molecules through the film is therefore slow. The total resistance (R) to the transfer of oxygen can be considered as being the summation of the individual resistances; i.e.:

$$R = R_G + R_I + R_L$$

However, because of the difficulty in quantifying the magnitude of the individual resistances, it is more usual to consider the mass transfer coefficients, K_L and K_G, where:

$$K_L = 1/R_L \text{ and } K_G = 1/R_G$$

Since the solubility of oxygen in water is low,

$$HK_G \gg K_L$$

where H is the Henry's law constant. This means that the transfer of oxygen is liquid film controlled.

The interfacial area across which transfer can occur will also affect the rate of oxygen transfer: the greater the area, the higher the transfer rate. This means that the rate of oxygen transfer (N_A) is calculated from

$$N_A = K_L A(C^* - C)$$

where A is the total interfacial area. Alternatively, this can be expressed as:

$$V\frac{dC}{dt} = K_L A(C^* - C)$$

which takes the more commonly used form of:

$$\frac{dC}{C^* - C} = K_L \frac{A}{V} dt = K_L a\, dt.$$

However, in most cases it is impractical to measure the value of the interfacial areas and therefore for all practical purposes the product of K_L and a are taken as a single constant (as is $K_L A$).

4.2.2   Factors affecting $K_L a$

Detergents. In general terms the addition of surface active material to aqueous solutions alters the interfacial properties of that fluid. In a simple aqueous solution, bubbles tend to coalesce fairly readily whereas when surface active agents are present coalescence is far less ready. It has already been established that, everything else being the same, the smaller the bubble size (i.e. the greater the interfacial area) the better is the mass transfer rate. This would suggest that detergents, which are invariably present in sewage, would enhance the transfer of oxygen in an activated sludge aeration tank by reducing the bubble size (Fig. 4.2). However, the effect of detergents on the mass transfer coefficient must also be considered. In reducing coalescence, surface active agents

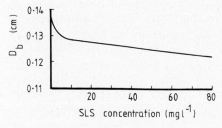

Fig. 4.2. The effect of sodium lauryl sulphate (SLS) on the bubble diameter (D_b). (From Aiba *et al.*, 1973.)

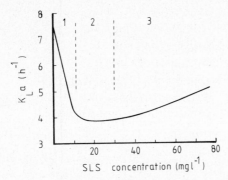

Fig. 4.3. The effect of SLS on $K_L a$. (From Aiba *et al.*, 1973.)

modify the bubble surfaces so that the surfaces become more rigid. This means that gas molecules find it more difficult to penetrate the surface, resulting in a decrease in K_L and therefore the rate of mass transfer. In assessing the effect of detergents therefore, these two opposing effects must be considered. An examination of the effect of detergents on $K_L a$ (Fig. 4.3) shows that three distinct areas can be identified:

Zone 1 The initial amounts of surfactant result in a rapid and significant (40–50 per cent) decrease in $K_L a$. This is due to the K_L effect being dominant.

Zone 2 The further addition of surfactant causes no variation in $K_L a$. The two effects are balanced.

Zone 3 Additional amounts of surface active material result in a slight increase in $K_L a$. The cause of this is the dominance of the bubble size factor.

In any activated sludge system therefore, it would seem likely that the variation in the precise value of the $K_L a$ associated with the aeration system will not easily be predicted and will depend on the amount of detergent in the incoming sewage.

Phenolics. This class of compound is also likely to be a contaminant of sewage particularly when it contains a significant proportion of industrial effluent. Simple phenolics have been shown to affect oxygen transfer rate, the degree of improvement increasing with the rate of aeration but being independent of the phenol concentration. The presence of *o*-cresol also enhances the rate of transfer. However, the effect is different at different concentrations with the optimum varying with the aeration rate (Fig. 4.4). *p*-xylenol has a variable effect causing an increase or decrease in the oxygen transfer rate depending on concentration and the intensity of aeration (Ganczarczyk, 1972).

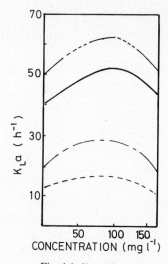

Fig. 4.4. $K_L a$ values for varying concentrations of *o*-cresol at different air flow-rates. (From Ganczarczyk, 1972.) -------- 6 m³ m⁻³ h⁻¹; —·— 10 m³ m⁻³ h⁻¹; —— 20 m³ m⁻³ h⁻¹; —-----— 30 m³ m⁻³ h⁻¹.

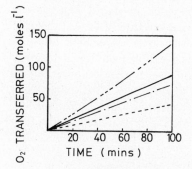

Fig. 4.5. The effect of fatty acids on oxygen transfer. (From Bell & Gallo, 1971.) ——Water at pH 7.5; —----— Water at pH 7.5 + 150 mg l⁻¹ fatty acid; —·—·— Water at pH 4; -------Water at pH 4 + 150 mg l⁻¹ fatty acid.

Fatty acids. Although fatty acids are not true surfactants they are absorbed at the air/liquid interface and, as such, are capable of affecting the gas transfer rates. However, the effect is pH-dependent. At a pH of 7.5 the acids are likely to be present in the form of soaps. These will improve the dispersion of air in the liquid phase and thus increase the surface area available for oxygen transfer. At lower values (pH = 4), the free acids will form fairly rigid monolayers at the air/liquid interface, reducing the oxygen diffusion across it and thus the overall rate of oxygen transfer (see Fig. 4.5; Bell & Gallo, 1971).

Table 4.1. *Values of alpha*

Source	α
Badger, Robinson & Kiff, 1975	0.63–0.94
Rees & Skellett, 1974	0.89–0.93
TWA (personal communication)	0.62–0.69
Lister & Boon, 1973	0.30–0.80
Eckenfelder & O'Connor, 1961	0.48–0.86
	0.53–0.64
Tewari & Bewtra, 1982	0.67–0.93

Alpha-factor. It can be seen from an examination of the preceding sections that a range of impurities in water can affect the mass transfer coefficient in a very variable and unpredictable manner. It is usual therefore to assess these in a single parameter, alpha, where:

$$\alpha = \frac{(K_L a) \text{ in waste}}{(K_L a) \text{ in clean water}}.$$

However, not all workers define alpha in the same way. Some use the $K_L a$ value of the raw effluent, some the value associated with mixed liquors and others that determined by the aeration of water to which standard anionic detergent (3–5 mg l^{-1}) has been added. The result is that a range of values (see Table 4.1) is available from the literature.

Alpha will also vary with the aeration system and, if a mixed liquor value is being used, with the length of time for which the sludge has been aerated. For example, alpha has been shown to vary from 0.3 at the beginning of the aeration period to 0.8 after 4 hours aeration for a domestic sewage treatment and from 0.45 to 0.79 (3 hours aeration) for the treatment of kraft mill waste.

Temperature. The transfer coefficient ($K_L a$) is dependent on temperature. The 'standard' is taken as being 20 °C and the conversion relationship is given by:

$$(K_L a)_T = (K_L a)_{20} (1.024)^{T-20}$$

However in assessing the transfer rate the effect of temperature on the saturation dissolved oxygen concentration (C^*) also needs to be considered. This effect is almost equal and opposite to the $K_L a$ effect and therefore for all practical purposes the role of temperature on dC/dt can be neglected (Table 4.2).

Table 4.2. *The effect of temperature on the oxygen transfer rate* dC/dt *over the temperature range typically found in sewage treatment, assuming* $C = 2$ *mg* l^{-1} *and* $(K_L a)_{20} = 5 h^{-1}$

Temperature (°C)	C^*	$(K_L a)_T$	$\dfrac{dC}{dt}$
14	10.29	4.34	35.95
12	10.77	4.14	36.27
10	11.28	3.94	36.60
8	11.84	3.76	37.01
6	12.45	3.59	37.49

Mean value for $\dfrac{dC}{dt} = 36.66 \pm 1.65$ per cent.

4.2.3 The effect of operational factors

Pressure. Since oxygen transfer involves a gas–liquid equilibrium relationship, pressure will be expected to have an effect on the process. Variations in pressure will in fact affect C^* (the saturation concentration) as shown:

$$(C^*)_P = (C^*)_{760} \frac{P-p}{760-p}$$

Beta-factor. The impurities in wastewaters will affect the value of C^* in much the same way as they do $K_L a$. This is taken into account by the use of the beta-factor where:

$$\beta = \frac{C^* \text{ in waste}}{C^* \text{ in clean water}}$$

If a precise value is not known, it is usually assumed that β is about 0.9.

Type of aerator. The two main types of aerator (diffused air and mechanical aeration) will have different characteristics in relation to the effect of impurities on oxygen transfer. As has been stated previously, the transfer rate is usually liquid film controlled. This means that the fine bubbles produced by diffusers are susceptible to the impurity effects which have been outlined in the preceding sections. Mechanical aeration on the other hand is a shearing process and as such is continually creating new interfaces. This almost total renewal of surfaces means that the overall transfer rate is far less dependent on the liquid film and those effects of impurities on that film.

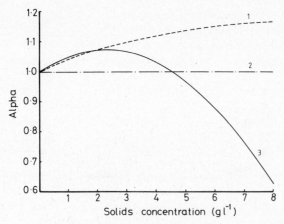

Fig. 4.6. Variation in alpha with solids concentration. (From Casey & Karmo, 1974.) 1 Activated sludge, A; 2 Non-flocculent solids; 3 Activated sludge, B.

The nature of the suspended solids. In part, the effect which suspended matter can have on oxygen transfer has already been discussed in that an alpha-factor related to the value of $K_L a$ in mixed liquor has already been mentioned. However, it has been shown that both the concentration and whether the solids are flocculent or non-flocculent will affect the alpha-factor (Casey & Karmo, 1974). For non-flocculent solids alpha is not altered by the solids concentration (Fig. 4.6). However, for flocculent solids, alpha is related to the solids concentration (c) by the expression

$$\alpha = 1 + k_1 c - k_2 c^2$$

where k_1 and k_2 are constants characteristic of the particular activated sludge. This is thought to be due to the influence of the solids on the bulk density and viscosity of the overall suspension. It may also be due to the effect that extracellular polymers excreted by the microbial flora, some of which will be partially soluble, will have on the air/water interface. This latter hypothesis could also explain the difference in alpha, mentioned earlier, that occurs as aeration progresses.

4.3   Aeration equipment

4.3.1   Introduction

In general, the theoretical aspects of oxygen transfer require that aeration equipment is designed so that, if an air-sparging system is to be used, the bubbles produced are as small as possible to give a high interfacial area/unit volume; in addition, if an air-entrainment system is to be used, the process should ensure a high rate of surface renewal. These requirements have resulted in two types of aerator, the

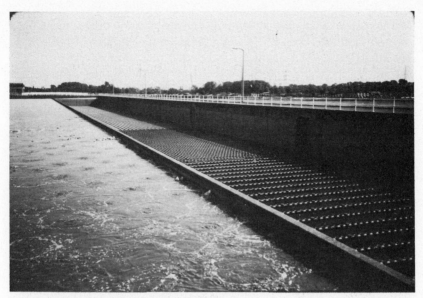

Fig. 4.7. Lay-out of fine-bubble diffusors.

fine-bubble dome diffuser and the surface aerator, being used in the
majority of activated sludge plants currently in operation. However,
other types of aerator do exist and are used.

4.3.2 *Fine-bubble aeration*

Dome diffusors are made in porous ceramic or plastic and are
connected to a central air main as shown in Fig. 4.7. Their design is
such that fine bubbles are produced and that the pressure drop across
the diffusor is not excessive. For a clean dome a typical figure for the
pressure drop would be about 0.4–0.7 bar (6–10 psi). The basic design
for a multiline diffusor lay-out is to have a spacing between the air
mains across the tank of 750 mm and a spacing of the domes along
each main of 300 mm; however, the actual lay-out of the air mains and
domes on the bottom of the aeration tank can be varied to suit the
process requirements of the overall system, the strength of the influent
and the location and number of inlets. Thus, a plug-flow system
treating a fairly strong waste might well have the domes close together
at the inlet end of the tank to achieve a high rate of oxygenation in that
region where a high rate of oxygen utilisation was occurring. Further
along the tank the dome spacing could be reduced to match the
decreasing organic load and thus the oxygen uptake rate. For example,
at the Oxford sewage works tapered aeration was achieved by
rearranging the existing diffusor domes in a 4:3:2:1 configuration

down the length of one of the aeration tanks (Lewin & West, 1978).
Comparison with an unmodified tank showed that the dissolved oxygen
concentration fell very slightly along the tapered unit (from 40 to 20 per
cent saturation), whilst in the control tank it rose from zero at the inlet
to about 70 per cent at the end of the tank. In other words tapering
achieved a better utilisation of the air supplied (Lewin & Henley, 1972).
Similarly, if denitrification were required, an anoxic region could be
achieved by using only sufficient domes to maintain the mixed liquor
solids in suspension.

The air is usually supplied by Rootes blowers, although for the larger
type of installation turbo-blowers may be used. Ideally these should
have a good 'turn-down' facility. That is to say there should be a
capability of reducing the intensity of the aeration during periods of
low organic load (e.g. at night-time). However, it is essential that the air
flow-rate per dome is not reduced below the recommended minimum of
$0.9 \text{ m}^3 \text{ h}^{-1}$. The provision of a continuously variable supply of air, in an
economic manner, means that the design of the air supply system must
be thought out with some care. The supply can be varied by using
combinations of variable speed motors, variable output blowers or
sequences of fixed speed blowers. The problem is to assess the cost both
in terms of capital expenditure and energy losses. Some of the possible
options and the problems associated with them have been previously
discussed by Clough (1982).

4.3.3   *Mechanical aerators*

Mechanical aeration devices fall into two main categories: those with
vertical shafts and those with a horizontal drive. In both cases the
intensity of aeration is controlled by the speed of rotation and the
depth to which the aerator is immersed. Aeration by horizontal shaft
systems tends to be used only in oxidation ditches and also serves as the
means of circulating the ditch contents at a speed sufficient to prevent
settlement of the mixed liquor solids (0.3 m s^{-1}). There are two main
types of horizontal rotor: the cage, or TNO, rotor which has a diameter
of 0.7 m and the Mammoth rotor which has a diameter of about 1.0 m
(Fig. 4.8). The former can only be used in ditches of up to 1.5–1.8 m
deep. In ditches of any greater depth their ability to maintain a uniform
suspension of solids within the ditch and to transfer oxygen efficiently
becomes impaired. This limits their suitability for the treatment of flows
from large population equivalents unless large areas of land are
available. The need to treat large loads and to do so in compact plants
led to the development of the larger type of horizontal rotor. Not only
was the diameter of the rotor increased but the blade configuration was
also modified. This resulted in improved oxygen transfer (Fig. 4.9). It
also meant that ditches with a depth as great as 3.5 m could be built.

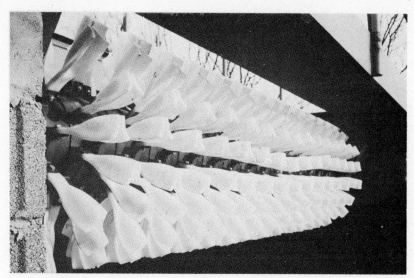

Fig. 4.8. Cage rotor (by courtesy of Manor Engineering Ltd).

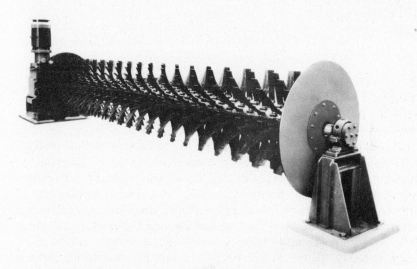

Fig. 4.9. Mammoth rotor (by courtesy of Whitehead and Poole Ltd).

However, Mammoth rotors also required that a system of baffles and guide-walls be incorporated in the tank design. These are used to reduce velocity differences within the ditch. Without them the surface velocity of the circulating liquors would approach that of the rotor tips and would therefore reduce the oxygen transfer rate (Stalzer & von der Emde, 1972).

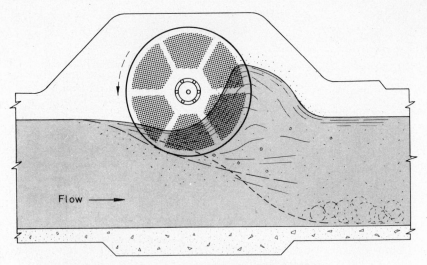

Fig. 4.10. Orbal disc aerators (by courtesy of Envirex Inc.).

Although the majority of horizontally driven aerators are either cage or Mammoth rotors, a third type does exist. This uses perforated discs, usually manufactured from high-strength plastic, attached to the horizontal drive shaft. Their diameter is 1.2–1.4 m and the perforations are 1.3 cm in diameter (Fig. 4.10). Aeration is achieved in two ways:

(i) by air, which is trapped in the perforations, being released as bubbles into the mixed liquor

(ii) by diffusion of air into the thin film of liquid which cascades down the disc whilst it is not submerged.

The rate of aeration can therefore be varied by altering the number of discs on the shaft. This means that aeration can be matched to the requirements of the biomass, as they change within the ditch, without recourse to variations in rotational speed. Disc aerators are usually driven at speeds of between 50 and 60 r.p.m. This is a narrower range than is used for the more usual type of horizontal aerator (50–90 r.p.m.). The range of immersion is also different. For disc systems it is 280–535 mm whereas for the cage and Mammoth rotors the range is 50–350 mm (Ettlich, 1978).

Aeration systems which have a vertical drive are more varied in design. Even so, they can all be considered as falling into two general classes based on their mixing characteristics (see Clough, 1974), In the one class, circulation is achieved as a result of a vortex being formed by the aerator. The Simcar aerator is typical of such systems which rely on vortex-induced mixing. Its normal rotational speed is 30–60 r.p.m. and the essential features of the impellor are its conical shape and the

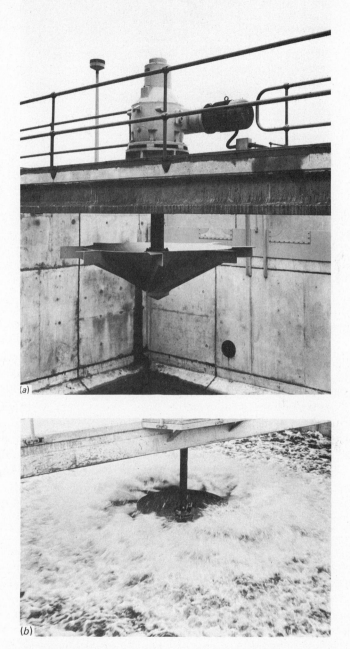

Fig. 4.11. *a* Simcar aerator (by courtesy of Simon Hartley Ltd.); *b* Aerator in operation.

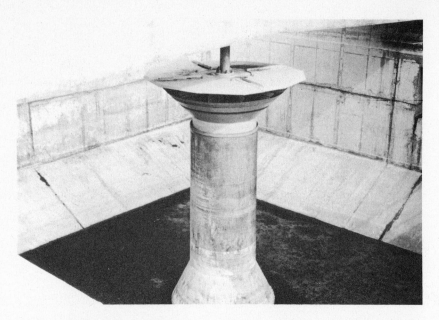

Fig. 4.12. Simplex aerator.

attached blade system (Fig. 4.11*a*). In the other, the impellor mixes the tank contents by acting almost as a centrifugal pump. This latter type is perhaps best typified by the Simplex system (Fig. 4.12). At the normal rotational speeds (30–60 r.p.m.) the conical impellor throws liquid away from the tank centre. Replacement liquid is then drawn up the draft tube from the bottom of the tank.

Both types of system achieve aeration by surface renewal and air entrainment. The rate at which oxygen is transferred depends, for any one design, on the degree to which the aerators are immersed in the liquid. This can be controlled either by an adjustable outlet weir which allows the liquid level to be varied or by mounting the aerator on a retractable drive shaft. This latter system is the more costly but it does reduce any hydraulics surges from the aeration tank.

4.3.4   *Other aeration devices*
Although surface aerators and fine-bubble diffusors together provide the majority of the installed aeration capacity at sewage treatment works, other designs exist and are used.

Jet aeration utilises a series of submerged ejectors connected to a central manifold which is usually arranged at right angles to the required flow of liquid. A pressurised supply of mixed liquor is discharged in the mixing chamber. The resultant pressure drop entrains air, which may or may not be under pressure (Fig. 4.13). A jet aeration

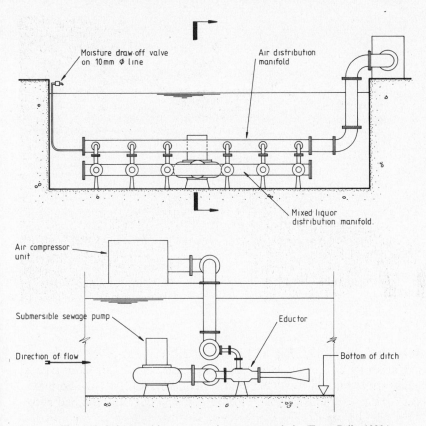

Fig. 4.13. Submerged jet aerator using compressed air. (From Pells, 1983.)

system using compressed air will provide a greater oxygen transfer efficiency than one using atmospheric air and in addition the use of a variable speed compressor means that the transfer can be ajdusted to suit the demand. Mixing of the aeration tank contents is achieved in two ways: horizontal mixing by the velocity of the air/fluid jet and vertical mixing by the rising plume of fine bubbles (Fig. 4.14). When jet aerators are used in oxidation ditches the horizontal velocity component is of considerable importance as it is this which is responsible for the circulation of the ditch contents and for ensuring that the settlement of solids does not occur. The circulation velocity that can be achieved varies with the air flow-rate but at rates of 0.57–1.13 m³ min⁻¹ velocities of approximately 0.3 m s⁻¹ have been recorded which are perfectly adequate.

Plunging-jet aerators rely on the fact that when a fluid jet is directed into water, air will be entrained and broken up into fine bubbles. Furthermore, if the jet is inclined at an angle and the point of release is

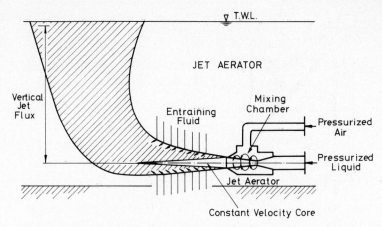

Fig. 4.14. Jet aeration (by courtesy of Pentech Division, Houdaille Industries Inc.).

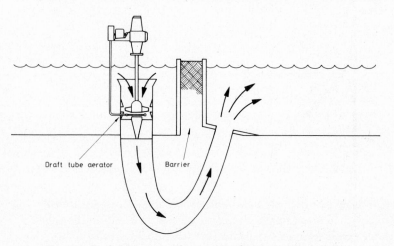

Fig. 4.15. Draft-tube aerator (by courtesy of Lightnin Mixers Ltd).

just above the water surface the kinetic energy of the jet will induce a velocity in the receiving water. This type of aeration system therefore consists of a high capacity, low-head pump connected to a manifold of jets placed across the required line of flow. The manifold should be capable of being rotated so that the jet impingement angle can be altered. In this way the mixing and aeration functions of the system can be varied to meet the overall process requirements. Both the theoretical and practical aspects of this type of aeration have been reviewed elsewhere (Dijkstra, Jennekens & Nooren, 1978), and since it is not a method in widespread use, the details of this review will not be reiterated here.

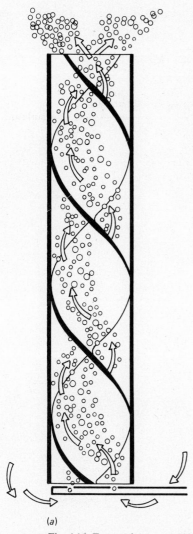

(a)

Fig. 4.16. For caption see p. 120.

Submerged turbine/sparger systems, although being a common process in industrial fermentations, have found little application in waste water treatment. One aeration method of this type that is worth commenting on and which is used in effluent aeration tanks is the process known as *draft-tube aeration*. Once again it is a process whose application tends to be restricted to the aeration of oxidation ditches. A wall is constructed across one arm of the ditch and the fluid circulation pattern completed by a draft-tube which passes under the barrier wall,

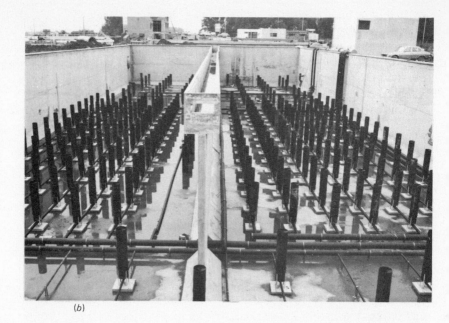

(*b*)

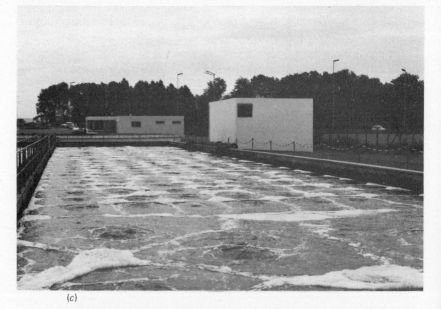

(*c*)

Fig. 4.16. Sub-surface static aerator. *a* Schematic diagram; *b* Empty basin showing main aeration and denitrification zones; *c* Activated sludge plant treating domestic sewage and coke oven effluent (all by courtesy of Polcon Environmental Control Systems Ltd).

extending in some cases to a depth of 6 m below the bottom of the ditch. The velocity of circulation is both achieved and controlled by an aerofoil impellor within the draft-tube (Fig. 4.15). Air is introduced immediately beneath the impellor and is taken down the draft-tube by the fluid flow. The transfer of oxygen is enhanced by shearing of the bubbles and by hydrostatic forces. The additional advantages claimed for this approach are that:

(a) All the ditch contents are mixed with the air
(b) The processes of circulation (i.e. mixing) and aeration are separated and may therefore be controlled individually to meet the operational requirements.

The final alternative method that will be discussed is the *sub-surface static aerator*, typified by the Helixor or Kenic systems. The basic design of the Helixor consists of a moulded polythene tube which is divided longitudinally by an internal helical section (Fig. 4.16). The tubes are anchored above an air main laid on the base of the aeration tank. Each Helixor tube (30.5 cm diameter) is aligned vertically above orifices in the main and the small bubbles emerging from these orifices and into the Helixor induce an upward, turbulent flow of liquid. The internal helix prolongs the period of contact between the air and liquid thus ensuring good oxygen transfer. Additional liquid is entrained by the jet as it leaves the tube so that the contents of the tank are well mixed. In a typical system, the aeration tank would be up to 6 m in depth and the height of the Helixor tubes would be 1.8 m. The air would be supplied by blowers at a pressure of 0.44 kg cm^{-2} and a rate of 19 l s^{-1} per tube. This would produce spiral velocities within the tubes in excess of 1.25 m s^{-1}. The number of Helixor units that would be used and their density per unit area would depend on the rate of oxygen transfer that was required (Bennett & Shell, 1976).

4.4 Aerator performance
4.4.1 *Introduction*

Whichever method of aeration is used, significant amounts of energy will be required to effect the transfer of oxygen. In some cases, this can amount to up to 80 per cent of the total energy budget for the treatment works. It is essential therefore that the design and operation of the aeration process is as near optimal as is possible or practicable, particularly in terms of energy efficiency.

Aerators must mix as well as transfer oxygen and although the energy requirements for mixing can, at times, be identified and quantified, in practical terms it is the total energy usage that is important. However, despite this dual function, the parameters used to define aerator efficiency are based on the oxygen transfer function. In fact they are all based on the overall oxygen transfer coefficient, $K_L a$.

4.4.2   *Measurement of transfer efficiency*

As has already been stated, the correct design and installation of the aerators is a key feature of the construction or uprating of an activated sludge plant. This statement presupposes three things: that the correct specification can be supplied, that the aerators are to be evaluated at the commissioning stage and that there is a reliable and generally acceptable testing procedure. The testing of aeration systems has been the subject of many studies and in order to establish a consensus of opinion, the US Environmental Protection Agency, in conjunction with experts from other countries, is currently attempting to define a standard methodology for the testing of aerators.

Within the UK, the techniques used may be considered as falling into two classes: the so-called 'steady' and 'unsteady' state methods. In the former the dissolved oxygen (DO) concentration is kept constant whilst in the latter it is permitted to change and the rate of change is measured. Whichever technique is to be used the precise measurement of the DO concentration is essential. The electrodes which are currently available are perfectly adequate for these purposes provided that they are calibrated accurately and frequently. It is also prudent to use more than one electrode in any large-scale testing; a minimum of four has been recommended (Boon & Chambers, 1984). These should be located around the aeration chamber and the oxygen transfer rate calculated from the data produced by each sensor. The individual rates should be within ± 10 per cent of the average value.

There are variations to the unsteady state method. The first of these applies to water which has a negligible oxygen demand – the so-called clean water test. Tap water, river water or a high quality final effluent may be used but it is advisable to wash and flush out the tank thoroughly before filling it. The DO electrodes should then be calibrated and placed in position and the aerators run for several hours. This enables the location of the electrodes to be checked and the rate of energy consumption of the aerators to be measured. A concentrated solution of sodium sulphite containing cobalt chloride (or nitrate) should then be distributed evenly throughout the tank. The amount of sulphite may be calculated from the stoichiometric quantity necessary to de-oxygenate the tank contents plus an excess of about 20 per cent. The amount of cobalt necessary should be sufficient to give a final concentration of 0.2 mg Co l^{-1}. The aerators may then be switched on and the increase in the DO concentration measured until the air saturation value is reached. This should take about $(6/K_L a)$ hours. Throughout the test period the power consumption of a mechanical aerator or the pressure and flow-rate of air being supplied to a diffused air system should be checked regularly to ensure that constant aeration is being achieved. It is also advisable to check the final DO concentration by chemical analysis.

For a mechanical aeration system the $K_L a$ value may be calculated from:

$$K_L a = \frac{1}{t_2 - t_1} \log_e \frac{C^* - C_1}{C^* - C_2}$$

For diffused air systems, the composition of the air will vary during its passage up through the tank. This variation can be accounted for by using an average saturation concentration (C_m^*) and a value for the saturation concentration at a pressure equivalent to the head of water above the aerator (C_i^*). The basic transfer rate equation therefore becomes:

$$\frac{dC}{dt} = K_L a(C_m^* - C)$$

and the equilibrium condition as

$$\frac{2C_m^*}{x_i + x_o} = \frac{C_i^*}{x_i} = H$$

where x_i = proportion of oxygen in the air entering the water, x_o = proportion of oxygen in the air leaving the water.

Combining these two equations with a mass balance gives:

$$K_L a = \frac{1 + K_L a(VH/2\rho Q)}{t_2 - t_1} \log_e \frac{C_i^* - C_1}{C_i^* - C_2}$$

where V = volume of water, in m^3, Q = air flow-rate, in $m^3 \, h^{-1}$, ρ = density of oxygen, in $g \, m^{-3}$ (Boon & Chambers, 1984).

Whichever type of aerator is being used the conditions being used to calculate $K_L a$ (i.e. t_1, C_1, t_2, and C_2) should be taken from within the range of 20–80 per cent of the saturation values.

The second variation of the unsteady state methods is that used for the measurement of the transfer rate into activated sludge. This ought to involve incorporating a value for the rate at which the biomass removes oxygen. However, the respiration rate of sludge is a very variable parameter, altering with the degree of longitudinal mixing and the composition and flow-rate of the sewage. A technique has therefore been developed which obviates the need for its use: the dual steady state technique. As a method it gives an appreciable error in the determination of $K_L a$ (up to 30 per cent) and as such is not widely used. A detailed description of the method has been given by Boon & Chambers (1984).

Both variations of the steady state method also have limitations. They are only valid for completely mixed systems and when used, as they are mostly, with mixed liquor require that measures be taken to ensure that the respiration rate of the sludge (r) is kept as near constant as possible. This means that the flow-rate and composition of the sewage needs to be controlled. Another essential criterion is that the DO concentration throughout the system is constant. The value of the DO should be greater than 40 per cent of the saturation value and, so as to facilitate respiration rate measurements, preferably greater than 60 per cent.

The steady state/respiration rate approach necessitates taking samples of the mixed liquor at quite frequent intervals (say every 5 min) for respiration rate measurements as well as recording the DO concentration. The overall mass transfer coefficient is then calculated from:

$$K_L a = \frac{r}{C_m^* - C}$$

The second steady state method depends on measuring the concentration of oxygen in the gases leaving the liquors being aerated. As such it can only be used with diffused air systems or with covered aeration tanks such as are used with some applications of oxygen to activated sludge (e.g. UNOX). The latter systems pose no problem. With diffused air plants a light hood is floated on the surface to enable the off-gases to be collected. However it must be remembered that the majority of diffused air plants are plug-flow systems and that the results will depend on the location of the hood. The $K_L a$ value for this method is calculated from:

$$K_L a = \rho \left[\frac{Q}{v} \right] \left[\frac{x_i - x_o}{C_m^* - C} \right]$$

Of the four methods that have been described, the one most commonly used in the UK is the unsteady state/clean water technique. UK practice would also require that surfactant (on average 5 mg l^{-1} of anionic material measured as Manoxol OT) be added to the water. This requirement is not so critical for the evaluation of mechanical aerators since changes in contaminants have been found to have little effect on the performance of these systems (Boon & Chambers, 1984). With diffused air, the composition of the test water can have a significant effect and it is therefore important to have a standardised approach to testing.

Whichever method is used a value of $K_L a$ is obtained. This is then used to calculate the oxygenation capacity (OC) where

$$OC = (K_L a)_{20} V C_i^* \text{ g h}^{-1}.$$

In turn, this is used to calculate the oxygenation efficiency in terms of the kg O$_2$ kWh^{-1}.

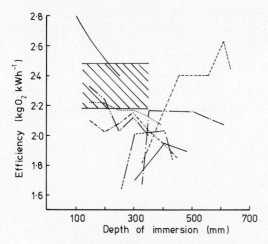

Fig. 4.17. The variation in clean water oxygenation efficiency with depth of immersion for vertical shaft aerators.

4.4.3   *Operational aspects*

The usual starting points in assessing an aerator are the manufacturers' claims for clean water efficiency. However, not all the reported data will specify precisely the techniques that have been used, particularly the concentration of added detergent and the volume of the vessel used in the trials. Ideally the latter ought to be the same as, or very similar to, the actual operational tank for which the aerator is being considered. If it is significantly different then the calculated efficiency can be grossly inflated or underestimated. The addition of surfactant is not always carried out and a 'clean water test' can mean that either clean water was used or clean water plus surfactant. However, it is generally accepted that for the full-scale testing of aerators, surfactant should be added to a final mean concentration of 5 mg l^{-1}. The second point in assessing an aerator is to test it against the claimed performance in its operational tank during the commissioning period. Any positive decision not to do this may be regretted at a later stage.

Any type of surface aerator will provide different rates of oxygen transfer and will draw different amounts of power as the depth of rotor immersion varies. It is therefore usual to assess the oxygenation efficiency (kg oxygen transferred kWh^{-1}) in relation to that immersion. An examination of this type of data (Forster, 1984) shows that for both horizontally and vertically driven aerators the efficiency/immersion relationship is described by quite a broad envelope with the greatest variation occurring at the lower immersion values (see for example Fig. 4.17). The significance of this can be seen when it is realised that there is an increasing use of dissolved oxygen control techniques which cause

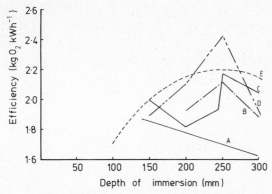

Fig. 4.18. The variation in clean water oxygenation efficiency with the depth of immersion for the Mammoth rotor. A Stanton & Hargreaves, 1979; B Rees & Skellett, 1974, water; C Rees & Skellett, 1974, water/detergent; D Manufacturers' claims; E Rachwal & Waller, 1982.

the level of the aeration tank to be lowered during periods of low load. Whilst this philosophy will reduce the wasteful transfer of oxygen on a 24 hour basis, it could, depending on the aerator characteristics, result in periods of low energy efficiency. This is obviously something to be considered both by the purchasers and designers of aeration equipment.

Good independent performance data for surface aerators is somewhat limited. However, some results are available for the Mammoth system. Fig. 4.18 shows the results of two separate evaluations (Rees & Skellet, 1974; Stanton & Hargreaves, 1979) together with the manufacturers' claimed performance and performance curves obtained from several works for both vertical and horizontal shaft aerators (Rachwal & Waller, 1982). In the most general terms, the results show that vertical shaft systems appear to have a slightly greater efficiency than horizontal shaft aerators. In the case of the Mammoth rotor the results show that, with the exception of the results reported by Stanton & Hargreaves, there is quite reasonable agreement between the various evaluations. This, if nothing else, ought to give confidence in the methodology employed to assess aerators.

Fine-bubble aeration systems have been the subject of a number of evaluations (e.g. Lister & Boon, 1973; Schmidt & Redmon, 1975; Houk & Boon, 1981). These evaluations have examined the effect of the configuration of the diffusers and the depth of liquid above the diffusers together with the performance characteristics during operational conditions. The results show that within the range of depths normally used in the UK (2.5–5 m) there is little variation in the intensity of aeration as the depth increases except for very close-packed diffuser configurations (Lister & Boon, 1973). The data have also shown that:

Table 4.3. *The effect of variations in the diffuser characteristics on the intensity of fine-bubble aeration*

Air flow-rate (m^3 h^{-1} per dome)	Packing density (diffusers m^{-2})	Aeration intensity (mg l^{-1} h^{-1})
1.7	11.1	193
1.7	4.4	70
1.7	2.2	29
1.7	11.1	193
0.85	11.1	108

From Boon, Chambers & Collinson, 1982.

    (a) For a given flow-rate of air per diffuser, the aeration intensity will decrease as the packing density of the diffusers (number per plan area of tank) decreases, and

    (b) For a given packing density the aeration intensity decreases as the air flow-rate per dome is reduced (see Table 4.3).

In general, fine-bubble systems have a higher clean water efficiency (kg kWh^{-1}) than mechanical systems – 1.5–3.6 compared with 1.2–2.4. However an examination of in-plant performance (Houk & Boon, 1981) has shown that transfer efficiencies only ranged from 1.08–2.13 kg kWh^{-1}. The reasons suggested for this include poor dissolved oxygen control, deviation from the design sludge loading rate and air supply systems whose flexibility was less than adequate. The cardinal rules for obtaining optimal efficiency may therefore be taken as (Boon, Chambers & Collinson, 1982):

    (a) Provide a flexible air supply system. This requires the use of more than one blower, one of which should have the facility of being controlled (variable speed; variable output)

    (b) Use dissolved oxygen probes to control the aeration intensity, possibly even linked to a micro-processor

    (c) Ensure that the air-flow is not reduced below the minimum recommended by the diffuser manufacturer. This will avoid inadequate mixing and the risk of diffuser clogging

    (d) Cleaning and maintenance schedules specified by the manufacturers should be followed

    (e) If a plug-flow system is to be used to achieve good sludge settleability the length to width ratio should not exceed 12:1

    (f) The optimal depth is between 4.5 and 6 m

    (g) Slime growths on diffusers can be minimised by reducing the BOD load at the inlet to the aeration tank. This can be achieved by good mixing of the incoming sewage and the return sludge.

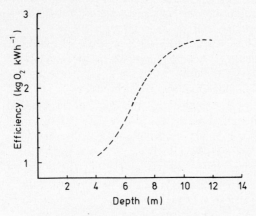

Fig. 4.19. The oxygenation efficiency of a jet aeration system in relation to the air flow-rate (by courtesy of Houdaille Industries Inc.).

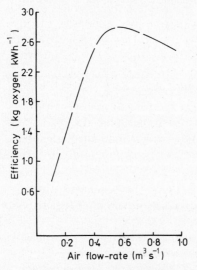

Fig. 4.20. The effect of draft tube depth on the oxygenation efficiency of draft tube oxidation channels (by courtesy of Lightnin Mixers Ltd).

The performances of the various alternative aeration systems have not been the subject of independent assessments. However, it is considered that it is unlikely that their efficiencies will be very different from those of surface aerators (Boon, 1983). Certainly the data available from the manufacturers (Figs. 4.19 and 4.20) provide no cause to believe otherwise (Forster, 1984).

4.4.4   *Control of aeration*

On a theoretical basis, the rate of aeration should be such that it is just in excess of the rate of oxygen removal by the microbial flora in the aeration tank. The overall oxygen requirements for any process, being operated within the range of sludge loading rates of 0.05 to 1.0 kg BOD kg MLSS^{-1} d^{-1}, can be calculated from one of two similar (and comparable) empirical equations. Both of these take into account the oxygen required for the oxidation of carbonaceous BOD and of ammoniacal nitrogen together with that required to satisfy the basal respiration of the mixed liquor solids. They also make an allowance for the oxygen that can be recovered from oxidised nitrogen (basically in the form of nitrate) if de-nitrification is being practised. The first of these was developed primarily for the operation of oxidation ditches (Johnstone & Carmichael, 1982) and has the form:

$$R = aB + 0.024Mr_{20}\,\theta^{(T-20)} + 4.34N_{\mathrm{H}} - 2.85N_{\mathrm{T}}$$

where R = daily oxygen requirements, in kg d^{-1}, B = BOD removed, in kg d^{-1}, M = mass of mixed liquor solids, in kg, r_{20} = basal (endogenous) respiration rate at 20 °C, in mg O$_2$ g MLSS^{-1} h^{-1}, T = operating temperature, in °C, θ = constant (taken as 1.07), a = constant (taken as 1.00), N_{H} = ammonia oxidised, in kg d^{-1}, N_{T} = total nitrogen removed, in kg d^{-1}.

The second equation was developed from data obtained, for activated sludge systems in general, from the UK and the USA (Boon *et al.*, 1982). Its form is:

$$R' = a'B + 2 \times 10^{-3}M + 1.47N_H + 2.83N_O$$

where N_O = nitrate produced in effluent, in g h^{-1}, a' = constant (taken as 0.75 for settled sewage and 1.0 for raw sewage); the other parameters have the units of g h^{-1} or g.

The basic difference between the two equations is that the former requires a specific input for the basal respiration rate. The significance of this will be discussed later. The real value of both equations is that they can be applied to any mode of operation – simple carbonaceous removal, nitrification and complete nitrogen removal. In addition, provided that the relevant data are available, the diurnal variations in oxygen demand can be calculated from the latter method. However, in practice if oxygen limitation is to be avoided, the demand must be calculated for a period equivalent to the hydraulic retention time (based on the flow of sewage *and* recycled sludge) of the mixed liquor in the aeration tank. Even so, this demand will relate to a completely mixed configuration. This is seldom the regime which is used in aeration tanks, plug-flow being preferred to achieve good settleability. In plug-flow tanks the gradation in demand will depend very much on the degradability of each element of influent which itself could vary on a diurnal basis if there is any significant industrial input to the sewerage system. The modelling of plug-flow systems is further complicated by the fact that the alpha factor can alter along the length of the aeration tank. The magnitude of this variation will obviously depend on the nature of the waste but it can also depend on the type of aeration system being employed; 0.3–0.8 for fine-bubble aeration and 1.2–1.0 for mechanical aerators have been reported for the inlet to outlet variation (Boon *et al.*, 1982). This would suggest that the use of this type of model for the complete control of aeration (i.e. linked to a micro-processor) is unlikely.

The normal control methods that are used in practice (if indeed any control is used) depend on dissolved oxygen measurements. These are usually obtained by the use of any of the electrodes currently available. Thus the mechanism of control is by adjusting the level of liquid in the aeration tank (and thus the rotor immersion) or by varying the air flow-rate to fine bubble diffusors. In most cases the control is based on simple on/off switching at predetermined upper and lower limits of dissolved oxygen concentration. In other words a step-wise process is used. However, in an attempt to show that aeration can be optimised, in terms of energy expended, without causing any detrimental effects to the overall process a study of a specially modified aeration tank is being undertaken at the Rye Meads sewage works by the Water Research Centre and Thames Water Authority. These modifications include a carefully designed diffuser configuration and, of particular reference to this discussion, the potential for continuously variable aeration intensity. The system is based on dissolved oxygen electrodes which are linked to programmable logic controllers. These control the operation of vent-valves on the aeration lines. This combination therefore allows the dissolved oxygen concentration in the various zones within the aeration tank to be maintained at a pre-set level (Boon *et al.*, 1982). The use of positive displacement Rootes blowers does mean that excess air is vented to the atmosphere. The design engineer wishing to carry this optimisation further is therefore faced with an interesting problem – what type and combination of blower to select so as to permit the delivery of a variable volume, constant pressure, supply of air without incurring high capital costs (Clough, 1982).

4.4.5   *Aeration and BOD removal*

An alternative way of assessing aerators is to examine F, the energy usage per unit mass of BOD removed; kWh (kg Δ BOD)$^{-1}$. The theoretical oxygen requirements for carbonaceous oxidation are taken as

$$R = aB + 0.024Mr_{20}\,\theta^{(T-20)}$$

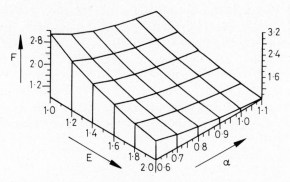

Fig. 4.21. The effect that variations in alpha and the aerator efficiency (E) can have on the energy efficiency (F).

and the energy utilisation as

$$F = R/E\alpha(OD) = R\phi$$

where OD is the oxygen deficit expressed as a fraction of the maximum deficit and E is the aerator efficiency (kg O_2 kWh^{-1}) (Johnstone, 1984). Considering the aerator in isolation from the other process variables, the key parameters are E and α. The effect that these can have on F can be demonstrated by assuming that:

$a = 1.0$

$r_{20} = 3.9$ mg g^{-1} h^{-1}

$T = 10\,°C$

$B/M = 0.1$ kg Δ BOD(kg MLSS)$^{-1}$

$OD = 0.8.$

Values of F can therefore be calculated for any values of E and α. These are shown in Fig. 4.21 for E values ranging from 1.0–2.0 and α values from 0.6–1.1. This shows that a very variable range of energy efficiencies can be obtained depending on the values of the other two parameters. The significance of this can fully be realised when it is remembered that α can vary with the degree of treatment that has been received and E can vary with the depth of immersion (for mechanical aerators). This means that there will be times within any day that E and α will conjoin to give significantly poorer energy efficiencies than might have been predicted. Conversely there will be periods when low F values prevail resulting in an average (on a daily basis) somewhere near the predicted value. However, if the peaks could be reduced then so could the daily average.

An alternative way of looking at the F, E, α relationship is to examine how the variables E and α need to be manipulated to produce a compliance with plant performance. Fig. 4.22 shows data from a wide range of plants presented in terms of energy efficiency (F) and the

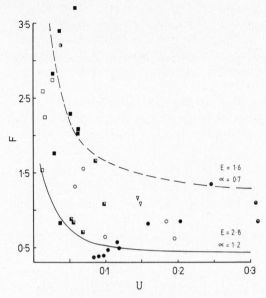

Fig. 4.22. The interrelationship between the energy efficiency (F) and the specific BOD removal (U; kg BOD removed per kg MLSS) for various plants, together with theoretical curves.

food:mass ratio based on BOD removal (U). Superimposed on these data are the theoretical curves based on $F = R\phi$ using values of E and α selected so as to form an envelope for the plant data. These results show either just how wide a variation in these two parameters must be occurring, or how poor the operational control of the plants is. Whichever is the case, there is obviously scope for improvement. The economic potential can be seen when it is realised that about 25 per cent of the 6×10^6 m³ of sewage treated daily in England and Wales receives treatment in surface aeration plant. Assuming a BOD removal of 150 mg l⁻¹ and an energy cost of 3.5 p kWh⁻¹, the annual saving would be of the order of £0.3 × 10⁶ if the F value could be improved by 0.2 at half the plants. An analogous situation exists in diffused air systems where it has been estimated that £0.5 × 10⁶ could be saved each year if the oxygen transfer efficiency at all plants could be maintained at a minimum of 2.0 kg kWh⁻¹ (Clough, 1982).

4.5   Scale-up of aerators

Using the correct scale-up procedure can be an important feature in the design of any reactor, be it chemical or biological. When considering aerators, scale-up needs to be applied only to surface aeration systems. However, no single method has been developed which can meet with the approval of all workers. Scale-up can be considered as covering two aspects: the effect of altering the rotor characteristics (i.e. diameter or speed of rotation) within any particular aeration basin, and the more usual problem of determining the characteristics of a fully sized impeller on the basis of small-scale tests. The objective in both cases is to achieve a similar oxygen transfer rate (taken as $K_L a$).

The former of these two cases can be modelled by a linear relationship between the mass transfer coefficient at 20 °C ($K_L a_{20}$) and the Froude number ($Fr = N^2 D/g$) of the impeller (Schmidtke & Horvath, 1977):

$$K_L a_{20} = aFr - b.$$

The coefficients a and b will vary from system to system and, as reported, the relationship is only valid for Froude numbers in the range of 0.08–0.34.

The second aspect of scale-up can be achieved by one of several procedures. Zlokarnik (1979) has concluded that scale-up should be done at a constant Froude number. An alternative viewpoint (Schmidtke & Horvath, 1977) is that the process of scale-up can be modelled by the relationships:

$$K_L a_{20} = aN^b D^c \text{ and } N_S = N_L \frac{D_L^{c/b}}{D_S}$$

where N = impeller speed, D = impeller diameter, subscript S refers to small aerator; subscript L refers to large aerator. It has also been suggested (Riet, 1979) that the concept of constant specific power (W m^{-3}) is an adequate basis for scale-up, whilst Pacz & Wassnik (1976), in discussing the implications of scaling-up under conditions of equality of Froude number, Reynolds number, and Power number, produce the relationship:

$$P_L = (k_1)^{\frac{7}{2}} P_S \text{ for vertical shaft aerators}$$

and

$$P_L = (k_1)^{\frac{5}{2}} k_2 P_S \text{ for horizontal rotors}$$

where P is the nett shaft power.

Although no one system has been developed, it is obvious from these various relationships that the rotor diameter and speed of rotation together with the applied power are the key parameters. What perhaps needs to be determined is whether there is any significant difference between the various approaches and what accuracy is needed when the scaling-up of aerators is being done.

4.6   The use of pure oxygen

There are some plants which use pure oxygen rather than air as the means of supplying the oxygen requirements of the microbial flora. In

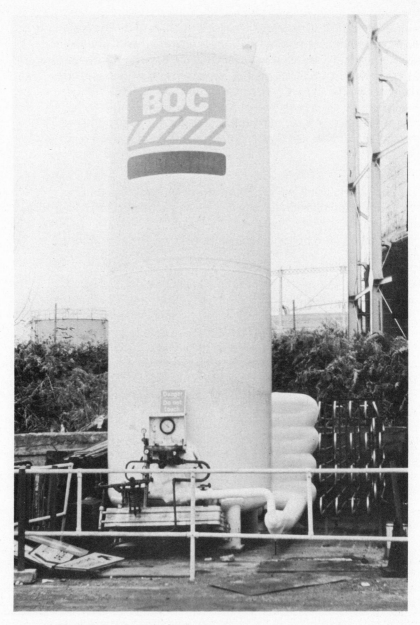

Fig. 4.23. Storage tanks for liquid oxygen.

the majority of cases these plants are activated sludge processes. However some fixed film reactors (fluidised beds; rotating disc filters) have also been operated as oxygenic systems. The rationale for using oxygen is that it results in an increase in the partial pressure of oxygen in the gaseous phase. This, in turn, brings about an increase in the deficit term – the driving force $(C^* - C)$ – in the oxygen transfer rate equation:

$$V \frac{dC}{dt} = K_L a(C^* - C)$$

and thus a corresponding increase in the rate of transfer.

The oxygen can be produced cryogenically on site or supplied to the work as a liquid and stored in insulated tanks. These can be permanent installations or temporary, skid-mounted, units (Fig. 4.23). Another approach is to produce the oxygen at the works using the process known as pressure swing adsorption (PSA). This system uses columns packed with a molecular sieve which, at pressures of 200–300 kPa, selectively adsorb nitrogen from air. The effluent gas therefore is oxygen enriched (typically it is 75–90 per cent oxygen). The adsorption process is reversible so that when the pressure is reduced to about 100 kPa the nitrogen desorbs and the sieve can be re-used. In a typical system, three columns would be used: one producing oxygen-enriched gas, one desorbing and one on stand-by. The rate of production of oxygen and the purity of the gas can be controlled by altering the time between each pressurisation/decompression cycle. Which of these systems is used will ultimately depend on a number of factors which will include location, scale, power availability, purity requirements etc.; however, in general, cryogenic plants are preferred for large installations – 20 tonnes per day plus. Smaller quantities can be provided by PSA separation or liquid oxygen, with PSA being advantageous for continuous, steady loads.

Oxygen can be used in one of two ways: in conjunction with conventional aeration or as the sole means of providing the necessary oxygen. The former case is an excellent method for coping with seasonal overloads (e.g. at seaside resorts) or for providing the additional capacity necessary for extending the operational life of a works which had, with time, become permanently overloaded. It also can be used to balance bacterial respiration in the initial part of the activated sludge lanes to avoid the need for stepped feed and to increase effective contact time. A further feature of oxygen plants is that it becomes possible to control the dissolved oxygen level to fine limits throughout the day – preventing unwanted nitrification etc.

Side-stream injection (the Vitrox process) is probably the most successful method of achieving this. The process requirements, apart

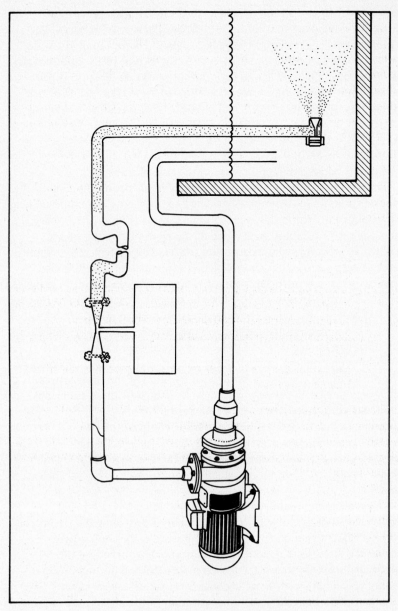

Fig. 4.24. The Vitox system (by courtesy of BOC Ltd).

from a supply of oxygen, are quite simple (Fig. 4.24); all that is
required is a pump, a venturi and dispersal jets. The pump delivers
liquid (settled sewage, final effluent or mixed liquor) into the venturi
where oxygen is injected. The pressure regime and turbulence at this
point is such that about 25 per cent of the gas dissolves. Further
dissolution takes place in the pipework so that 50 per cent of the gas is
dissolved before the mixture is discharged through the jets. The action
of the jet breaks up the remaining liquor. The jet energy also provides
excellent mixing. The recorded capacity of the Vitox system for
transferring oxygen has been as high as 3 kg kWh^{-1} (Kite & Garrett,
1983).

The use of pure oxygen as the sole source of the oxygen needed by
the aerobic processes can be achieved in several ways (Boon, 1976).
These can be summarised as:

(i) The use of a covered aeration tank with conventional
mechanical aerators operating in an atmosphere of oxygen or
oxygen-enriched air.

(ii) The use of special diffusers which produce very fine bubbles of
oxygen at the bottom of an open aeration tank. The design of
the diffusor/mixing system is aimed at achieving maximum
dissolution of the gas and thus no excessive loss of oxygen at
the surface.

(iii) The circulation of biomass through an external down-flow
bubble oxygenator.

In examining these three types of process only the oxygen transfer
characteristics will be discussed at this stage; an assessment of the
process performances is given in Chapters 3 and 6. The aerators used in
conjunction with covered tanks are the vertical shaft mechanical surface
aerators that have already been discussed and therefore need no
additional comment. A recent report (Blachford, Tramontini &
Griffiths, 1982) has shown that this configuration of the oxygen
activated sludge process (OASP) will utilise better than 85 per cent of
the oxygen being fed to the aeration tank. The same workers also
commented on the energy requirements of the process. This took
account both of the energy required to separate the oxygen from air
using a PSA unit and the energy used to mix, aerate and pump the
sludge. The results show quite a wide variation: 1.8–4.1 kWh kg^{-1} BOD
and ammoniacal nitrogen oxidised. The high figures were in fact
associated with low oxygen requirements and the fact that the PSA unit
did not have an effective means of reducing the output of oxygen
(turn-down). As such, therefore, they ought to be discounted in any
assessment of the energy efficiency of the overall system. However, it
does highlight the need for including an effective turn-down facility in
the design of this type of OASP.

The diffuser system used in the open tank OASP is a rotating disc. Oxygen is fed down the hollow drive shaft and passes into the mixed liquor through an annulus of diffusion medium. The entire disc is rotated slowly and the combined effect of the diffusion medium used and the hydraulic shear produced by the rotation is to produce very small diameter bubbles – about 150 μm compared with 2 mm from conventional dome diffusors. The transfer efficiency of the process is claimed to be better than 90 per cent for flows of up to about 130 per cent of the design flow.

The third alternative uses an oxygenator which is separate from the main tank. As marketed commercially, the oxygenator is a downflow bubble contactor. The oxygen is injected into the sludge/sewage mixture immediately prior to the oxygenator, the amount being determined by DO measurements made before the point of injection. There is a degree of instantaneous dissolution but the majority of the oxygen transfer is achieved within the downflow contactor.

External oxygenators of this type have also been used in conjunction with oxygenic, fluidised beds (Hoyland & Robinson, 1983). In one such system the gas and liquid streams are introduced into the top of the oxygenator column at a velocity sufficient to maintain, at least in the upper region of the column, a substantially continuous froth of close-packed bubbles extending across the entire cross section of the column. The froth consists of bubbles with a relatively uniform size and gas accumulation at the top is prevented by the velocity of the inlet stream. Bubble-free liquid is withdrawn from the bottom of the column. The interfacial area of 1000–3000 m^2 m^{-3} results in a high approach to equilibrium and a utilisation which approaches 100 per cent (Boyes *et al.*, 1982).

5   Site and process selection

5.1   Introduction

Although society accepts that its sewage must be treated, it usually
demands that the treatment is done at a site as remote as possible from
the community and at a minimal cost. The site selection for a new
sewage treatment works is therefore of considerable importance. Not
only must the environmental impact be minimal but also the
operational costs (i.e. pumping to the works, pumping within the works
and sludge disposal) must be kept as low as possible. This latter aspect
quite frequently also involves the tailoring of the various unit processes
to suit the conditions of the site selected. Therefore, the following
factors need to be taken into consideration during the site selection
process:

> The population; alternative locations (e.g. a regional works);
> the location relative to development (e.g. the availability of
> services, access, the fall available across the site, the receiving
> waters); the possible energy requirements; the nature of the
> sewage (and in particular its industrial content); the scope for
> sludge disposal; the availability and value of land; and the site
> conditions (e.g. flooding risk, nature of foundations).

5.2   Population

The size of the population to be served by any new works is probably
one of the most important factors in the selection of the bio-oxidation
process, as some systems are more appropriate than others to specific
population ranges (see Table 5.1). The determination of the population
to be served, both existing and proposed, requires liaison with the
Planning Authorities, and in estimating future populations it is usual to
design for a period 10 years in advance of the completed construction.
Furthermore, it must also be remembered that a treatment works which
has been extended by an appreciable amount or the provision of a
substantial new works may well enable a Planning Authority to revise
their own proposals and allow development, particularly from industry,
which had previously been considered unsuitable. As this could take up
surplus capacity and make a treatment works overloaded ahead of

139

Table 5.1. *Bio-oxidation processes related to the optimum populations to be served*

Process	Typical population ranges
Septic tanks	0–300
Package plants	50–4000
Filters	100–100 000
Extended aeration (oxidation ditch)	100–20 000
Extended aeration (Carrousel)	10 000–100 000
Activated sludge	10 000–2 000 000

schedule the importance of a regular dialogue between Planning and Water Authorities cannot be stressed too strongly.

5.3   Regionalisation of sewage treatment

Historically, sewage treatment works have been associated with individual communities so that in essentially rural areas there is a numerical predominance of small works (Fig. 5.1), all of which require regular routine servicing and maintenance. This can be an expensive

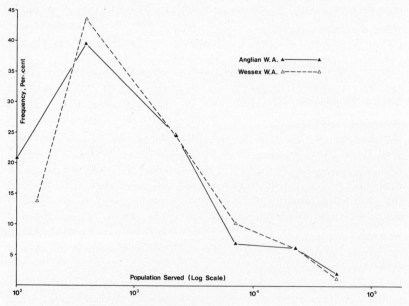

Fig. 5.1. Distribution of sewage works sizes.

deployment of man-power so that, in the long term, regionalisation of sewage treatment is the measure most likely to result in operational economies and efficiency. In every case therefore where an extension, or new works, is being planned, the scope for a regional scheme ought to be considered. This will mean examining the planning proposals, the sewer systems and existing treatment works in a wide area around the site for which the new works or extension is being designed.

5.4   Location relative to development

To minimise its environmental impact a sewage treatment works should ideally be sited well away from housing, to reduce any nuisance from flies, and down-wind of the prevailing winds to minimise problems caused by odours. As this is not always possible, consideration must be given to screening the works from view, and if natural features do not provide such screening, then it may be necessary to plant trees. However, when houses and a treatment works are in close proximity, trees may act as a gathering point for flies, particularly for *Psychoda*. Although a variety of tree species will present a more environmentally pleasing screen than one comprised totally of evergreens, the use of deciduous trees should be avoided as the falling leaves can cause filter blockages resulting in poor performance. Noise may also become a problem when a treatment works is too close to housing and under these circumstances some form of audio-screening may become necessary to prevent the works being classified as a statutory nuisance under Section 58 of the Control of Pollution Act, 1974. In an urban area, a more suitable location would therefore be on an industrial estate.

In operational terms, any proposed site would need to have good and easy access and, as it is not uncommon for the transport of heavy loads to be required, the access roads should have a hard surface. It is also an advantage if the site has, either readily available or without undue expense, the facilities of electricity, water and telephone links. The site itself should wherever possible be one to which the developed area can drain by gravity and there should be sufficient fall across the site to enable the principal processes to operate without pumping. In addition, the quality and quantity of the receiving watercourse is important in the site selection. For example, if the treatment works can be moved closer to a large watercourse, the standard of treatment may not need to be as intense as it would have to be if the discharge were being made to a relatively small stream.

Table 5.2. *Bio-oxidation processes related to the fall required for their operation*

Process	Typical fall required (m)
Filtration	5
Activated sludge	2.5
Extended aeration	1.5

5.5   Energy requirements

Over the past half century the cost of energy, relative to that of capital, has dropped appreciably and this has favoured processes such as activated sludge which use energy rather than capital. However, 1973 saw the onset of expensive energy and although the increased cost of capital means that the relative cost of energy has changed little, the energy awareness of recent years has created a situation in which the design of a treatment works should also minimise the energy requirements.

On a large plant, energy can be obtained from digester gas, and in some cases practically all the energy requirements of the works can be derived from this source. Obviously the gas yield is a function of the population served and it is generally considered that power-generation from sludge gas is uneconomic below a population of 200000 due to the cost of manning a generating station.

The type of plant with a minimum energy requirement would be a biological filtration unit located on a sloping site. Under these circumstances, it could be possible to run single-stage filtration without power, except possibly that required for sludge pumping. The energy required for any particular site will depend on the processes being proposed (Table 5.2). If there is negligible fall across a site, the pumping which will be necessary may well offset the advantages of filtration, especially as the raising of plant above ground level may well increase its cost. Thus, for a large works located on a site with little fall, activated sludge would normally be the first choice.

5.6   Nature of the sewage

Domestic sewage will contain carbon, nitrogen and phosphorus in such proportions that it is readily amenable to bio-oxidative treatment. In addition, its flow to the works is such that excessive hydraulic shocks are not usually experienced. However, if the area to be drained contains

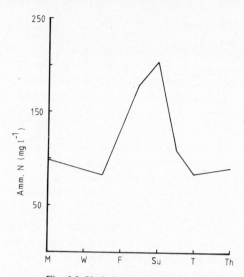

Fig. 5.2. Variation in the ammoniacal nitrogen concentration in the raw sewage arriving at a small rural works.

a significant industrial or recreational development, significant shock-loads can be expected. Industrial effluents, even when controlled (see Chapter 11), are likely to contain toxic materials, and even when this is not the case they can be nutritionally unbalanced or very strong. In addition, the discharge of process water may well be restricted to the working day or possibly even to part of it if batch processes are being used. Recreational sites (e.g. caravan parks and marinas) will not only be prone to give a seasonal variation in load but also to shock loads when chemical closets are emptied. Load variations of this type can also be experienced at holiday resorts and even motorway service stations. Fig. 5.2 shows the variation in the ammoniacal nitrogen concentration in the sewage arriving at a small rural works during a typical week in the summer months. The week-end peak of some 200 mg l^{-1}, which was due to the heavy use of toilet facilities at a nearby service station, resulted in an excessive oxygen demand being exerted by the sewage; one which was in fact in excess of the aeration capacity of the works.

These variations in flow, load and type of effluent must be considered at the planning stage and may in fact determine which unit processes are to be used. For example, bio-filters are normally regarded as being more suitable for the treatment of dairy wastes than activated sludge. Under these circumstances a compromise needs to be reached between the process dictated by the type of sewage and that indicated by the site conditions and energy requirements.

5.7   Sludge disposal

Another important policy decision will be the means of treating and disposing of sludge, and the value or scarcity of land may well affect this decision; for example, the areas of land required for drying beds can be as much as the area required for the remainder of the processes. These circumstances could therefore favour the selection of mechanical de-watering. In addition, the method of disposal will affect the choice of treatment; sludge that is merely being tipped can be mechanically de-watered whereas sludge being disposed of to agricultural land frequently requires heated digestion. Finally, of course, the cost of treatment and disposal must be considered (for example see Chapter 7).

5.8   Land availability

It should be normal policy to endeavour to purchase land by negotiation rather than by compulsory powers and if this is to be done it may be necessary to adjust the site location to suit the requirements of the landowner. The value of the land will affect the choice of process only in as much as activated sludge processes use less land than filtration, but with small works this difference is not significant.

5.9   Site conditions

In some cases land subject to flooding may be the only land that is available for the construction of a treatment works. However, if a site is the preferred site from all points of view apart from its liability to flooding, it may still be used if it is economic to take the necessary precautions (e.g. the raising of levels or the construction of banks).

Ground conditions will also affect the cost of construction and therefore can affect the choice of plant. Normally the most economical ground is one which has a good bearing value but is not too difficult to excavate (e.g. marls). Poor ground conditions (e.g. alluvium) may result in all structures having to be piled; certainly this would be necessary for activated sludge or filtration plants. However, if an oxidation ditch or some other extended aeration system were being adopted, piling might not be required if some flexibility were included in the construction. When piling has to be used, special attention is needed when flexible jointed pipe-lines connect to the piled structure. There is a risk of shear at this point. One method of avoiding this type of failure is to provide a hinged reinforced concrete slab secured to the piled structure at one end but free to subside at the other. This will largely relieve the pipe-line of shear at the critical point.

5.10   **Process optimisation**

With almost any site, whether it has been selected rationally or merely because it is the only one available, there is a need to consider how effectively the operation of any of the unit processes being considered can be optimised. Process optimisation at a sewage treatment works can be thought of in several ways. For example, at the design stage it is usually the costs that are optimised with process selection being the variable which is selected to achieve this target. At the operational stage, it is the process variables which have to be altered or controlled so as to obtain the highest quality of effluent at the lowest operating cost. These various types of optimisation can also be achieved in more than one way. The techniques that have been used range from kinetic modelling to the use of empirical performance relationships and must even include the application of intuition, inventiveness and experience. Some aspects of optimisation are discussed elsewhere: for example, the control of aeration and the utilisation of energy (Chapter 4) and the way in which mass flux theory can enable settlement tanks to be used most effectively (Chapter 6). This discussion will therefore highlight other aspects of optimisation, both from the theoretical and practical viewpoint.

5.10.1   *Mixing*

Mixing is an important feature of the operation of an activated sludge aeration tank. Two types of mixing can be considered: contact mixing, which ensures that dissolved oxygen, the sludge solids and the sewage are always fully mixed within any element of the tank, and longitudinal mixing which affects how any element of the mixed liquor is dispersed within the tank as a whole. Good contact mixing is important if 'dead-spots' and sludge deposition are to be avoided. The significance of selecting the most suitable longitudinal mixing regime is perhaps more subtle. The two extremes are a completely mixed tank and a plug-flow system. The former affords an instantaneous dilution of the feed and, as such, minimises the effect that shock loads or high strength (or potentially toxic) industrial wastes can have on the sludge flora. However, this type of mixing regime is more likely to suffer from sludge settlement problems than one which has a greater degree of plug-flow (Tomlinson, 1982). It may therefore be worthwhile contemplating whether to design (or select) an aeration basin which has the flexibility of being altered from one regime to the other according to operational needs. The simple expediency of installing penstocks to alter the flow pattern would enable this alteration to be made (Fig. 5.3). An alternative would be to make use of the 'contact-tank' concept described by Rensink, Donker & Ijwema (1982). With this method the return

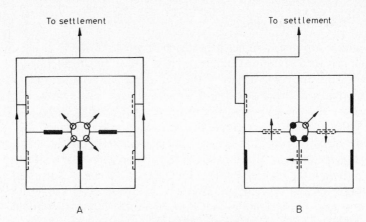

Fig. 5.3. A potentially flexible lay-out of a four-pocket aeration tank. A: Penstocks and weirs set to give a completely mixed configuration. B: Penstocks and weirs set to give a plug flow regime.

sludge and sewage are passed through a small plug-flow contact tank prior to entering the main aeration zone. Whilst this latter option could be installed at any time, it is probably easiest to do at the design/initial construction stage.

The degree of longitudinal mixing can be described in terms of the Dispersion Number (DN) (see Tomlinson & Chambers, 1979; Chambers, 1982) which, for the two extreme cases of plug-flow and complete mixing, has values of 0 and ∞ respectively. An alternative approach is to use the 'tanks-in-series' concept. That is to say a real tank would be described in terms of the theoretical equivalent number (j) of equal-sized completely-mixed tanks. However, both methods at the moment require that tracer studies be made on the full-scale tank. Longitudinal mixing can therefore only be assessed retrospectively. As a general guideline, the target conditions for achieving good settleability are DN < 0.1 and $j > 10$–15.

5.10.2   *Theoretical modelling*

The derivation of theoretical models for use in process optimisation has been a popular pastime for a number of years (see Miscellaneous Authors, 1975; James, 1978); however, as yet, they do not appear to have made any real impact on design and optimisation as practised in the United Kingdom. Most of these models have their basis in a combination of the Monod equation, the microbial growth rate and a mass balance across the reactor at steady state conditions. Using this approach, Middlebrooks & Garland (1968) developed two equations to describe the kinetics of extended aeration systems:

$$\frac{\beta \Delta S}{M} = \frac{1}{Y} + \left[\frac{K_\mathrm{D}}{Y}\right]\beta\theta$$

$$\frac{\beta\theta}{1 + \beta\theta K_\mathrm{D}} = \frac{1}{\mu_\mathrm{m}} + \left[\frac{K_\mathrm{s}}{\mu_\mathrm{m}}\right]\frac{1}{S_1}$$

where β = ratio of mixed liquor solids to effluent solids, ΔS = influent BOD − effluent BOD, S_1 = effluent BOD (mg l⁻¹), M = mixed liquor solids (mg l⁻¹), θ = hydraulic retention time (d), Y = yield coefficient (kg solids kg⁻¹ BOD), K_D = specific decay rate (d⁻¹), μ_m = maximum specific growth rate (d⁻¹), K_s = saturation constant (mg l⁻¹).

These equations have been used to compare the values of the kinetic constants of a pilot-scale extended aeration plant with those for two full-scale plants, and they have also been tested for a pilot-plant treating an industrial waste (Yang & Chen, 1977). The main problem with this, or almost any other, kinetic model is the prerequisite for steady state conditions, something which seldom, if ever, occurs in the operation of sewage treatment works. The significance of this can be seen by examining the values of the kinetic constants that were obtained for a series of oxidation ditches using the Middlebrooks & Garland equations. These show that, although the equations gave relatively sound statistical correlations for the data from any one plant, the values of the individual constants varied significantly from plant to plant (Table 5.3). This means, therefore, that before any kinetically based model can be used, the values of the constants will need to be determined. This situation obviously limits the applicability of kinetic models to a 'green-field' situation. It is suggested therefore that as a

Table 5.3. *Kinetic constants calculated from data obtained from full-scale oxidation ditches*

System	Ditch volume (m³)	K_D (d⁻¹)	Y (g g⁻¹)	μ_m (d⁻¹)	K_s (mg l⁻¹)
TNO-rotor	1000	0.007	0.757	0.010	0.49
	2080	0.003	0.154	0.004	0.18
Mammoth rotor	828	0.043	0.367	0.091	2.04
	2600	0.017	0.235	0.049	2.10
	3280	0.275	3.140	0.315	0.30
	5000	0.030	0.143	0.041	0.70
Carrousel	6200	0.002	0.126	0.006	0.46

From Forster, 1982.

general rule the use of kinetic models is not a profitable exercise either for the design or the operational control of full-scale plant. However, kinetic studies at the laboratory-scale or even pilot-scale level can have considerable value in terms of basic research.

5.10.3   *Pragmatic modelling*

Within the United Kingdom, the main example of this concept is the Sewage Treatment Optimisation Model (STOM) that has been developed jointly by the Construction Industry Research and Information Association (CIRIA) and the Water Research Centre (Anon., 1981). The basis of STOM is a series of equations which describe the performance and the costs (both capital and operating) of the individual processes likely to be used in sewage treatment. The basic cost relationships were obtained statistically from data derived from full-scale plants throughout the United Kingdom (Anon., 1977), whilst the performance relationships were based on empirical or semi-empirical equations. STOM, by combining these equations within a single computer program, allows the design engineer to assemble a series of process trains and examine which option will produce the required quality of final effluent at the minimum cost. Alternatively, STOM can be used to forecast the cost and performance of any particular process train. STOM therefore provides a uniform basis for design and design assessment. Also, since most of the performance and cost data can be altered or replaced with other equations, the model does not reduce the need for the user to be both creative and experienced.

5.11   **Summary and conclusions**

It can be seen therefore that the processes involved in site and process selection can be both lengthy and involved. There are a number of aids that can be used to facilitate these procedures, two of which are worth mentioning. The first of these is Critical Path Analysis which divides the management function into two distinct phases: planning and scheduling. Planning is the deciding of *what* should be done whereas scheduling is the determining of *when* it should be done. In addition, a critical path network can be a useful tool for presenting preliminary plans to senior management.

Technical decisions, such as a choice of site or process, involve choosing between alternative solutions to the problem, but a correct comparison can only be made when the various choices are assessed on a consistent basis. One of the best ways of doing this is to define the consequences of each solution in money units and then reduce all future cash expenditure to a common basis using Discounted Cash Flow methods. Thus each disbursement is converted, by a relatively simple compound interest calculation, to a sum of money to which each is equivalent at a given date. This is usually the first date of the study as the cost of the preliminary report must also be included. The conversion formula is:

$$P = \sum_{n=0}^{n=N} \frac{E_n}{(1+r)^n}$$

where P = the present worth of a series of disbursements made over N years, E_n = the cash disbursement made in the nth year, r = the discount or interest rate. It must be realised however that there will be associated with each alternative a number of factors which cannot be given a monetary value. These are often related to the environmental impact (e.g. smell problems or loss of visual amenity) and may enhance or detract from an alternative. In cases where the economic analysis shows only a marginal difference the assessment of these intangible factors is of vital importance.

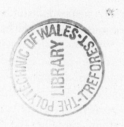

6 Operational aspects

6.1 Introduction

In discussing the performance of wastewater treatment systems, the first thing that needs to be defined is the composition of the substrate – of sewage. This is all but impossible to do since no two sewages are alike. The presence of infiltration water will dilute the sewage whilst the input of industrial wastes will make it stronger and, at times, add components which can be inhibitory, non-degradable or capable of exerting a high rate of oxygen demand. Even what is predominantly domestic sewage can vary in composition within a year under certain circumstances; for example, at holiday resorts where, during the 'season', not only will the population be increased very significantly but also the large number of hotels and restaurants being used will cause an increase in the organic content well in excess of the normal *per capita* allowance. However, in most cases the wastewater will be defined in terms of its biochemical oxygen demand (BOD), suspended solids (SS) and ammoniacal nitrogen (Amm. N) concentrations. Typical values for sewage in the UK are shown in Table 6.1. When industrial wastes are known to be present, it is also advantageous to define the sewage in terms of the BOD/COD ratio, since this provides an assessment of the treatability of the waste and the likely residual organic matter that will be discharged in the final effluent. Table 6.2 shows how this ratio can vary.

Another feature which will affect the nature of the sewage arriving at

Table 6.1. *Typical average values for the constituents of sewage*

Source	BOD (mg l^{-1})	SS (mg l^{-1})	Amm. N (mg l^{-1})
Forster, 1969	269	328	24
Eves, 1981[a]	324	381	32
Mayman *et al.*, 1981[b]	361	401	34
Lowe, 1982[c]	320	345	—
Eno & Pollington, 1975[d]	352	379	41

[a] 12-year average; [b] 5-year average; [c] 3-year average; [d] 5-year average.

Table 6.2. *BOD and COD values for various industrial effluents*

Effluent	Source	BOD (mg l⁻¹)	COD (mg l⁻¹)	COD/BOD
Lurgi gas liquors	Neufeld, 1984	5 600	12 500	2.23
Cane sugar	McNeil, 1984	1 400	2 000	1.43
Molasses stillage	McNeil, 1984	70 000	102 000	1.46
Brewery	Ruffer & Rosenwinkel, 1984	775	1 220	1.57
Slaughter-house	Hopwood & Rosen, 1972	1 791	3 145	1.76
Settled sewage	Water Research Centre, 1978	—	—	1.96
Settled sewage	Mayman *et al.*, 1981	215	391	1.82

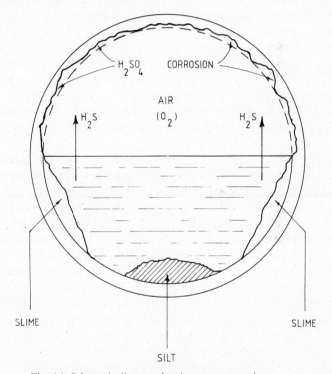

Fig. 6.1. Schematic diagram showing sewer corrosion.

a treatment works is the type of sewer leading to the works. Essentially there are two types: the gravity sewer and the rising main (sometimes referred to as a pressure main or a pumped sewer). The former flows downhill under gravity and with most flow conditions the sewer pipe is only part filled. This means that the air space above the liquid confers an aerobic environment to the sewage. Rising mains run uphill with the sewage being pumped. As a result, they invariably flow without an air space and, since microbial action will very rapidly utilise any oxygen present initially, anaerobic conditions will prevail. When this occurs, sulphate is often converted to sulphide by the sulphate-reducing bacteria (e.g. *Desulphovibrio* spp.). This is particularly pronounced under low flow conditions or if the sewer is long.

The presence of sulphide can have two main effects. If the sewerage system combines both gravity and pressure sewers such that anaerobic conditions precede aerobic, the sulphide formed in the anaerobic part of the system can become oxidised to sulphuric acid within the aerobic phase with a resultant corrosion of the sewer structure (Aldred & Eagles, 1982) (Fig. 6.1). Alternatively, if sulphide-containing anaerobic sewage ('septic sewage') is discharged at the inlet of a sewage treatment works, hydrogen sulphide can be liberated to the atmosphere and give rise to odour complaints.

6.2   Odour control

From the point of view of the neighbouring community, one of the major difficulties in the operation of a sewage treatment works is smell. The control of odours is made particularly difficult by the fact that the detection, both in qualitiative and quantitative terms, of the smells that result from the various stages of sewage treatment is very subjective. Science has yet to devise an instrument more sensitive than the human nose. Therefore, although tests have been devised to measure or describe the effect of specific chemicals (Matthews, 1976), the detection in general of 'smells from the sewage works' which result from a miscellany of compounds depends on the sensitivity and, in some cases, the psychological response of the people living in the vicinity of the works. The problem is further complicated by the fact that the odour threshold of compounds can vary considerably from person to person, even depending on their age and sex. Also, in some cases the quality of the odour can change with the concentration of the chemical. Several expressions have been developed to describe the effects of odoriferous compounds, the most basic of which is the Absolute Threshold Concentration (ATC). This is defined as the geometric mean of the minimum detectable concentrations identified by members of a sensory testing panel. Values of these concentrations for various compounds are given in Table 6.3.

The compounds causing smells which emanate from a sewage works are usually the result of the anaerobic decomposition of organic matter. Typical of these are mercaptans; heterocyclic nitrogen compounds such as skatole; hydrogen sulphide; short chain aliphatic amines and organic

Table 6.3. *Absolute threshold concentrations for various compounds*

Compound	Odour description	ATC (p.p.m.)
Ethyl mercaptan	Decayed cabbage	0.00032
Dimethyl amine	Fishy	0.0470
Skatole	Faecal	0.0012
Butyric acid	Sweaty	0.0010
Diallyl sulphide	Garlic	0.00014
Valeric acid	Sweaty	0.00062
Dimethyl sulphide	Decayed vegetable	0.0100
Hydrogen sulphide	Rotten eggs	0.0011
Crotyl mercaptan	Rancid	0.00003

From Neufeld, 1975 and Henry & Gehr, 1980.

acids (e.g. butyric and valeric acid). Good housekeeping will go a long way towards minimising the problem of complaints about smells – for example, by keeping a few centimetres of water over stored sludge odour emissions can be reduced. However, there are certain processes that can be readily associated with the emission of odours (Henry & Gehr, 1980). These are:

(i) The works inlet, particularly if this is at the top of a rising main. Problems can also be experienced after a lengthy dry period when the first flush of storm water is received, bringing with it the anaerobic solids which had been deposited during the low flow conditions.
(ii) The handling of screenings
(iii) Sumps and wet wells
(iv) Grit removal plants
(v) Sludge treatment and handling processes.

Odours can also result from operational problems associated with the bio-oxidation stage, for example, an under-aerated activated sludge system or a bio-filter which is not fully wetted. In addition to these problems, a works manager frequently has to cope with smells coming from within sewers, at points remote from the treatment works, which are caused either by anaerobiosis or by specific smelly compounds discharged as trade effluent.

Within the UK there is no statutory requirement to control smell. However, if the smell can be shown to constitute a nuisance, abatement notices can be sought under the Common Law or legislation such as the Public Health (Recurring Nuisances) Act, 1969 and the Health and Safety at Work Act, 1974 (see Matthews & Boon, 1978). Nuisance can be subjective and is hard to define, although the Health and Safety

Executive use $\frac{1}{30}$th of the threshold limit value. In other parts of the world emission standards for smells have been established (Ando, 1980), although there is no indication that these standards relate to the potential nuisance of the odours. Thus, for example, in California the threshold levels of the specified odorous compounds have been determined and a limit of 100 times the threshold level has been set as the maximum concentration for emission (Koczkur & Stone, 1974).

Within the UK, methods have been suggested for the quantification of odour emissions (North, 1979; Keddie, 1982). Odour emission rates have been reported for one situation (North, 1979) and this work has been extended to estimate 'fall-out zones' – the maximum distance at which complaints might be received (Keddie, 1982). Both methods involve assessing the degree of dilution that a polluted air sample requires before 50 per cent of a sensory panel will just not detect an odour.

There are essentially three methods for odour control (see Henry & Gehr, 1980):

(a) Direct oxidation
(b) adsorption or
(c) masking of the odorous compound.

In addition, it may be possible to minimise smells by the more effective use of trade effluent control measures (e.g. requiring the discharge temperature to be lowered or restricting compounds which are specifically odorous or which can react with other trade wastes in the sewers to produce smells), or by the controlled deflection of the prevailing wind (e.g. by trees).

One of the oxidants used for controlling odours from sewage treatment works is ozone (Anderson & Greaves, 1983). However, its use means that the process causing the smell must be enclosed so that all the contaminated air can be channelled through a single exhaust point. Two different techniques have been adopted for contacting the ozone-rich air with the smell-laden air: a dry method and a wet method (Table 6.4), the former being the more common. The advantages claimed for the wet contacting technique are that contact times are reduced and so ozone usage and therefore running costs are minimised. Also, any hazards from potentially explosive gas mixtures are eliminated. A further advantage of using ozone, whichever method is employed, is that as well as destroying the odour-producing compounds, the biocidal properties of the ozone cause a reduction in the concentrations of bacteria in the air discharged from the plant. One disadvantage is that all the materials of construction must be capable of withstanding the strongly oxidising conditions imposed by the ozone. Traditionally this has meant using stainless steel but this is expensive

Table 6.4. *Operational examples of odour control by ozone*

Source of odour	Air volume (m^3 min^{-1})	Contacting method	Contact time (s)	Ozone yield (kg d^{-1})
Septage and grit treatment	70	O_3/air	13	0.9
Sludge storage	417	O_3/water/air	—	—
Grit treatment	1920	O_3/air	25	8
Screening and grit treatment	850	O_3/air	6	11
Entire works	833	O_3/water/air	—	48

and the resultant structure is heavy. The problem can be overcome by using fibre glass and PVC.

Aeration, which can be considered as a type of oxidation, can be used to overcome odour problems. If the source of the smell is a rising main which is long enough to bring about anaerobic conditions, an obvious solution is to ensure that anaerobic conditions do not occur. Aeration with air has been examined in a number of cases, using blowers supplying 0.354 m^3 min^{-1} at 20 kPa, although all the mains investigated were less than 0.18 m in diameter (Todd, 1974). The broad conclusions that can be reached from this work were that (i) whilst aeration did lower the sulphide levels, particularly if lime was added to the sewage, it did not completely eliminate the problem, and (ii) the efficiency of aeration used alone was inversely related to the ambient temperature. The main problems with the use of air are its limited solubility and the fact that it must be dissolved as a mixture with nitrogen. This latter point can be a particular nuisance in rising mains, as residual nitrogen (i.e. in the gaseous form) can prevent the operation of syphons or can cause water hammer. With larger long rising mains it is probable that the amount of oxygen which could be dissolved in water from air would be insufficient to prevent the onset of anaerobiosis before the top of the main. An alternative to the use of air is the injection of oxygen into a rising main. Depending on the pumping head, this would increase the dissolved oxygen concentration to several times the normal air saturation concentration, thus delaying anaerobiosis for a longer period. From an investigation into this technique (Boon & Lister, 1975) it is possible to calculate the daily weight of oxygen that must be dissolved to prevent the concentration of dissolved oxygen falling below 0.5 mg l^{-1}, the value above which no sulphide is formed. Studies on a test main, which was 2700 m long and had a diameter of 0.4 m, showed that the injection of oxygen was capable of removing the odour nuisance from sulphide, whereas earlier tests using air had only been partially effective (Boon *et al.*, 1977; Skellett, 1978).

Oxygen can also be used to reduce odours within the treatment works itself (Garrett & Jeffries, 1983). Under these circumstances, the oxygen is transferred by a Vitox system (see Chapter 4).

Oxygen deficiencies in bio-oxidation systems can also cause odours. In one activated sludge plant the lack of oxygen was traced to inadequate mixing which in turn was leading to a deposition of solids in the aeration basin. These became anaerobic and then released odours. The problem was overcome by altering the mixing pattern so that turbulence sufficient for regular bottom scouring was achieved. Not only did this stop the smells but it also improved the BOD removal (Bhatla, 1975).

Hydrogen peroxide is a more specific oxidant that can be used to control those odours produced by dissolved sulphides (e.g. Cole, Paul & Brewer, 1976; Sims, 1980). At a more or less neutral pH the hydrogen sulphide is oxidised to elemental sulphur:

$$H_2S + H_2O_2 \rightarrow S + 2H_2O$$

The commercially available peroxide, which is usually between 35 and 50 per cent, can be added directly to gravity mains, rising mains or processes within the treatment works itself either by a simple drip feed or a metering pump. Although a fast reaction is said to be achieved with the stoichiometric dose, practical experience indicates that in sewers, slightly larger doses (H_2O_2:sulphide up to 3:1) are needed. Chlorination can also be used to control odours although, since it is debatable whether the reductants are the odour-producing molecules or the bacteria whose action produces those molecules, the classification of the role of chlorine should perhaps be disinfection rather than oxidation. Nevertheless, the importance of chlorination should not be underestimated. It is frequently used as one of the more 'instant' techniques for odour control. However, it must be recognised that chlorination can also produce chlorinated organics which may well be non-biodegradable.

If the odour-contaminated air can be channelled through a single exhaust vent, the odoriferous molecules can be removed by adsorption (Shahalam, 1982). In theory, either wet or dry adsorption can be used. In practice, since most of the odorous compounds produced at sewage works are not very soluble in water and since water is the most practical scrubbing medium that can be used at such sites, wherever adsorption is used, it is more common to operate the dry system. However, it is possible to effect some degree of odour control by 'fixing' the odour compounds and thus preventing their emission. This has been done, in the case of a sludge storage and handling system, by the use of ammonia to increase the pH (Neufeld, 1975). Alternatively, odours can be reduced by minimising evaporation from a unit. One technique which is claimed to be successful in this role is the use of hollow plastic balls floating as a close-packed layer on the surface of open sludge-tanks (Baum, 1975). Of the dry adsorbents that are available, activated carbon is probably the most readily acceptable although other materials (e.g. zeolites, alumina) have been investigated. Activated carbon, which in general will adsorb volatile organics whose molecular weight is greater than 45, has been used successfully to deodorise air from trickling filters, primary clarifiers and humus tanks. However, at high odour concentrations frequent regeneration is necessary, and since this is accomplished by passing steam through the carbon bed it is energy intensive, and consideration should be given whether to regenerate or merely to incinerate the carbon at the end of its active life (see, for example, Huang & Wilson, 1979).

Two types of deodorants or odour-masking chemicals can be distinguished. In one case the masking agent has a smell whose characteristics and intensity make it impossible to detect the original offensive odour. In the other case, which is usually known as odour counteraction, the smell of the active component counteracts that of the malodorous compound in some way, either at the molecular level or as a sensory interaction. Natural compounds (e.g. oil of juniper which reacts with butyric acid) that can be used for this purpose have now been supplemented by synthetic compounds (e.g. esters, ketones). This has enabled a greater range of smell problems to be dealt with by this technique, particularly when a blend of chemicals is used as the deodorising formulation. It is claimed that counteraction is more acceptable than masking because: (a) the masking odour can be more annoying than the original smell to some people, and (b) the two odours could disperse at separate rates. Whichever system is chosen the formulation can essentially be used in three ways:

(a) batch surface spraying
(b) continuous direct feed
(c) random aerial spraying.

Surface spraying is probably best used at unmanned treatment works where the smell is coming either from sludge storage tanks or stabilisation lagoons. Assuming an application rate of about $0.6 \text{ g m}^{-2} \text{ d}^{-1}$, the overall costs, excluding labour, for deodorising will be of the order of £0.06 m^{-2} of lagoon surface. Sludge tankers could also be treated by direct spraying – the cost per treatment for a 9 m^3 (2000 gallon) tanker will be about £0.15–0.20. Direct feed deodorising is used mainly for counteracting smells from preliminary and primary treatment units, usually by drip-feed systems which add the deodorant directly to the raw sewage. The usual rate of application is 5 mg l^{-1} which means that the cost is around £0.01 per m^3 of effluent treated. However, on some installations difficulties have been experienced in controlling the rate of drip and as the alternative feed system involves the expense of metering pumps it might be easier, for operational purposes, to consider controlling the smell by aerial spraying.

Two types of aerial spray installation are used, although both operate with spray nozzles mounted on lances. These lances are usually about 10–12 feet high. The difference between the two systems is the spray nozzles; in one case the spray is of pressurised liquid (i.e. diluted deodorant), in the other it is an air/liquid mist. With the latter system, lances would probably be spaced at 23 m intervals (Collett, 1972) and usually fed at between 0.6 and 2.2 l h^{-1} depending on the formulation and the operational dilution; the cost would be £0.03–0.05 h^{-1} per lance. Electrical/pumping costs would also have to be considered and this would obviously depend on the number of lances being operated. As an approximation it could be considered that a 2237 W (3 h.p.) pump would be sufficient to operate five lances. In the case of the pressurised liquid system, the lances should be more closely spaced, 9 m being the usually recommended distance. The technique for starting the operation of aerial sprays will depend on the type of treatment works involved (i.e. whether it is a manned works or not), the direction and the frequency of the prevailing winds in relation to housing, and the origin of the smell. Essentially there are only two options – a manual method and an automatic system operated by the wind direction.

It can be seen therefore that there are a variety of techniques available to a sewage works' manager for controlling smells. However, their effectiveness is measured only in terms of the response of the general public, and more particularly that of their noses. In some cases, the techniques that are employed have more of a psychological effect than an actual odour-controlling effect.

Whilst there are methods that can be brought into operation once a problem has developed, there are steps that can be taken as early as the works design stage to minimise odour problems. For example, sumps and storm water wells can be designed so that they can be emptied completely. In a similar way, planners should appreciate odour problems and attempt to ensure that the sprawl of housing development does not engulf a treatment works. Forethought and good housekeeping are as important as oxidants and masking sprays in controlling odours.

Table 6.5. *Performance of primary tanks*

Source	Parameter	Raw sewage (mg l⁻¹)	Settled sewage (mg l⁻¹)	Removal (%)
Eves, 1981	BOD	324	177	46
	SS	381	123	68
	Amm. N	32	32	—
Mayman *et al.*, 1981	BOD	361	205	43
	SS	401	128	68
	Amm. N	34	36	—
Eno & Pollington, 1975	BOD	352	203	42
	SS	379	122	68
	Amm. N	41	40	—
Lowe, 1982	BOD	320	174	46
	SS	345	144	58

6.3 Primary settlement

The operation of primary settlement tanks is an essential and often neglected part of the overall treatment sequence. As a process, taken in isolation, its purpose is to remove solids. However, in doing so, primary tanks also effect a degree of BOD removal. Typical performance data for primary tanks are shown in Table 6.5. A number of techniques have been suggested to enable performances to be predicted (see Anderson, 1981). Two are worth mentioning: that reported by Tebbutt & Christoulas (1975) and that used in the STOM model (Water Research Centre, 1981; see Chapter 5). The former enables the removal efficiency (E) to be calculated as:

$$E = A \exp-\left(\frac{B}{S_i} + C \times O\right)$$

where S_i = raw sewage suspended solids (mg l⁻¹), O = over-flow rate (m³ m⁻² d⁻¹), $A = 0.955$, $B = 265$, $C = 0.0021$. The STOM model calculates the suspended solids concentration in the settled sewage (S_o) as:

$$S_o = \frac{14}{\theta} S_i^{\alpha} V^{\beta}$$

where θ = constant, often taken as 1.0, α = constant, often taken as 0.4, β = constant, often taken as 0.4.

Both these expressions are empirical and both contain constants which have a varying degree of general applicability since their magnitude depends on the settlement characteristics of the solids, the

Table 6.6. *Comparison of predicted and actual*
suspended solids concentration in settled sewage

| Source | Predicted S_o (mg l^{-1}) | | Actual S_o (mg l^{-1}) |
	Tebbutt & Christoulas (1975)	STOM	
Cotton, 1973	242	135	146
Eves, 1981	207	137	123
Kellock, 1973	207	102	111
NWWA (a)	158	67	72
(b)	158	77	145

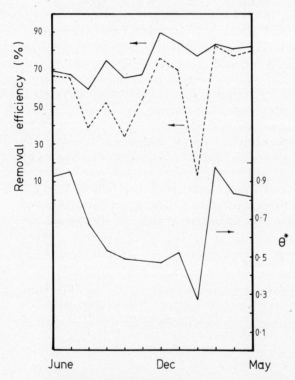

Fig. 6.2. Predicted (——) and actual (-----) performance of a primary
settlement tank showing the values of θ necessary to permit the two
performances to coincide.

design of the tank and the frequency with which the tank is desludged. The danger of using these models without first re-calculating the values of the constants can be seen from the data in Table 6.6 which compares actual and predicted concentrations of the suspended solids in settled sewage. It is also interesting to note that even with one set of primary tanks wide variations can occur. Fig. 6.2 shows the variation in predicted (STOM) and actual removal efficiencies for a twelve month period, together with the values required for θ to enable the predictions to give the actual values (assuming $\alpha = \beta = 0.4$).

What then causes variability in performance? A fairly recent survey (Lockyear, 1980) has enabled this question to be answered, at least in part. One feature is the seasonal variation in the quantity of solids reaching the primary settlement tanks. The survey by Lockyear showed that the maximum concentration of primary sludge was more likely to occur in the spring. This was attributed to the higher flow-rates in the sewerage system scouring solids from the sewers. In addition, if excess secondary sludge is being co-settled in the primary tanks, an increased solids production can be expected in the winter months since less of the carbonaceous matter will be oxidised to carbon dioxide.

The settlement behaviour of secondary sludges, particularly activated sludges, will also influence the primary/secondary co-settling mixture. If the settlement characteristics of the secondary sludge are poor then problems are likely to occur in the primary tank (see Lowe, 1982). The shape of the tanks will also affect the removal efficiencies, circular tanks being more efficient than rectangular ones (Lockyear, 1980). The most common cause of problems in the operation of primary tanks is associated with pipework blockages. This tends to happen if the sludge becomes too thick and the diameter of the desludging pipes is narrow. By examining the sludge pipe diameters (d) and the maximum solids concentration achieved by the various primary tanks surveyed (C^*) in relation to the occurrence of desludging problems, Lockyear suggested that if $d > (2.88C^* - 4)$ then few problems should be expected. In certain specialised cases the blockages can be the result of specific types of solid material. For example, the presence of fine coal tailings was the main cause of blockages at one works (Eno & Pollington, 1975).

An underloaded primary tank can create as many difficulties as one which is overloaded. Underloading can be the result of poor design, the need to cope with wide fluctuations in flow or simply the fact that the works was designed for a population equivalent which has yet to appear. Whatever the reason, a low hydraulic loading results in excessive retention times within the primary tanks. This in turn leads to anaerobiosis and odour (usually hydrogen sulphide) problems. The evolution of gas from anaerobic primary tanks can also carry sludge to the surface where it will float and eventually pass to the secondary processes, adding an unnecessary load to these systems. This can be controlled by using only the number of settlement tanks that is appropriate to the flow of incoming sewage (Mayman *et al.*, 1981) and by ensuring that the tanks are desludged frequently.

6.4   Trickling filters

Filters have been in use for over 70 years and today their performance is all but taken for granted. Certainly, if properly designed and loaded within the design limits, they are a process capable of oxidising both carbonaceous and nitrogenous material. However, an examination of their performances shows that the degree of treatment achieved is very variable (Table 6.7). The regular occurrence of poor performance is usually due to overloading, either because of the age of the plant or because significant amounts of trade effluent are present in the sewage. The data presented in Table 6.7 have been selected to illustrate that both good and bad performances do occur. A better perspective can be obtained from the data reported by Booth (1984). These were an analysis of the performances, from 1977 to June 1983, of the trickling filters being operated by one division of the Wessex Water Authority. The analysis did not include those works serving populations of less than 100. It also neglected works which were required to produce only a partially treated effluent. The survey thus covered 90 works. The results (Fig. 6.3) show that more than 60 per cent produced effluents whose long term average BOD was less than 15 mg l^{-1}, that the suspended solids concentration produced by 49 per cent was less than 25 mg l^{-1} and that 58 per cent produced practically fully nitrified effluents (< 5 mg Amm. N l^{-1}). In other words, trickling filters can perform as well as any type of sewage treatment process.

Having said that it must also be explained that certain problems do

Table 6.7. *Performance data for trickling filters*

Design DWF (Ml d^{-1})	Actual daily flow (Ml d^{-1})	BOD 95 percentile	SS values	Amm. N (mg l^{-1})
1.8	2.0	46	59	16
3.0	1.7	36	37	16
3.4	3.7	45	63	18
13.6	14.4	77	75	—
19.0	22.6	47	64	16
—	42.5	13	22	4
—	0.05	20	26	7
—	2.9	22	38	4

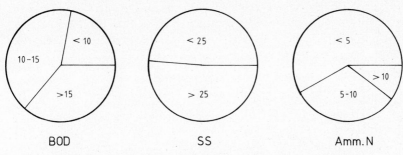

Fig. 6.3. The distribution of final effluent quality. (From Booth, 1984.)

exist in the operation of trickling filters. For example, all filters tend to
suffer from 'spring sloughing'. This is an unloading of the excess
biofilm that has accumulated during the winter months as a result of
the reduced activity of the predators within the film (see Hawkes &
Shepherd, 1971). Thus the humus tanks (final settlement tanks) are
subjected to a much higher solids loading than at any other part of the
year. The degree to which this can be accepted or tolerated depends on
how near those tanks are to their hydraulic limit, but in most cases
there will be a noticeable increase in the solids discharge with the final
effluent (Fig. 6.4).

Another problem which is characteristic of filters is the presence of
flies. A detailed survey of the problem and the associated literature has
been published elsewhere (Painter, 1980) and only key points will be
emphasised here. Fly larvae form a significant part of the filter ecology
and yet the adult flies emerging as a swarm can present a definite
nuisance either to works operators or houses/factories that are close to
the works. Generally, complaints come from property closer than
1.6 km. In the event of flies creating a nuisance the first step should be
to identify the species involved. This enables two things to be done. The
characteristics of the life cycle (and therefore the frequency with which
the problem will arise) can be determined, using published constants
and the prevailing temperatures (see Woods, Williams & Croydon,
1978), and then a control strategy can be developed.

Nuisance tends to be most common when one species is dominant.
Therefore, one means of control is to increase the diversity. In this way,
competition will keep the numbers of each population low. For
example, considering just two of the main species, a heavy growth of
biofilm will inhibit the numbers of Chironomids (midges) but will
enhance Psychodid species. Decreasing the biofilm thickness by using
ADF or by changing the periodicity of dosing will therefore allow the
Chironomid population to compete with the Psychodids. There are
inherent disadvantages in this approach since the Chironomids have

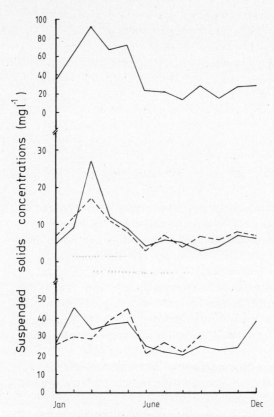

Fig. 6.4. Suspended solids concentrations in the final effluent from three trickling filter works, showing the increased concentrations in spring.

two unfortunate characteristics: they fly well and they swarm (for mating) which is noticeable. Psychoda do neither of these. Alternatively, the wetting of the filter surface can be improved. On most filters there are, almost invariably, areas which are seldom wetted (e.g. the ends of rectangular filter beds) and it has been shown that Psychoda spp. emerge through dry media (Otter, 1966). However, these are long term approaches and it may be necessary to instigate some measure of control in the short term. This means the use of insecticides. The adult fly can be attacked if there are identifiable 'resting points', such as a tree screen around the works or areas of long grass, that can be sprayed when emergence is expected. If this is not possible, then the larvae must be treated (see Harbott & Penney, 1983). On the basis of the survey made by Painter (1980) it would appear that there is a somewhat limited choice and it must also be remembered that (a) most species can develop a tolerance to toxic agents, and (b) the requirements of the Health and Safety Executive must be considered. In addition, however the insecticide is being applied, pollution of the receiving watercourse must be avoided. Flies only constitute a nuisance to the general public if property development is allowed to encroach sufficiently close to a treatment works for flies to reach those properties. The best method of control therefore is to ensure that there is an adequate and permanent 'buffer zone' around treatment works. All too often this has been neglected.

Sewage treatment works are not the most beautiful of sights and trees are often used to create an 'out of sight, out of mind' philosophy. However, when the main secondary process is a trickling filter, trees, and in particular deciduous trees, can be a self-inflicted operational hazard in that the volume of leaves shed in the autumn can cause significant blockages of the surface voids. The moral must therefore be, if trees are essential for visual screening – plant coniferous species.

The regularity of maintenance must also be considered when performance is being assessed; in particular, the cleaning of distributors. If this is not done, blockage of the jets will create a sufficient pressure within the distributors to 'blow-off' the end-caps. If this occurs, the settled sewage will be applied only to the periphery of the filter and performance will deteriorate. During the 1983 Water Industry Strike in the UK this did occur in at least one Region with the trickling filters being the first process to break-down. The recent development by the Water Research Centre of an automatic cleaning device for jets (see Hoyland & Ronald, 1984) could not only prevent this problem in the unfortunate event of another strike but could also reduce the running (maintenance) costs of trickling filters; this is because it has been estimated that the time spent ensuring that the distributor jets are clear constitutes some 10–15 per cent of the total manual labour time at trickling filter works (Booth, 1984). An alternative approach is to use fine screening (1.5–5 mm apertures) either between the primary settlement tanks and the filters or as an alternative to primary settlement (Hoyland & Ronald, 1984). As well as reducing the potential for nozzle blockages; during the strike period no blockages occurred at two works employing fine screening (Booth, 1984); the use of fine screens as an alternative to primary settlement is also claimed to be a more economic option (Hoyland & Ronald, 1984).

As has already been stated, overloading is one of the major problems with the operation of filters. This can be the result of spasmodic (e.g. seasonal) discharges of high strength trade effluents to the sewerage system or it can result from the natural increase in the population being served since the filter was originally built. The latter situation may be aggravated by a deterioration of the media through weathering. Overloading can be accommodated to a certain extent by the use of

Table 6.8. *Performance data* (*average values*) *for a parallel operation of stone and plastic media*

	Stone		Low-rate plastic	
	ICI data	Wessex WA data	ICI data	Wessex WA data
BOD (mg l^{-1})	7	10	9	17
SS (mg l^{-1})	22	5	20	18
Amm. N (mg l^{-1})	4	2	11	9
Nitrate-N (mg l^{-1})	30	25	20	16
Organic loading rate (kg BOD m^{-3} d^{-1})	0.01		0.16	
Hydraulic loading rate (m^3 m^{-3} d^{-1})	0.05		0.72	

From Hemming & Wheatley, 1979.

re-circulation or alternating double filtration (see Chapter 3). If this is not possible or has already been used, it may be possible to reduce the effect of the overload (i.e. filter ponding) by replacing the upper part (*c*. 0.4 m) of the filter with new media. Indeed it has been suggested that the replacement media ought to be high voidage plastic rather than stone. However, plastic media will only be properly wetted if the irrigation rates are in excess of 6 m^3 m^{-2} d^{-1} and these rates tend to be incompatible with the stone media which would constitute the bulk of such a hybrid filter. A better way of dealing with the problem is to use a plastic media filter as a high-rate primary filter with the existing stone systems being used to polish the effluent. Alternatively, the flow can be split so that the existing stone filters only treat their original design load with the excess being treated on a low-rate plastic media tower. Results from this latter option indicate the potential for this approach (Hemming & Wheatley, 1979). Table 6.8 reports the analytical data obtained, at one of the works discussed by Hemming & Wheatley, both by the Regional Water Authority responsible for the works (routine measurements over an extended period) and by the contractors (an intensive site survey lasting five days).

Plastic media towers are also used as high-rate filters and as such their performance, which is best described by the envelope shown in Fig. 3.8, varies with the organic loading rate and the treatability of the waste. Although it is dangerous to generalise, in most practical applications a single tower would be loaded so as to effect a removal of 55–60 per cent of the applied BOD. A typical application for domestic sewage is the use of a high-rate filter loaded at the rate of

2.0–2.5 kg m^{-3} d^{-1} to achieve a 60 per cent removal. The residual BOD
is removed on the existing stone-packed trickle filter. The introduction
of the high-rate filter therefore enables the loading of the original filter
to be reduced from about 0.3 kg m^{-3} d^{-1} to a more acceptable 0.12.

Single towers can also be used for the treatment of industrial waste.
However, because they are almost invariably of a much higher strength
than domestic sewage, a more usual configuration is a sequence of
towers. With either method, if a relatively complete treatment is
required the effluent from the high-rate filtration is 'polished' with a
conventional process (either a stone-packed filter or activated sludge).
For example, a three stage sequence has been used to reduce a BOD
from 10 000 to 600 mg l^{-1} and thus enable it to be treated by activated
sludge. The loadings applied to the three towers, which were of an
equal size, were 4.29, 2.36 and 0.94 kg m^{-3} d^{-1}.

One of the problems which is often claimed to beset high-rate filters
is the generation of odours. In some cases, these can be caused by a
combination of the sewerage system and the filters. In other words, the
odour potential is generated by anaerobiosis within the sewers (see §6.2)
and this potential is realised within the filters when the high upflow of
air (relative to a conventional filter) strips the volatile, odoriferous
compounds from solution. The control of this version of the problem
should therefore be applied before the filtration stage. However, the
filters themselves can create odours (Smith & Yates, 1980) although the
mechanism for their doing so is still supposition.

6.5   Activated sludge

As has already been described (Chapter 3), the activated sludge process
can take many forms. In discussing their performance however, the
main differentiation that will be made is between conventional and
extended aeration. Any activated sludge should have two specific
properties: the ability to oxidise the substrate being fed to it and the
ability to settle readily. These properties must therefore be the prime
yardsticks for measuring performance.

The degree to which activated sludge units can oxidise the pollutants
in domestic sewage can be seen from the data in Table 6.9. These show
that in general activated sludge can remove BOD and can also oxidise
ammoniacal nitrogen to a considerable degree. This agrees with the
survey made by Booth (1984) which was mentioned earlier (§6.4). Of
the activated sludge plants covered by the survey, 83 per cent reduced
the BOD to less than 10 mg l^{-1} and 75 per cent produced effluents
whose ammoniacal nitrogen concentrations were less than 10 mg l^{-1}.
The oxidation of ammonia requires that an adequately sized colony of
nitrifying bacteria exists in the sludge. Since the nitrifiers are slow

Table 6.9. *Activated sludge performance data assessed in terms of final effluent*

Type of plant	Daily flow ($m^3 d^{-1}$)	BOD (mg l^{-1})	SS (mg l^{-1})	Amm. N (mg l^{-1})
CDA	239712	6	17	2
CDA	51970	22	20	5
EAC	25000	5	9	3
CSA	22500	11	11	13
EAM	6000	7	8	3
CSA	5750	29	40	6
CSA	4400	5	9	2
CSA	120	26	34	30

CSA: Conventional plant, surface aeration; CDA: Conventional plant, diffused air; EAM: Extended aeration, Mammoth system; EAC: Extended aeration, Carrousel system.

growing species this means that a long sludge age is required. Under the conditions (pH and temperature) which normally prevail in an aeration tank, it is generally agreed that the minimum sludge age compatible with nitrification is about 10 days. It has been suggested (Marais, 1973) that this minimum sludge age (SA^*) is dependent purely on the temperature (T) since the aeration tank pH will, except in exceptional or specialised cases (see §6.8), approximate to 7:

$$SA^* = 3.05 \times (1.127)^{20-T}$$

Jones & Sabra (1980), in a recent study, have produced results which agree well with the Marais equation. Extended aeration plants and most conventional plants that are well managed will operate with sludge ages that are greater than the required minimum. However, conventional plants, by their nature, do not have sludge ages which are as long as those of extended aeration plants and there will therefore be some occasions when the temperature will dictate an SA^* value greater than that being used. When this happens nitrification is reduced.

The total removal of nitrogen can be accomplished, if required, by permitting a well nitrified effluent to pass through an anoxic region (DO < 0.5 mg l^{-1}) in which the effluent, the sludge and an additional carbon source are well mixed (see Chapter 3; also Jank & Bridle, 1983). Although it is probably more common to do this with extended aeration systems, and in particular oxidation ditches, it is quite feasible to achieve denitrification in a conventionally loaded plant. Fryer & Musty (1983) have reported the use of an anoxic zone at the inlet end of plug-flow diffused-air aeration tanks. The objective of this anoxic zone was to reduce the concentration of nitrate-nitrogen ($NO_3 - N$) to

Table 6.10. *Performance of an anoxic zone in a plug-flow diffused-air aeration tank*

	Nitrate-nitrogen (averages)	
	% Removal	Effluent concentration (mg l⁻¹)
June	57	16.0
July	52	14.5
August	42	16.5
September	56	13.0
October	60	13.5
November	61	16.5
December	53	14.5

From Fryer & Musty, 1983.

Table 6.11. *Nitrogen concentration (mg l⁻¹) in a Carrousel system*

	Influent	Effluent		
	Amm. N	Amm. N	NO_2-N	NO_3-N
1978–79	23.8	1.3	0.2	6.2
1979–80	15.4	2.7	0.4	6.1
1980–81	16.6	2.3	0.3	7.2

From Rachwal *et al.*, 1983.

less than 20 mg l⁻¹ and thus prevent the problem of denitrification and rising sludge in the final settlement tanks. Based on denitrification rates, which were found to vary from 2.0 to 2.9 mg NO_3-N g MLSS⁻¹ g⁻¹ at 11 and 18 °C respectively, an anoxic zone having a retention time of about 90 minutes was found to be necessary. This represented about 30 per cent of the aeration tank volume. The anoxic conditions were achieved by removing about 90 per cent of the diffusors in the required zone. This left a sufficient input of air to achieve mixing and to prevent any deposition of sludge but not enough to cause any measurable concentration of DO. The results that were reported (Table 6.10) relate to the overall plant performance and include an element of nitrate removal in the final settlement tank. However, the occurrence of rising sludge was reduced significantly showing the effectiveness of the anoxic treatment.

Table 6.12. *Nitrogen concentrations (mg l⁻¹) in complex ditch systems*

	Influent	Effluent	
Ditch type	Total – N	Amm. N	Total – N
Double ditch	20–35	0.7	6.7
Triple ditch	20	1.7	2.0
Multi-channel	25	3.1	6.7

Table 6.13. *Settlement properties of activated sludge*

		Settlement index		
Type of plant[a]	Type	Max.	Min.	Mean
CDA	$SSVI^{b}_{3.5}$	113	72	87
CSA	SVI^{c}	351	111	266
CSA	SVI	540	270	310
CDA	SVI	100	53	72
EAM	$SSVI_{3.5}$	104	36	66
EAC	$SSVI_{3.5}$	218	16	73

[a] For abbreviations see Table 6.9. [b] Stirred sludge volume index. [c] Sludge volume index.

The technique of nitrogen removal in oxidation ditches is well documented (see Forster, 1983; Rachwal *et al.*, 1983) and is relatively easy to achieve. However, the control of DO within a single ditch system is essential if results comparable to those shown in Table 6.11 are to be achieved (see Chapter 3). It is also possible to effect nitrogen removal with more complex ditch configurations such as the multiple ditches or multiple channels (Table 6.12). With the former system the anoxic conditions are achieved by reducing the rotational speed of the aerators whilst with the latter, the number of discs being used on the aerator shaft (see Fig. 3.15) is reduced.

The settlement properties of activated sludge (Table 6.13) have traditionally been measured by the sludge volume index (SVI). In the UK, this is best done in a 1 litre measuring cylinder. This is filled with sludge which is then allowed to settle for 30 minutes (or occasionally for 60 minutes). The volume occupied by the solids (SV) is recorded as a percentage of the total volume and the SVI calculated as:

$$SVI = \frac{SV\ (\%)}{\text{Suspended solids concentration}\ (\%)}.$$

A high (> 150) SVI value represents bad settlement. This is referred to as bulking. Occasionally the SVI is expressed as the sludge density index (SDI) where SDI = 100/SVI. In recent years there has been considerable debate, perhaps even controversy, over the validity of the test and its applicability to the operation of sewage treatment works (e.g. Dick & Vesilind, 1969; White, 1975). The main criticisms are that the SVI varies, in an inconsistent way, with the concentration of solids being used and that the settlement characteristics measured by the test depend on the dimensions of the test vessel. This dependence is also a function of the solids concentration and is the result either of the streaming of liquid up the walls or by 'bridging' by the solids. Because of these inconsistencies, it has been suggested that whilst the SVI is a suitable yardstick for the day-to-day control of any one plant, its use for comparisons between plants or for scale-up is dubious (Dick & Vesilind, 1969).

The alternative is the stirred index (SSVI). This is measured in a column (10 cm OD × 50 cm) fitted with a stirrer which rotates at 1 r.p.m. (White, 1975). The SSVI is measured in the same way as the unstirred index. It is usual to make two measurements: on the mixed liquor and on the return sludge (RS); and then extrapolate or interpolate to a standard concentration of 3.5 g l^{-1}, assuming a linear relationship between SSVI and the solids concentration. This value of 3.5 was chosen in part because many activated sludge plants operate either with MLSS or with RS concentrations of about this value and partly to suit correlations with solids loadings and hindered setting velocities which were poor at lower concentrations (White, 1975). This latter point is perhaps not the best reason for selecting 'standard' conditions and certainly the value of 3.5 ought not to be thought of as sacrosanct. Indeed, it is interesting to examine the relationship between SSVI and the initial solids concentration for sludges from two systems, one a pilot-plant and the other a full-scale works (Design DWF = 9650 m^3 d^{-1}) (Fig. 6.5). These data show a very variable relationship and one which has the potential for giving a comparative assessment of settleability which varied with the solids concentration. For example, with Works A, sample (i) would appear to have very much better settlement properties than sample (ii) at 2.5 g l^{-1}, whereas the situation is totally reversed when examined at 4.5 g l^{-1}.

One must therefore ask which index should be used and even whether the SVI and SSVI measure different properties of the sludge. The SVI has been shown to bear no unique relationship to some of the macro-physical properties of the sludge, such as yield strength, plastic viscosity or settling rate (Dick & Vesilind, 1969). However, it is linearly related to the surface charge carried by the particles and has a realistic relationship with the size of the particles and the bound water content

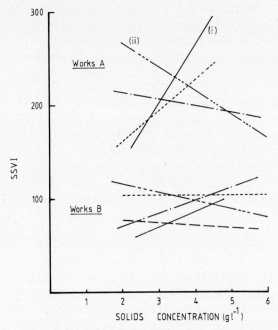

Fig. 6.5. The relationship between SSVI and solids concentration.

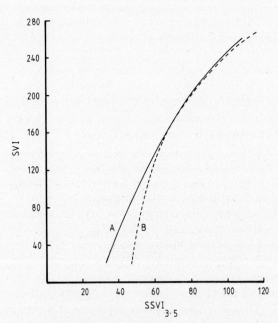

Fig. 6.6. The relationship between SVI and SSVI. A: Regression line for pilot-study data; B: Bosman & Kalos, 1978.

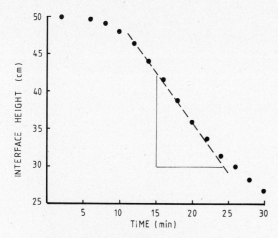

Fig. 6.7. Sludge settlement profile in the SSVI test, showing the measurement of initial settlement velocity.

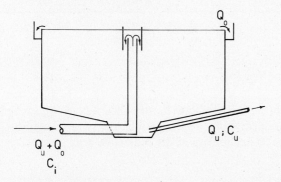

Fig. 6.8. Schematic representation of a settlement tank.

of the sludge (Forster & Choudhry, 1972; Forster & Lewin, 1972), in other words, the micro-physical properties. The relationship between stirred and quiescent indices has been described by Bosman & Kalos (1978). This is shown in Fig. 6.6 together with the regression line for some 150 results obtained over a 9-month pilot-plant study. Both curves show what can only be described as the insensitivity of the stirred index, and it could be argued that the data again suggest that the indices are a measurement of different characteristics.

From this discussion it is obvious that the quantification of sludge settleability still requires further work. Neither index has a total acceptance, although the older SVI is probably used more widely. However, an extension of the stirred test, the initial settlement velocity (v) Fig. 6.7), has an extremely useful role, both in design and operation, by way of mass flux theory. If the flow of solids per unit cross-sectional

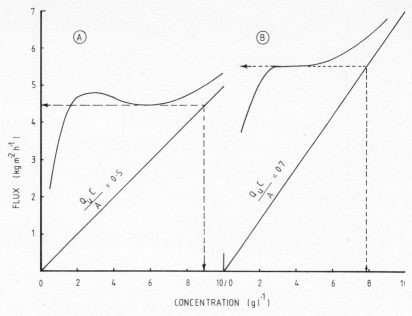

Fig. 6.9. Total flux/solids concentration curves. A: underflow rate = 0.5;
B: underflow rate = 0.7.

area of the settlement tank is considered, the solids flux (F, kg m^{-2} h^{-1})
consists of two components: one due to gravity, the other caused by the
withdrawal of sludge from the base of the tank (Fig. 6.8).

$$F = VC + \left[\frac{Q_u}{A}\right] C$$

Typical flux/concentration curves are shown in Fig. 6.9. In Fig. 6.9A
the compound flux curve shows a distinct minimum. This corresponds
to the maximum flux (F_L) that can be applied to the tank under the
prevailing conditions. The concentration of solids in the underflow can
be obtained by extrapolating the horizontal tangent to intersect with
the withdrawal flux line ($Q_u C/A$) and dropping a perpendicular from
this point. In Fig. 6.9A, the value of 8.9 g l^{-1} shows that the tank is
operating effectively as a thickener. However, to avoid the overflow of
solids, the applied flux (F_A) must be kept at a value less than F_L. If the
applied flux does exceed the limiting value, solids will be retained in the
tank ('hold-up') and, in time, these solids will be discharged with the
effluent at a rate of ($F_A - F_L$). The pressure on the tank can be relieved
by increasing the underflow rate. This can eventually lead to the
replacement of the minimum in the flux curve by an inflection (Fig.
6.9B). Also as Q_u is increased the underflow concentration will decrease
as the tank's ability to act as a thickener is reduced. Indeed, under

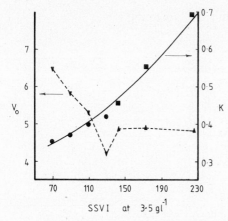

Fig. 6.10. Variation of V_0 and K with the SSVI.

extreme cases there is a need to check whether the tank's potential as a clarifier has been impaired. This can be done by solving the basic flux equation for the inlet concentration of solids and the mixed liquor settlement rate (V^*) and then applying the condition that $F_A \leqslant F_L$; i.e.

$$\frac{C_i(Q_o + Q_u)}{A} \leqslant V^* C_i + \left[\frac{Q_u}{A}\right] C_i$$

$$Q_o A \leqslant V^*.$$

This means that when high recycle rates are being used, the overflow rate must not exceed the settling velocity of the mixed liquor solids.

Initial settling velocities may also be calculated (White, 1975) from $V = V_0 \exp(-KC)$, and it has been shown that although V_0 and K will vary with the SSVI, they are constant for SSVI bands (e.g. 80–99; 100–119) (Rachwal *et al.*, 1982). This has enabled the maximum solids handling capacities (for the tanks investigated) to be determined and, from these, a set of operator guidelines to be established. These stipulate the maximum MLSS that should be used for any return sludge flow-rate or SSVI (up to a value of 140). The validity of this concept has been confirmed and its range extended to include badly bulked sludges (SSVI up to 250). This work (Forster, 1982) showed that whilst K varied smoothly with the SSVI, the V_0/SSVI curve had a discontinuity at an SSVI value of about 120 (Fig. 6.10). It was also suggested that the initial settling velocity (V) could be calculated from the SSVI (at 3.5 g l^{-1}) (S) and the MLSS concentration (C) using:

$$V = 5 \exp[-0.2498C \exp(0.0046S)].$$

A comparison of the maximum solids handling capacities calculated by

Table 6.14. *A comparison of mass flux analysis*

$Q_u = 189$ m^3 h^{-1}; $A = 755$ m^2

SSVI$_{3.5}$	Maximum solids handling capacity (kg m^{-2} h^{-1})	
	Forster, 1982	Rachwal *et al.*, 1982
60	4.18	4.1
80	3.82	3.8
110	3.37	3.4
125	3.14	3.1
170	2.56	—

this equation and by Rachwal *et al.* (1982) shows a good agreement between the two methods (Table 6.14).

Being able to predict settlement velocities and thus to provide operating guidelines is not always sufficient to prevent the effects of sludge bulking. Certainly this facility will not change the settlement characteristics of a bulked sludge. Bulking is a microbially induced problem and two separate theories have been offered to explain the phenomenon. One suggests that bulking is caused by a dominance of the activated sludge flora by filamentous species (Sezgin, Jenkins & Parker, 1978); the other that bulking is the result of an increased surface charge on the component particles brought about by changes in the sludge surface chemistry (Forster, 1968). However, although these two theories have been maintained as separate concepts, it is most likely that the real cause of bulking somehow combines the two philosophies, as suggested in Fig. 6.11.

Whatever the outcome of this debate the three types of control measure that are currently in use are aimed specifically at reducing the number of filamentous species, although their effect on sludge surfaces has never been considered. Jenkins *et al.* (1982) report the successful use of chlorine (up to about 15 kg tonne^{-1} MLSS d^{-1}) to reduce bulking, the rationale for this being that the chlorine destroys filamentous bacteria in preference to the flocs which usually confer good settlement. The other two measures rely on changes being made to the geometry of the aeration tank. The technique described by Tomlinson & Chambers (1979) involves using an anoxic zone at the inlet of the aeration tank. The retention time in this zone should normally be 30–40 minutes but its effectiveness in controlling settleability cannot be predicted. It is also not known why the anoxic conditions affect the sludge in this way. Nevertheless it is a technique that works, as confirmed by Price (1982),

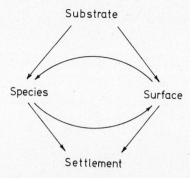

Fig. 6.11. The S-sequence as an explanation of bulking.

who describes the improvement that was achieved (SSVI from 155 to < 100) at a medium-sized treatment works (average daily flow of 3600 m³ d⁻¹).

The fact that those aeration tanks with significant plug-flow characteristics tend to produce better setting sludges than those which have a large degree of complete mixing has been noted by several workers (e.g. Tomlinson, 1976; Kroiss & Ruider, 1977). Several applications and implications of this fact are described in the book edited by Chambers & Tomlinson (1982) and readers are referred to this text for details of performance. One suggestion for the success of plug-flow tanks is that the sludge experiences a high floc-load (kg BOD kg⁻¹ MLSS) at the inlet of the tank. This concept has been extended to the use of a specific but small mixing zone (either within the aeration tank or as a separate unit) in which return sludge and incoming sewage are contacted prior to the main aeration (see several authors in Chambers & Tomlinson, 1982).

Bulking as a problem can both be tolerated (by the use of operator guidelines) and, to a certain extent, controlled. However, there is still a need to understand the physiology of the component bacteria, both filamentous and floc-formers, so that the various *ad hoc* control measures can be optimised.

Another microbially induced problem which affects activated sludge plants is the formation of stable foams (Fig. 6.12). These are caused by *Nocardia*, *Rhodococcus* and *Microthrix* spp. (Lemmer & Popp, 1982; Dhaliwal, 1979). The amount of foam on an aeration tank can vary from 2–3 cm to 50–60 cm and the foam itself is comprised of an almost pure culture of the organism involved at a concentration of 5–6 g (dry solids) per 100 g of foam. The foam appears to have little effect on the performance of the aeration tank (other than a visual one) but it does seriously affect the operation of the final settlement tanks and sludge sumps. The conditions which initiate foaming are not known and

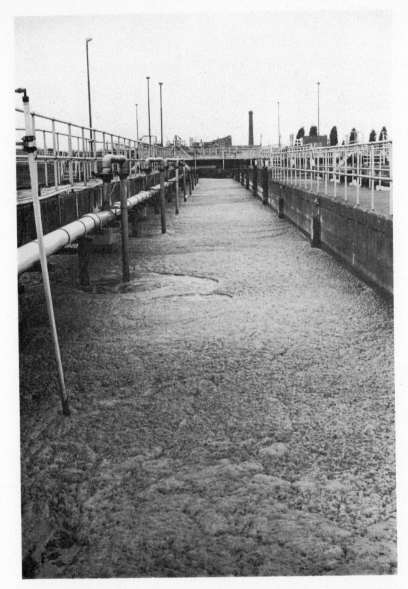

Fig. 6.12. Stable foam on an aeration tank.

existing control measures (high-pressure sprays; hypochlorite or physical removal) are only short-lived in their effectiveness and are time-consuming and costly.

The amount of sludge produced by an activated sludge plant is as important as the settleability of the sludge. However, the precise value

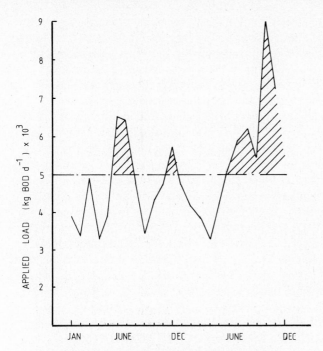

Fig. 6.13. Overloading of an activated sludge plant.

of the amount of secondary sludge produced (the yield factor) is often obscured by the fact that excess activated sludge is usually pumped to the primary tanks to be co-settled (and eventually wasted) with the primary solids. Published data for the quantity of sludge produced at activated sludge sites range from 0.6 to 1.3 kg dry solids kg BOD removed[-1]. This is a range which is comparable with that derived theoretically by Johnstone *et al.* (1983) for oxidation ditches whose feed-stock contained inert solids. The reason for there being such a wide range is that (a) the degree to which 'endogenous' respiration will reduce the amount of solids formed varies from plant to plant (with the retention time) and (b) the amount of inert material entering both the primary and secondary tanks varies from works to works.

As with any sewage treatment plant, it is not uncommon for the organic load being applied to the aeration tanks to exceed the design capacity of the system – meaning the aerators. This tends to happen gradually as the population expands, as new sewerage systems are introduced or as the *per capita* load increases with increased affluence. Initially, although noticeable, the overload can be handled. However, eventually the magnitude of the excess becomes intolerable (Fig. 6.13). When this happens the plant must be uprated. This is something which takes time; major civil engineering work cannot be done overnight.

There is therefore a need for short-term remedial measures. One of the most effective, both in terms of performance and cost, is to increase the aeration capacity with liquid oxygen using the Vitox technology (see Chapter 4). The achievements of the Vitox method in uprating a 33 Ml d^{-1} plant have been described in detail elsewhere (Robinson, Varley & Kimber, 1982). This report showed that the plant modifications based on Vitox (which included the uprating of some of the surface aerators), purely for carbonaceous oxidation, reduced the BOD from an average of 168 to one of 14 mg l^{-1}. The effective additional oxygenation capacity was 7.7 tonnes d^{-1}. The capital cost of the modification was £188000 (1980, Q3). The cost of a conventional system having a similar oxygenation capacity was estimated as £1.25 million (Toms & Booth, 1982). A second part of the works was uprated with Vitox to provide nitrification for a portion (10.5 Ml d^{-1}) of the flow. This used oxygen at the rate of 4 tonnes d^{-1} and produced an effluent with an average BOD of 21 mg l^{-1} and an ammoniacal nitrogen concentration of 7.3 mg l^{-1} (feed BOD/Amm. N = 168/43) (Robinson *et al.*, 1982). It is from these data that the versatility of Vitox can be judged.

The uprating of an activated sludge system has also been described by Guarino *et al.* (1980). These workers used air-driven rotary biological contactors which were installed in existing aeration tanks. In this way, additional biomass was provided without the need for the provision of a comparable oxygenation capacity and, because this biomass is 'fixed', additional clarifiers were not required. Uprating could therefore be achieved without major civil engineering work being necessary. The report by Guarino and his co-workers covers the early development of the uprating and the testing of various modes of operation and, although the data that are presented indicate the potential of this approach, the performance of the final fully modified system operating under full load conditions must be awaited before a final judgement can be passed.

The final point that needs to be mentioned is the energy required to operate an activated sludge unit. This really means the energy for aeration. This has already been discussed in Chapter 4. However, it is worth reiterating the findings of the joint WRC/EPA survey (Houk & Boon, 1981) that a significant number of diffused air plants have aeration units whose efficiencies are less than optimal. Similar results are currently being found for surface aeration systems.

6.6   Rotary biological contactors

The performance of RBC systems depends (like most other bio-oxidation processes) on the temperature, the strength of the

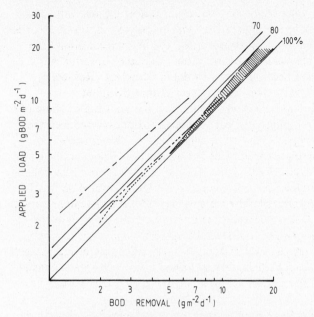

Fig. 6.14. Relationship between the applied BOD load and the removal rate for RBCs. —·—·— Cheung & Mack 1982; ———·——— Poon *et al.*, 1981; ------ and ------------ Pike *et al.*, 1982.

feed-stock, and the rate at which the treatment is expected to proceed; i.e. the loading rate or reaction time (see Lehman, 1983). Cheung & Mack (1982) have shown that, in terms of BOD removal, there is a critical hydraulic retention time of 3 hours and that any further increase in the retention results in little or no improvement in performances. The same workers have also shown that as the applied organic loading rate (expressed in terms of g BOD m^{-2} d^{-1}) increases above about 5, the deviation from 100 per cent efficiency becomes more pronounced. The performance characteristics of RBCs are frequently expressed as applied loading/removal rate curves. However, in some cases (e.g. Cheung & Mack, 1982; Poon *et al.*, 1981) linear relationships are used, whilst in others (Pike, 1978) a geometric one is reported. Fig. 6.14 shows the geometric relationships used by Pike for 70, 80 and 100 per cent efficiencies. Superimposed upon these are data from other performance studies. These show that the usual performance efficiency is better than 80 per cent. It was also found that the data, from what is probably the best reported field study in the UK (Pike *et al.*, 1982), are just more appropriate to a geometric relationship (coefficient of determination, R^2, = 0.997) than to a linear one ($R^2 = 0.995$).

Whilst performance efficiencies are important, it is also necessary to know the performance in terms of the BOD of the final effluent. Most

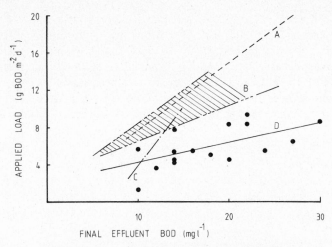

Fig. 6.15. Relationship between applied load and the effluent BOD produced by RBC reactors. A: Steels, 1974; B: Cheung & Mack, 1982; C: Poon *et al.*, 1981; D: Pike *et al.*, 1982.

of the recent studies have been carried out in America and report only soluble (i.e. filtered) BOD values. Fig. 6.15 shows the data obtained from an examination of a 50 population-equivalent plant (Pike *et al.*, 1982). Performance relationships reported by other workers are also shown on this figure and demonstrate that there is a significant difference between the UK data and that of RBCs operated elsewhere. On the basis of the results obtained in the UK, the disc loading compatible with the production of a 20:30 effluent is 6 g m^{-2} d^{-1} (see Bruce & Merkens, 1975 and Fig. 6.15). Most other data indicate that higher loading rates could be used. Indeed, Poon and his co-workers recommend that a loading rate of 7.8 g BOD (soluble) m^{-2} d^{-1} is the maximum that is compatible with an effluent standard of 30 mg BOD (total) l^{-1}.

The oxidation of ammonia is also an important feature in assessing the performance of any biological reactor. The degree of nitrification that is achieved by RBCs would appear to be dependent on several factors. Antonie (1978) has shown that the removal of ammoniacal nitrogen is related to the hydraulic loading rate, whilst Cheung & Mack (1982) have reported that full nitrification can only be achieved when the organic loading rate is less than 5 g BOD m^{-2} d^{-1}. The work reported by Hitdlebaugh & Miller (1981) highlighted two aspects of nitrification by RBCs, showing that the process was oxygen limited in summer months (raw sewage temperature = 26 °C) and that a good BOD removal was necessary prior to nitrification. Failure to achieve this meant that the amount of disc surface available for colonisation by the nitrifying species was significantly restricted. This is confirmation of the data produced by Hao & Hendricks (1975) who showed that at hydraulic loading rates of greater than 0.06 $m^3 m^{-2} d^{-1}$ low ammoniacal nitrogen removal was associated with poor reductions in BOD. The role of temperature on the nitrification process has also been noted by Pike *et al.* (1982) who showed that the specific removal rate (y, g Amm. N removed $m^{-2} d^{-1}$) was related to the temperature of the feed (T) such that:

$$y = 1.165^{(T-15)} \times 0.812.$$

Although these facts do not enable a precise assessment, or prediction, of performance to be made, they do quantify individually the factors which common sense suggests ought to control nitrification.

De-nitrification can also be achieved with disc systems (e.g. Cheung & Krauth, 1980). However, for the vast majority of cases where RBCs are used in the UK, this facility is not required.

6.7 The Deep Shaft process

The Deep Shaft process has been the subject of many reports (e.g. Hemming *et al.*, 1977; Bignal, 1982). However, in assessing the performance of this process only the results of two independent evaluations will be used. Both of these were made by Regional Water Authorities in the UK. The first of these had a quite specific objective for the process: to treat a sewage with a maximum flow of 277 $m^3 h^{-1}$ and an average BOD of 1060 mg l^{-1} such that the BOD of the final effluent did not exceed 60 mg l^{-1}. The shaft, which had a diameter of

Table 6.15. *Performance data for the Deep Shaft process*

Study period	Determinand	Concentration (mg l^{-1})		
		Max.	Min.	Mean
1980	Influent BOD	1350	400	909
	Effluent BOD	192	45	106
	Effluent BOD (filtered)	110	8	40
	Influent SS	1416	340	763
	Effluent SS	208	72	149
1982	Influent BOD	1643	872	1118
	Effluent BOD	101	25	56
	Influent SS	1020	364	641
	Effluent SS	230	37	104

From Collins & Elder, 1980, 1982.

Table 6.16. *Performance data for the Deep Shaft process*

Determinand	Concentration (mg l⁻¹)	
	Range	Mean
Influent BOD	120–775	423
Effluent BOD	19–63	34
Effluent BOD		
(filtered)	3–16	7
Influent SS	172–1330	690
Effluent SS	29–120	64

From Cox *et al.*, 1980.

1.86 m, is 130 m deep. After passing through the shaft, the mixed liquor is de-gassed with a vacuum of 0.3 bar and finally the solids are separated in a clarifier having a hydraulic retention time of 4.1 hours at maximum flow. Two sets of data are available from which the performance can be judged. One is daily data covering a fourteen day period (Collins & Elder, 1980), the other is presented in the form of weekly averages for a 6-week study period (Collins & Elder, 1982). A *précis* of these data is presented in Table 6.15 and shows that despite being able to remove a large proportion of the influent BOD (which is atypically high due to discharges of trade wastes), the overall performance is marred by the concentrations of suspended matter in the final effluent. Since the settlement properties of the sludge in the SVI test were good ($\leqslant 70$ on the basis of the 1980 report), it was assumed that an inadequate disengagement of gas in the form of micro-bubbles was occurring.

The second study (Cox *et al.*, 1980) was made with a smaller shaft, 0.126 m diameter × 61 m. The average flow-rate of the screened and de-gritted sewage was 1 m³ h⁻¹ and the BOD load applied to the shaft over the three-month trial period averaged 10.2 kg d⁻¹. Two methods were used to achieve gas disengagement: a vacuum tower (0.2 bar) and a bubble stripping tank. The results (Table 6.16) are not dissimilar to those reported by Collins & Elder in that whilst a good removal of BOD can be achieved by the shaft, the concentration of suspended solids in the effluent is higher than would have been anticipated on the basis of batch settlement tests (SSVI at 3.5 g l⁻¹ = 31–46). The only explanation offered for this was that, as the overall system was in fact of a pilot-scale size, wall effects and short-circuiting within the clarifier were to blame rather than incomplete de-gassing.

Taking both sets of data into consideration the Deep Shaft process still seems to be something of a mystery. It is capable of removing BOD with very short contact periods (less than 2 hours) and has the very obvious advantage of being compact in terms of land usage. The production of excess sludge is low. Collins & Elder quote 0.6 kg kg BOD removed^{-1} and Cox *et al.* give a figure of 0.85. These compare very favourably with the sludge production figures for oxidation ditches, probably the most efficient of the conventional systems, which can range from 0.3 to 1.2 kg kg BOD removed^{-1} (Johnstone, Rachwal & Hanbury, 1983). However, it has not been possible to relate performance to any of the more usual criteria such as the food:mass ratio, the sludge age or the hydraulic retention time (Collins & Elder, 1982). In addition, the process would appear to have a problem with solids in the final effluent. However, this should not be a problem with the second generation Deep Shaft system which operates in conjunction with a plug-flow aeration tank (Anon., 1983; see also Chapter 3). Despite the reservations that have been expressed about the level of solids in the final effluent, over 20 Deep Shafts are currently in operation throughout the world (mainly in Japan and Canada).

6.8 Oxygen activated sludge systems

The use of pure oxygen (or oxygen enriched air) in conjunction with the activated sludge process is now a well documented concept. However, the use of oxygen activated sludge plants (OASPs) in Europe and the UK is somewhat limited (see Steen & Johnson, 1978). Although there are several variations on the OASP theme (Anon., 1975; also Chapter 3), the one most widely used is that with a covered aeration tank and surface aerators. In the UK this means the UNOX system; however, while much of this discussion on the performance of OASPs will be based on data from UNOX systems, data from other types of process will also be included.

Performance must be judged both in terms of the operational criteria (e.g. removal of pollutants; production and handling characteristics of the sludge) and the economics of the process (energy usage and plant size). Data for the removal of BOD (Fig. 6.16) show that, as with any bio-oxidation process, the efficiency of BOD removal depends on the applied loading rate. However, the relationship between the removal efficiency and loading rate would appear to be quite a wide band. The data that have been included originate from a full-scale plant (Blachford *et al.*, 1982), which was designed to treat a dry weather flow of 4500 m^3 d^{-1}, and a series of pilot-plants (Banks, 1976; Hegemann & Bischofsberger, 1976). The pilot-plant data reported by Wood *et al.* (1976) are also included although the relationship from this evaluation

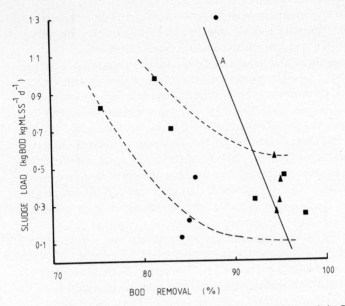

Fig. 6.16. Relationship between the sludge loading rate and the BOD removal achieved by OASPs. A Wood *et al.*, 1976; ■ Blachford *et al.*, 1982; ● Banks, 1976; ▲ Hegemann & Bischofsberger, 1976.

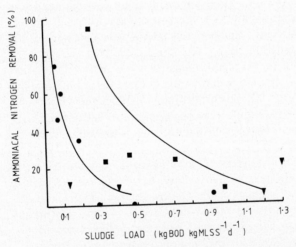

Fig. 6.17. Relationship between the sludge loading rate and the removal of ammoniacal nitrogen by OASPs. ■ Blachford *et al.*, 1982; ▼ Banks, 1976; ● Wood *et al.*, 1976.

was significantly different from the trend which developed from the other results. Figure 6.16 shows that although no formal relationship can be derived to describe the performance of OASPs, they are obviously capable of affording a high standard of treatment, although the loading rates which have been used and which give the higher efficiencies ($\geqslant$ 90 per cent) are not always significantly higher than those used in conventional activated sludge plants (see Table 3.8).

The oxidation of ammoniacal nitrogen (Fig. 6.17) also follows a trend rather than a formal relationship, although it has been suggested that Monod kinetics might be used to predict the rate of nitrification (Wood *et al.*, 1976). On the basis of the data shown in Fig. 6.17, it must be concluded that an OASP, operated on its own, and at the higher sludge loading rates for which it is really best suited, is unlikely to produce a fully nitrified effluent. Indeed the UNOX plant at Palmersford, which was the first full-scale OASP to be built in the UK, was designed as a two-stage system with the UNOX reactor being used to oxidise carbonaceous BOD and the second air-aerated tank being used for nitrification. There would appear to be two related reasons for the relatively poor performance of a covered oxygenic tank, as far as nitrification is concerned. Firstly, the fact that the tank is covered means that the carbon dioxide evolved during the metabolism of the BOD is not stripped from solution by the action of the aerators. This tends to lower the pH of the mixed liquor. Secondly, the sludge age in OASPs is frequently insufficient to enable an adequate colony of nitrifying bacteria to be maintained. The relationship between the minimum sludge age (*SA*) compatible with nitrification and the pH (*P*) and temperature (*T*) was derived by Downing (1968):

$$[1/SA] = [0.18 - 0.15\,(7.2 - P)]\exp[0.12\,(T - 15)]$$

Taking the data from the Palmersford plant (Blachford *et al.*, 1982) and the pilot-plant evaluated by Thames Water Authority (Wood *et al.*, 1976), it is possible to compare the sludge age required for nitrification with that actually being used (Table 6.17). This shows both the degree to which the pH is depressed and the difference between the two sludge ages. The actual sludge age within an activated sludge plant is related to the applied load. However, for the OASP it would appear, both from the work on the Palmersford plant (Blachford *et al.*, 1982) and the data reported by Stamberg, Bishop & Kumke (1972), that to achieve the type of sludge age required for nitrification (i.e. > 10 days) the applied loading rate would need to be of the order of 0.3 kg BOD kg MLSS^{-1} d^{-1} (as indicated by Fig. 6.17). Alternatively, the carbon dioxide effect can be overcome by control of the mixed liquor pH. This has been shown to be effective, on pilot-scale plant, using a control pH value of 7.5 (Wyatt, Brown & Shabi, 1977). The addition of sodium hydroxide to

Table 6.17. *A comparison of sludge age and nitrification in the OASP*

Source	Temperature (°C)	pH	Sludge age (d) Actual	Required	Nitrification (%)
Blachford *et al.*,	16	6.4	2.8	14.8	26.5
1982	12	7.2	1.3	8.0	8
	18	6.4	9.8	11.6	94.6
	10	7.0	1.4	12.2	21.1
Wood *et al.*, 1976	11.3	6.5	16.4	20.8	60
	14.4	6.3	5	23.9	35
	17.3	6.3	1.3	16.9	NIL
	20.2	6.2	1.4	17.9	5

this control value increased the nitrification efficiency from 24 to 72 per cent.

Although these discussions about BOD removal and nitrification might appear to suggest that the OASP offers no distinct advantage over air-aeration, on the basis of the applied load, it must be remembered that the rate of oxygen transfer in an OASP is such that a higher concentration of biomass can be maintained. Thus, for any particular loading, the OASP will be a more compact reactor.

An essential feature in maintaining high concentrations of biomass in the UNOX reactor (aeration tank) is good sludge settlement. It has always been claimed by manufacturers that oxygenated sludge has better settling properties than aerated sludge and certainly there are data to support this claim (Nash *et al.*, 1977; Hegemann & Bischofsberger, 1976). However, this is not universally true. For example, the work reported by Blachford *et al.* (1982) shows that oxygenation and aeration can produce very comparable settling behaviour. Their data also show that an OASP can produce quite a badly bulked sludge (maximum SSVI = 619). The pilot-plant study made by Wood *et al.* (1976) also showed that the settlement of OASP sludge was not as good as previously reported and in fact was very similar to the conventionally aerated plug-flow plant which was being operated in parallel with it. The debate about settlement and the use of oxygen is a long standing one. Indeed little has changed since the arguments were reviewed in 1976 by Parker & Merrill. This is a valuable critique of the situation, as it existed in the mid-1970s, with the authors making the point that in many cases comparison had been made between adequate OASPs and inadequate conventional plant. This point seems to have been either forgotten or neglected. It does seem essential to determine not only whether OASPs do promote

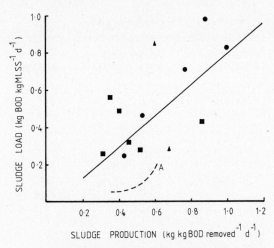

Fig. 6.18. Relationship between the sludge loading rate and the sludge production of OASPs. ■ Hegemann & Bischofsberger, 1976; ▲ Boon, 1976; ● Blachford *et al.*, 1982; A Johnstone *et al.*, 1983.

superior settlement but also, if they do, why they do so. However, any investigation of this type must bear Parker & Merrill's caveat in mind.

The amount of surplus sludge produced by any biological process is always a significant aspect of performance because of disposal costs. Data from OASPs (Fig. 6.18) show that the amount of sludge produced, expressed as kg dry sludge solids (kg Δ BOD)$^{-1}$ d^{-1}, depends on the applied loading rate. Similar relationships have been reported elsewhere (Steen & Johnson, 1978; Blachford *et al.*, 1982). These workers also compared the sludge production by oxygenic and air-aerated systems and showed that OASPs produce significantly less sludge. Fig. 6.18 also includes the theoretical relationship derived by Johnstone *et al.* (1983) for oxidation ditches, having no inert solids in the influent (almost analagous to settled sewage), operating at a temperature of 10 °C. This also shows that a conventionally aerated system (albeit a specialised case) would, in theory, produce more sludge than an oxygenic process (about 100 per cent within the range considered).

Despite the number of OASP installations throughout the world (> 200, mainly in North America and Japan), published data for energy usage is remarkably sparse. In addition, the data that are available (Table 6.18) show wide variations. Both at the New York plant (Nash *et al.*, 1977) and the Palmersford works (Blachford *et al.*, 1982) these variations were due to a lack of 'turn-down' facility with the oxygen generation equipment; 'turn-down' being the ability to

Table 6.18. *Energy usage by oxygen activated sludge plants*

Source	Design DWF (m^3 d^{-1})	Energy usage (kWh kg BOD removed^{-1})
Nelson, 1979	273000	1.42
Nash et al., 1977	76000	0.79–2.96
Blachford et al., 1982	4500	1.8–4.1

Table 6.19. *Estimated energy usage by oxygen activated sludge plants*

Source	Oxygen usage (kg oxygen kg BOD removed^{-1})	Estimated energy usage (kWh kg BOD removed^{-1})
Banks, 1976	1.1–1.9	1.04–1.80
Hegemann & Bischofsberger, 1976	0.8–1.1	0.76–1.04
Kashiwaya & Yoshimoto, 1980	1.04–1.34	0.98–1.27
Guarino et al., 1974	1.54[a]	1.46

[a] Value predicted for design load.

reduce the energy consumption of the PSA units (see Chapter 3) when less oxygen is required by the mixed liquor. The inability to reduce energy consumption in this way means that the figures reported are not only variable but are also unrealistically high on occasions. Boon (1976) has reported that, based on UK data, the energy requirements for the generation of oxygen are about 0.35 kWh kg oxygen^{-1} for cryogenic production and 0.35–0.60 for a PSA plant, whilst for the dissolution of oxygen (at DO = 0.0 mg l^{-1}) about 0.30 kWh kg^{-1} are needed. Thus, for the worst conditions, the total energy usage would be 0.9 kWh kg^{-1} and this figure would need to be increased by 5 per cent if a high (5 mg l^{-1}) dissolved oxygen concentration were being used. It is therefore possible to make an estimate of the energy usage from the oxygen utilisation data (Table 6.19). Considering both sets of data (i.e. Tables 6.18 and 6.19) the average energy usage is 1.46 kWh kg BOD removed^{-1}. In the absence of more precise data (i.e. performance figures from an OASP treating its design load and having full 'turn-down' facility) it is therefore suggested that this figure should be taken as typical of the energy usage of OASPs. If this is in fact correct, it is a value which compares quite favourably with that reported (1.3 kWh kg^{-1}) for an oxidation ditch operating at its design load (Rachwal et al., 1983).

It can be seen therefore that the use of oxygen in conjunction with

activated sludge does create a process of considerable value. Certainly it
is more complicated to operate and strict safety precautions (including
automatic monitoring and alarms) are essential. However, it does offer
the facility of a compact, high-rate treatment both for domestic and
industrial wastes. The only real problem with its performance is the
oxidation of ammonia, but there are many applications where full
nitrification is not required.

6.9   Tertiary treatment

Although the processes used for tertiary treatment cannot really be
thought of as being of a biotechnological nature, they are a part of
wastewater treatment. As such, therefore, a brief description of the
more important processes is included, whilst for greater details readers
are referred to a more specialised text (IWPC, 1974).

Tertiary treatment is a further treatment of effluent from the
biological stage to remove suspended matter (and thereby, BOD) so as
to comply with a standard more stringent than 30:20. It should not be
thought of as a means of upgrading a substandard works. Because of
the cost involved, consideration should be given to the avoidance of
tertiary treatment by means of augmentation of low river flows, direct
oxygenation of the river, when required, or adoption of a process such
as extended aeration which normally produces a better effluent than
30:20.

6.9.1   *Methods of tertiary treatment*

(a) *Lagooning* to give further settlement. Detention period should be
less than 50 hours and the depth about 1 m to restrict growth of algae
in summer. Baffling, scum boards, and a series of compartments should
be used to prevent short circuiting and escape of rising sludge. A
further advantage is the buffering effect of lagoons. For an inflow
having a quality of 30:20, loading should be at 3500–5000 m^3 ha^{-1} d^{-1};
for a feed-stock of worse quality, this should be reduced to about
1500 m^3 ha^{-1} d^{-1}.

(b) *Grass plot irrigation* may be by means of channels or spray guns.
Loadings of 2000 m^3 ha^{-1} d^{-1} should be suitable for average conditions
(this is on the total area, including plots resting), but could be doubled
or halved according to circumstances, e.g. soil structure and rainfall.
The plots may be underdrained and should slope at 1 in 60 to 1 in 100
towards the collection channels. At least two plots should be provided
for intermittent use.

(c) *Microstraining or microscreening* is only appropriate when the
secondary effluent is within the 30:20 standard. Maximum loading of
the fabric varies from 300–700 m^3 m^{-2} d^{-1} depending on the grading of

Table 6.20. *Performance of tertiary treatment units*

Method	Percentage removal			
	Suspended solids	BOD	Coliform bacteria	Approximate cost (£ per 1000 m³)
Grass plots	70	50	90	0.38
Shallow lagoons (detention 3–4 days)	40	40	70	0.29
Deep lagoons (detention 17 days)	80	65	99	0.54
Slow sand filters	60	40	50	1.92
Rapid gravity sand filters	80	60	30	0.67
Upward-flow sand filters	70	55	25	0.46
Microstrainers	70	40	15	0.75
Upward-flow gravel bed clarifier	50	30	25	0.63

the fabric (90–390 apertures per mm²). As a general guide, mesh apertures having a diameter of around 23 μm would give an effluent quality of about 10:10; those of a larger size, say 35 μm, would produce a 15:15 effluent. Continuous backwashing with 2–5 per cent of the filtrate is necessary. At least two units should be installed to facilitate maintenance.

(d) *Slow sand filters*, loaded at 3.5 m³ m⁻² d⁻¹ are expensive in capital and operating costs, normally making them uneconomic.

(e) *Rapid downward flow filters*, loaded at 250 m³ m⁻² d⁻¹ at maximum flow are preferably provided with automatic backwashing (2–3 per cent of total throughput at a rate of 10 l m⁻² s⁻¹). The wash water contains sand and must be returned to the works inlet upstream of grit extraction. The sand used has 0.8 to 1.7 mm diameter; the bed is up to 1.5 m deep.

(f) *Upward flow sand filters* are very suitable for larger applications, loading up to 400 m³ m⁻² d⁻¹ being usable. Washing of the filter is carried out by increasing the flow to 900 m³ m⁻² d⁻¹ and this wash water must be diverted to the works inlet during washing and for a few minutes afterwards.

(g) *Upward flow clarifiers* using pea gravel or wedge wire may be used at loading rates (3 × DWF) up to 42 m³ m⁻² d⁻¹ for biological filter effluent or 30 m³ m⁻² d⁻¹ for activated sludge effluent. Backwashing is carried out by lowering the water level below the bed, with hosing down if required. At least two units are therefore required. The surface of the medium should be at least 150 mm below TWL and preferably 300 mm below.

(h) *Tilted plate clarifiers* of proprietary types can be used for small installations. Temperature differences are critical and operating costs high.

A general comparison of the performances of the various processes is given in Table 6.20.

7 The handling and disposal of sewage sludge

7.1 Introduction

While the treatment of domestic and industrial wastewater removes, either totally or in part, one problem of environmental pollution, it also creates another – sludge. The treatment and disposal of this solid waste is such a problem that it has been suggested that the design of effluent treatment works should be centred around the sludge disposal part of the works (Gale, 1972). In the past, estimates of the magnitude of the sludge disposal problem have varied quite appeciably, but the Jeger Report (Ministry of Housing and Local Government, 1970) gives a figure of 1.1 million tonnes (dry solids) as the figure for sludge production in England and Wales; this is in good agreement with the figure of 1.24 million tonnes for the UK given in a survey by the Department of the Environment (1978). Not only does this latter report show how sludge is disposed of in the four countries (Table 7.1), it also shows how the 0.93 million tonnes (75 per cent) which does go to land is distributed (Table 7.2). Essentially this shows that in England and Scotland, disposal to arable land and tips is the more favoured method, that in Northern Ireland tipping predominates and that in Wales the majority of sludge goes to grazing and arable land.

In most discussions on sludge disposal the material is too often discussed under the general description of 'sewage sludge' and yet, as has been pointed out by Wood (1975), there is no such material; rather

Table 7.1. *Disposal of sludge (dry solids) in 1975 in the UK*

		England	Wales	Scotland	N. Ireland
Sludge to land	⎫	0.853	0.028	0.041	0.009
Sludge to sea	⎪	0.186	0.009	0.058	0.003
Sludge incinerated	⎬ (million tonnes)	0.027	—	0.001	—
Total sludge production	⎭	1.066	0.037	0.100	0.012
Population covered by survey (million)		40.94	1.36	2.76	0.46

194

Table 7.2. *Weights (million tonnes of dry solids) disposed of to various types of land in* 1975

		England	Wales	Scotland	N. Ireland
Grazing	Undigested	0.0513	0.0070	0.0004	0.0007
	Digested	0.1281	0.0040	0.0053	0.0021
Arable	Undigested	0.1708	0.0045	0.0102	—
	Digested	0.1196	0.0062	0.0065	0.0025
Horticultural	Undigested	< 0.0085	0.0002	0.0008	—
	Digested	0.0171	—	—	—
Forestry	Undigested	—	< 0.0002	—	—
	Digested	Negligible	—	—	—
Land reclamation	Undigested	0.0256	< 0.0002	0.0033	—
	Digested	0.0342	—	—	—
Land tip	Undigested	0.1879	0.0054	0.0110	0.0028
	Digested	0.1025	< 0.0002	0.0033	0.0013
Allotments	Undigested	—	—	< 0.0004	—
	Digested	0.0085	—	< 0.0004	—

there is a wide variety of sludges arising from sewage treatment. These variations result from the different origins of the sludge (i.e. primary, activated, humus or mixtures), the different types of conditioning process (i.e. digestion, chemical addition), the different techniques used for de-watering (i.e. filtration, air drying) and the various methods of storage. When all the combinations are considered it can be seen that an almost infinite number of gradations is possible. The difference this makes on the composition of the sludge can be seen from Table 7.3. As well as these chemical differences the various types of sludge will be different microbially. In particular, it is the pathogen content which is of concern when sludge disposal is being considered (see §7.5).

The processes which are available for the treatment and disposal of sludge are shown in Fig. 7.1. In selecting a sequence of processes for a treatment works, be it a new site or a major extension, consideration must be given to the amounts of sludge being generated (see Chapter 6), the disposal routes available for the final product and the costs. Not all the options given in Fig. 7.1 will be discussed in detail. However, adequate references to additional reading will be provided for those which are not.

Table 7.3. *Nutrient composition of different sludges*

Type	Source	Treatment	Analysis (dry weight basis)		
			Nitrogen	Phosphorus	Potassium
			as % N	as % P_2O_5	as % K_2O
Primary + humus	Domestic + food industry	Al-chlorohydrate/press	3.4	3.1	0.12
Primary + activated	Mainly domestic	Heated digestion	6.2	4.2	0.58
Primary + humus	Domestic	Drying beds	2.2	0.9	0.08
Primary + activated	Domestic	Drying beds	1.1	0.4	0.06
Primary + activated	Domestic + industrial	Lime-copperas/press	2.7	2.9	0.02
Primary + humus	Domestic + food industry	Polymer/press	2.1	0.4	1.10
Primary + humus	Mainly domestic	Cold digestion/belt press	2.7	2.3	0.24

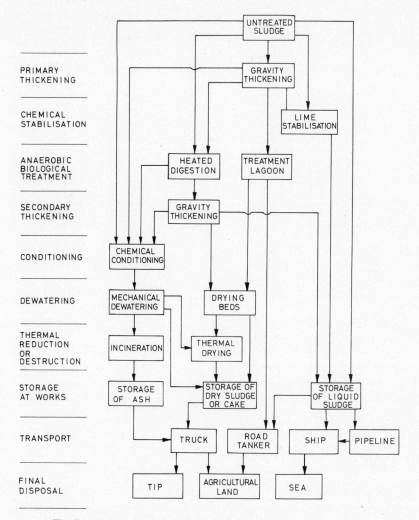

Fig. 7.1. Options for the handling of sewage sludge.

7.2 **Thickening**

7.2.1 *Simple gravity thickening*

Sludge, as it is wasted, is not very concentrated. One of the initial processes must therefore be one which reduces the volume of liquid being handled. Gravity thickening can achieve this objective simply and effectively. The basic requirements of the process are a tank or tanks where the sludge can be held for sufficient time (perhaps several days) to allow gravity to effect a separation of solids from some of the water. If the process is being operated in a continuous manner it is usual to

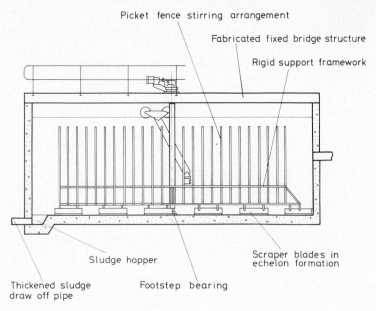

Picket fence stirring arrangement

Fabricated fixed bridge structure

Rigid support framework

Sludge hopper

Scraper blades in echelon formation

Thickened sludge draw off pipe

Footstep bearing

Fig. 7.2. Typical picket fence thickener.

have circular tanks with rotating 'picket fence thickener' (Fig. 7.2). The picket fence consists of a series of vertical rods with spacings of about 100 mm and the rotational speed is such that peripheral velocities of between 0.5 and 3.0 m min^{-1} can be obtained. The use of a picket fence:

(a) releases gas bubbles
(b) prevents bridging by the solids
(c) forms void channels which aid water release.

Thickeners of this type can also be operated as batch processes. The performance of gravity thickeners (whether they be operated on a batch or a continuous basis) will depend very much on the type of sludge being handled; the best performance is achieved with sludges which are affected by ageing.

The theoretical aspects of thickening and the mechanisms whereby the process occurs have been reviewed in detail by Lockyear (1977). The basic conclusion of this and earlier reviews is that the compressed force of the particles in the sludge blanket (in the upper region of the tank) causes thickening by squeezing water out of the sludge at the bottom of the tank. The design of thickeners is somewhat arbitrary and can involve the under-flow concentration, the depth of sludge blanket and the solids loading rate, with batch thickening tests being used to provide the design basis (see Lockyear, 1978). Recent work has also shown how the thickenability of sludges can be predicted by simulating the compressive forces of the sludge blanket in a low-speed centrifuge (Lockyear & White, 1979). Nevertheless, there would appear to be considerable scope for the development of an optimised design procedure.

Lagoons are a simple and widely used method for thickening and stabilising sludges. Indeed, one water authority in the UK thickens some 63 000 tonnes (dry solids) annually in this way. However, the criteria for the design and operation of lagoons are even more arbitrary than for thickening tanks. A possible danger with the use of lagoons is that they can become semi-permanent storage units and, since water can permeate into the underlying soil and the solids content be reduced by microbial action, their capacity for storage can be significant. The danger lies not in their use for storage but in the fact that a surface crust can develop a substantial growth of vegetation which hides the presence of the semi-liquid sludge. A lagoon of this type must therefore be securely fenced and adequate warning signs provided.

7.2.2   *Other methods of thickening*

Although gravity thickening is the most common method for achieving an initial reduction in the water content of sludges, other techniques are available and are used. These are flotation and centrifugation. The types of centrifuge that are available and their use both to thicken and to de-water sludge have been reviewed recently (Institute of Water Pollution Control, 1981), and an appraisal of the use of flotation is provided by Melbourne & Zabal (1977) and Maddock & Tomlinson (1980). With both flotation and centrifugation, it may be appropriate to condition the sludge (see §7.3.2) before treatment.

7.2.3   *Sludge rheology*

As the solids concentration of sludge increases, the rheological properties of the suspension become increasingly non-Newtonian. Sludges must therefore not be thickened to a concentration at which they cannot be pumped. For primary sludge this situation is reached at a solids concentration of about 12 per cent.

Although there is a general acceptance that sludge is non-Newtonian, an examination of past work shows a conflict of information, with sludge being described as a Bingham plastic, a pseudo-plastic and a Herschel–Bulkley fluid (see Forster, 1981). There is also disagreement in the literature as to whether or not sludges are thixotropic. In addition, there is little information about the way in which the properties of the sludge particles can influence the rheological characteristics. The role of the suspended solids concentration has been examined (Johnson, 1981). It has also been shown that the surface charge and the surface polymers responsible for the charge are involved (Forster, 1982). This idea is substantiated by the work reported by Rose-Innes & Nossel (1983). Their work also showed how rheological measurements made in the laboratory could be used to design pumping systems. Similar data are available in the reports by Johnson (1981) and Frost (1982).

7.3   De-watering

7.3.1   *Drying beds*

De-watering, as opposed to the removal of water during thickening, refers to processes which give a cake-like product in which the solids concentration is at least 15 per cent. Drying beds are perhaps the simplest method for de-watering sludges. They are constructed of sand (25 mm) laid on pea gravel (100 mm) which in turn is laid on drainage tiles. The floor should slope (not less than 1 in 60) towards the outlet chamber. Sludge is applied to a depth of 150–300 mm (Fig. 7.3) and de-watering occurs by drainage and to a certain extent by evaporation. The removal of the solid cake, which could have a solids concentration perhaps as high as 40 per cent, is done mechanically (at large works) or manually. The performance of drying beds depends on the type of sludge being applied, the loading rate that is used and the weather. However, it is not unreasonable to expect 3–5 applications a year although in the UK these may have to be confined to the 6–7 months of the year when drying conditions are good.

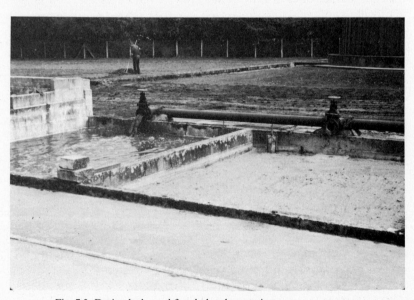

Fig. 7.3. Drying beds used for sludge de-watering.

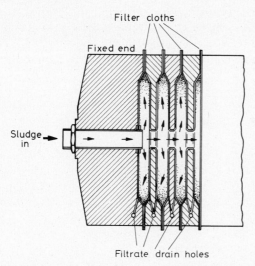

Fig. 7.4. Schematic diagram of a filter press.

7.3.2 *Filter presses*

Filter presses are probably the most widely used process (in the UK) for de-watering sludges. They consist of a series of plates, suspended from a side-bar or an overhead beam, which are recessed so that chambers are formed between them (Fig. 7.4). Filter cloths are fitted over the surface of each plate which are then closed against each other and held in position either by screws or hydraulically. The sludge is then pumped into the unit. The pumps that are used also provide the pressure which drives the filtration; the maximum pressure is of the order of 690 kPa. When the flow of filtrate stops, the pressure is released, the plates are separated and the cake removed. It is usual to locate presses on the first floor of a building so that the cake can be dropped directly into containers for removal. If necessary, the press components are washed (high pressure water jets) and the cycle is repeated. It has been reported that, using lime and copperas as the conditioner, the cloths required washing every 20 cycles, and that when an organic polyelectrolyte was used washing was required, on average, every 30 cycles (Pullin, 1981).

Filter pressing is a batch process which consists of three stages: pressure build-up, filtration at maximum pressure and cake release. The entire cycle can take between 3 and 14 hours depending on the type of sludge, the type of cloth and the type of pump. It has been said (Gale, 1975) that choosing the right cloth for a particular application is something of an art. However, at the same time, Gale did indicate some of the points that need to be considered. These include the solids

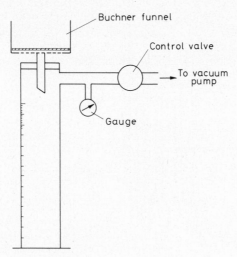

Fig. 7.5. Buchner funnel apparatus for the measurement of the specific resistance to filtration.

content of the filtrate, the susceptibility to 'blinding' (which occurs when small particles pack into the spaces between the fibres in the filter cloth and thus prevent the passage of water), and the readiness with which the cake is released. According to Gale, cloths with an open weave produce a filtrate with a higher solids concentration than cloths with a tight weave. However, open weave cloths are less susceptible to blinding. Also, for any particular weave, both the retention of solids and the tendency to blind increase with the type of yarn, the order being monofilament, multifilament, then staple fibres. The type of sludge and the way it has been conditioned will also govern which type of cloth is most suitable. For example, the work described by Pullin (1981) reports that although polypropylene cloths were suitable for a sludge conditioned with lime and copperas, undefined changes in that sludge, together with a change in the type of conditioner (an organic polymer), meant that a multi-filament cloth had to be used.

The rate of filtration is given by:

$$\frac{dv}{dt} = \frac{PA^2}{\mu(rVc + RA)}$$

At constant pressure, this can be written as;

$$\frac{t}{V} = \left[\frac{\mu rc}{2PA^2}\right]V + \frac{\mu R}{PA}$$

where V = volume of filtrate at time t, P = applied pressure, A = filter are, μ = filtrate viscosity, c = solids concentration, R = resistance of filter cloth, r = specific resistance of sludge. The derivation of this

Table 7.4. *Typical values for the specific resistance to filtration of various sludges*

Type of sludge	Specific resistance ($\times 10^{11}$ m kg^{-1})
Primary	1000–1500
Humus	500–3000
Activated	1000–4000
Digested	1000–2500
Primary/activated and lime/copperas	14

equation (Coackley, 1960) makes no allowance for any compressibility of the cake. In the laboratory, the simplest way of measuring the specific resistance of the sludge (i.e. its filterability) is to use a Buchner funnel, a graduated receiver for the filtrate and a vacuum which can be controlled at the standard test value of 49 kPa (Fig. 7.5). More sophisticated systems have been described (e.g. Department of the Environment, 1972; Wuhrmann, 1977) but it is debatable whether they achieve a more correct value and, if they do, whether it is necessary. Any of the methods require that the filtrate volume and time be recorded so that (t/V) can be plotted against V. The slope of the resultant line is given by $(\mu rc/2PA^2)$ and since values are known for all the other components, r can be calculated. Table 7.4 shows typical values of r for various types of sludge.

It is generally considered that a value for the specific resistance of greater than $10–50 \times 10^{11}$ m kg^{-1} is indicative of poor filterability. In practical terms, this means that the solids concentration in the final cake would be low or that long press times would be required. The filtration characteristics of a sludge can be improved by conditioning. This usually involves the addition of chemicals which increase the degree of flocculation of the sludge particles. The cake that is formed from conditioned particles tends therefore to have a more ready passage of water. Conditioning also reduces the possibility of blinding, mentioned above, in which the passage of water is prevented by small particles clogging the filter cloth. The chemicals that are used for conditioning include aluminium chlorohydrate; poly-aluminium chloride (PAC); copperas (ferrous sulphate); ferric chloride; lime; and organic polymers. Of these, ferric chloride is more commonly used in America than in the UK; PAC is still a relatively new compound and lime and copperas tend to be used together, the lime being added after the copperas. There is currently a very wide range of organic polymers available with a range of molecular weights, forms (i.e. powder or liquid) and ionic affinities (cationic, anionic and non-ionic). The critical

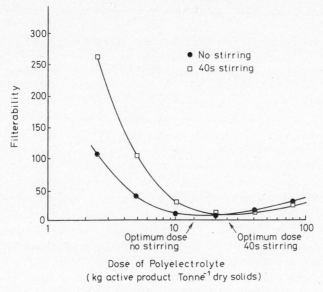

Fig. 7.6. Typical effect of polyelectrolyte dosage on sludge filterability.

features in the structure of these compounds are their molecular weight and their charge density. The significance and proper application of these properties are discussed in a recently published 'Users' Manual' (Lockyear, Jackson & Warden, 1983) which also provides a comprehensive listing of the polymers available in the UK together with details of testing equipment and procedures for dosing the sludge with the polymers. It must be remembered that most of the chemicals used for conditioning have properties that require care to be taken during their handling.

Whatever type of conditioner is used (i.e. inorganic and organic) it is essential that the correct dosage is used. As can be seen from Fig. 7.6, if too much chemical is added, the filtration characteristics can start to deteriorate, and even if this does not happen the addition of chemicals beyond the point of optimum effect is both wasteful and costly. The capillary suction time (CST) apparatus provides a simple and rapid method for determining the most appropriate dose (Baskerville & Gale, 1968). In its simplest form (Fig. 7.7) it consists of a rectangle of absorbent paper (Whatman No. 17; 90 × 70 mm) sandwiched between two pieces of Perspex. The upper piece contains a hole for the sludge reservoir and is also fitted with three stainless steel electrodes located in two concentric circles. These electrodes are connected to an amplifier and stop-clock. When sludge, which has been sheared under standard conditions, is added to the reservoir, filtration occurs as a result of the

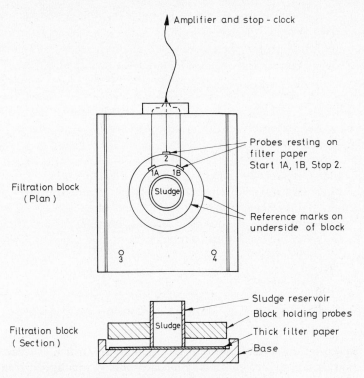

Amplifier and stop-clock

Filtration block
(Plan)

Probes resting on
filter paper
Start 1A, 1B, Stop 2.

Reference marks on
underside of block

Filtration block
(Section)

Sludge reservoir
Block holding probes
Thick filter paper
Base

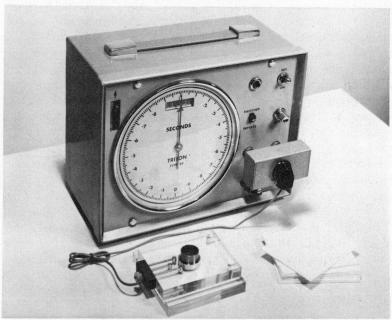

Fig. 7.7. Apparatus for the measurement of CST. *a* Schematic diagram of the
filtration unit; *b* the complete system.

capillary suction pressure of the paper and the filtrate diffuses outwards. The two electrodes located on the inner circle detect the filtrate front and start the clock. When the front reaches the third electrode the clock is stopped. The time recorded, the CST, is proportional to the specific resistance of the sludge, for a given solids concentration and filtrate viscosity. A more advanced system, the multi-radii CST (Baskerville & Lockyear, 1980), enables the capillary suction concept to be used to measure the specific resistance to filtration. However, the calculation requires the pressure at which the filtration was conducted (the capillary suction pressure) to be quantified. Baskerville & Lockyear assumed a value of 49 kPa and showed a very reasonable agreement between results from the CST method and the conventional Buchner funnel method.

The dosage of any conditioner is usually expressed as a percentage of the dry solids concentration. Although the dosage will vary with the type of sludge, typical values are:

> Raw sludge – lime (20%)+copperas (10%)
> Digested sludge – lime (30%)+copperas (40%)
>   – aluminium chlorohydrate (5–8%)
>   – polymers (1–8%)

The performance of filter presses is also quite variable. Indeed, it could be said that there is no single yardstick by which the performance of one plant can be judged against another. The pressing time, the dryness of the cake and amount of solids that can be handled are all measurements of performance. All of them however, depend on the type of sludge, the type and amount of conditioning and even the age of the sludge (Williamson & Wheale, 1981). Therefore, whilst it is possible (and sensible) to examine how sludge handling practices at any one plant affect the operational costs of filter pressing at that plant, attempts to compare performances of different plants (and different sludges) could be misleading. Table 7.5, which gives generalised data on filter performance, should be examined with this caveat in mind. It must also be remembered that the use of chemical conditioning agents increases the mass of solids which require disposal; for example, lime and copperas can account for 50 per cent of the solids in the final cake.

A recent development, the membrane press, is claimed to produce a cake with a higher solids content in a shorter time (Edmondson & Brooks, 1978; Pietila & Joubert, 1981). With this system every other plate can be inflated with air pressure (up to about 800 kPa). This is done during the press cycle before a firm cake is formed. The data presented by Pietila & Joubert show not only the benefit in terms of press times and cake yield but also that the amounts of conditioning chemicals can be reduced and that the various aspects of the process

Table 7.5. *Performance of filter presses with various sludges and conditioning agents*

Type of sludge	Conditioning agent	Solids concentration (%) Initial	Cake
Primary	Lime and copperas	4.0	35
Primary/humus	Lime and copperas	6.5	35–39
Digested	Aluminium chlorohydrate	4.6	30
Digested	Lime and copperas	4.6	37
Digested	'Zetag 57'	4.1	30
Primary/activated	Aluminium chlorohydrate	2.5	30
Primary	Aluminium chlorohydrate	5.0	34
Primary/humus	Aluminium chlorohydrate	7.0	40

can be modelled mathematically. The cost of installing membrane plates, however, is high and it is therefore desirable to assess the economic aspects very carefully before considering their installation (Bruce & Lockyear, 1982).

An alternative way of optimising the operational costs of filter pressing has been described by Hoyland, Day & Baskerville (1981). This work showed that, after the filling period, the pressing of conditioned sludges has two distinct stages: the first in which the filtration curve is parabolic, and the second in which it is exponential. In the former phase, the sludge cake is still growing and the rate of filtration is controlled only by the specific resistance. In the second phase, filtration takes place by cake compression with the rate being controlled both by the specific resistance and the ability of the cake to flow longitudinally within the press chamber. By developing the mathematics of filtration during the exponential phase, Hoyland *et al.* show that:

$$\frac{dV}{dt} \propto V_\infty - V$$

where V is the filtrate volume ($m^3 \ m^{-2}$). This means that, during the latter part of a normal pressing cycle, the rate of filtration is related linearly to the filtrate volume irrespective of the conditions being used or the sludge properties (Fig. 7.8). It is therefore possible to predict the point that has been reached in any filtration cycle by plotting (dV/dt) against V as pressing is proceeding and then determining V_∞ by extrapolation. By being able to predict the degree of completion (V/V_∞), sludge cakes can be produced which are neither too 'hard' nor too 'soft'. The accuracy of these predictions can be improved by the use of micro-processors which could also be used to control the automation of the pressing cycle.

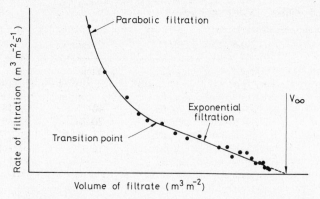

Fig. 7.8. Rate of filtration in a filter pressing. (From Hoyland, Day & Baskerville, 1981.)

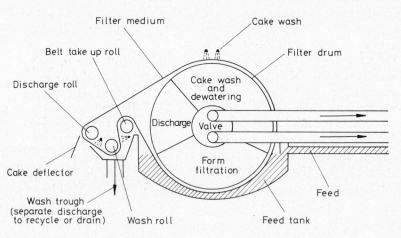

Fig. 7.9. Rotary vacuum filter.

7.3.3 *Vacuum filtration*

De-watering of sewage sludges may also be achieved by vacuum filtration. The most widely used system is the rotating-drum filter (Fig. 7.9). The drum consists of a series of cells or compartments which run the length of the drum and which can either be pressurised or placed under vacuum. The filtration medium can be a cloth, a wire screen or closely packed wire coils lying with their long axis in the direction of the rotation. The speed of rotation would typically be about 5 mm s^{-1} and the vacuum used would be between 40 and 90 kPa. Conditioned sludge would be fed into the filter reservoir so that as the drum passed through the reservoir, a mat of wet sludge became attached to the filtration medium as a result of the vacuum being applied to the

Table 7.6. *Performance of vacuum filters*

Type of sludge	Lime/ferric chloride		Polymer	
	Yield ($kg\ m^{-2}\ h^{-1}$)	Cake (% solids)	Yield ($kg\ m^{-2}\ h^{-1}$)	Cake (% solids)
Primary	20–60	25–38	40–50	25–38
Primary/humus	20–30	20–30	20–30	20–30
Primary/activated	21–31	14–19	15–20	11–13
Activated	12–17	10–15	10–15	10–15
Digested primary	20–40	25–32	35–40	25–32

submerged cells. Filtration continues, under this vacuum, as the drum rotates. Just before a complete revolution is completed, the vacuum is released so that the cake (3–10 mm in thickness) can be discharged. In some applications, pressure may be applied to the compartment at the discharge point to assist the cake removal.

The advantage of vacuum filtration is that it is a continuous process. However, as a general rule, the cake produced by vacuum filtration contains more moisture than that produced by pressing (see Table 7.6 compared with Table 7.5). A useful appraisal of the operation of vacuum filtration has been provided by Nelson & Tavery (1978). This includes a 'trouble-shooting' guide and an equipment inspection program. Although vacuum filters are used in the UK (see for example Sleeth, 1970; Nice, Pullen & Robinson, 1978), the majority (75 per cent) of the sludge that is de-watered is processed by filter pressing or belt (Bruce & Lockyear, 1982).

7.3.4 Belt presses

A belt press consists of two continuous belts (a porous filter belt and an impervious press belt) and a series of rollers (some to drive and guide the belts, some to provide compression and shear). The main variation in the design of belt presses lies in the configuration of the compression zone. In some cases, this follows a highly convoluted path (so as to remove extra water), in others the belts have a simple, horizontal drive (see Fig. 7.10).

Conditioned sludge is fed evenly across the width of the filter belt. Initially, filtrate drains from the sludge under gravity. As the belts pass between the rollers, pressure and shear is gradually applied to the sludge by the action of the rollers on the press belt and water is squeezed from the sludge. The amount of de-watering that occurs depends on the retention time (i.e. the belt speed) and the clearance between the two belts. Both of these can be adjusted to suit operational

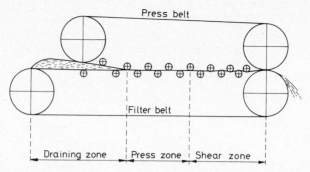

Fig. 7.10. Schematic diagram of a belt press.

Table 7.7. *Performance data for belt presses treating mixed primary and humus sludge*

Solids concentration (% DS)		Polymer dose	
Feed	Cake	(g kg⁻¹ DS)	Source
7.6	22.8	2.52	Moore, 1983
9.4	24.5	2.29	
6.1	21.8	3.15	
4.2	20.5	2.79	DOE, 1975
5.84	23.6	2.18	

conditions. Evaluations of the belt press (Department of the Environment, 1975; Moore, 1983) show that cakes with a solids concentration of around 25 per cent can be achieved (Table 7.7). In both these cases the feed was a mixture of primary and humus sludges which had been conditioned with organic polyelectrolytes (1.3–7.7 kg tonne⁻¹ dry solids).

7.3.5   *Other methods*

Methods other than those which have been described can be used for de-watering sludges. Centrifuges, for example, will produce a cake with a solids concentration of around 25 per cent (see Sidwick, Butler & Ruscombe-King, 1975) and the Rotoplug system (Berger & Warren, 1966) gives similar results (Symes & Michaelson, 1977). However, these alternative systems are not used widely in the UK. In other parts of the world they would appear to have a greater popularity (e.g. Egglink, 1975).

Table 7.8. *Typical values for the strength of the liquors produced by de-watering processes*

| | BOD | SS | Amm. N | |
Treatment		(mg l⁻¹)		Source
Filter press	2550	192	274	Nice *et al.*, 1978
Filter press	1750	350	184	Pullin, 1981
Vacuum filter	414	3000	355	Sleeth, 1970
Belt press	800	250–1500	—	Moore, 1983
Centrifuge	3000–4000	360–4000	—	Sidwick *et al.*, 1975
Rotoplug	3840	3700	—	Hamilton, 1969

7.3.6 Conclusions

Most types of sludge produced at a sewage treatment works can be de-watered to a greater or lesser degree. However, this will almost invariably require the use of conditioning agents which in turn will affect the treatment costs. Two points need to be emphasised. Firstly, the degree to which the sludge is de-watered may well affect the disposal of the sludge. For example, press cake cannot readily be disposed of to agricultural land. Secondly, de-watering produces a liquid fraction with a BOD which can at times be quite significant. These liquors must be returned to the works inlet for treatment and it is essential that an allowance is made for the organic load that they will produce. Typical BOD values for these liquors are shown in Table 7.8.

7.4 Digestion

The digestion of sewage sludges has two objectives: to stabilise the solids so that they do not become objectionable on storage or when applied to agricultural land, and to reduce the level of pathogens and parasites in the sludge.

7.4.1 Anaerobic digestion

About half the population in the UK is served by sewage treatment works using anaerobic digestion. This is a process in which the putrescible organic matter in the sludge is reduced by 30–50 per cent by being converted to carbon dioxide and methane. This conversion takes place in two very generalised stages (Fig. 7.11). The first converts large molecules (polysaccharides, proteins etc.,) to small ones, predominantly acetate. The second step is the break-down of the acetate to methane and carbon dioxide. The types of bacteria involved and the step-wise biochemistry are discussed in §1.5.

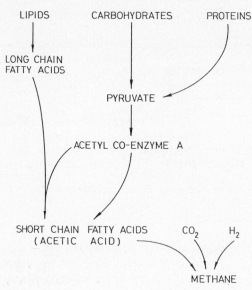

Fig. 7.11. Simplified metabolic pathways for the degradation of biopolymers to methane.

The process requirements are an absence of oxygen, a pH of 7–7.5, good mixing, an elevated temperature and an adequate solids retention time. Mixing is an important feature as it enhances the release of gas, minimises stratification, scum formation and grit settlement, and assists in maintaining a uniform temperature. A variety of different systems have been used, but essentially they can be divided into two types: mechanical devices (either internal or external) and gas re-circulation (see Brade & Noone, 1981; Rundle & Whyley, 1981). Mixing efficiencies can be assessed by the use of tracers. For example, tritium will effectively label the aqueous phase and gold-198 will enable the movement of the solids to be followed. A survey within one water authority region showed the power requirements for mixing varied from 1.5 to 20.5 W m^{-3} (Brade & Noone, 1981). The temperature at which digestion takes place can vary widely. Cold digestion is practised (Lowe & Williamson, 1983), as is thermophilic digestion (Garber, 1982). However, the majority of the digestion plants which are operated in the UK use the mesophilic range (30–35 °C). This means that heat exchangers are an integral part of the digester. The heat exchange medium is usually water which has been heated by burning some of the digester gas. An alternative is direct steam injection.

Most digesters at British treatment works consist of two tanks: a primary digester which is covered, fully anaerobic and heated, and a secondary unit which is a tank, uncovered and unheated, where a

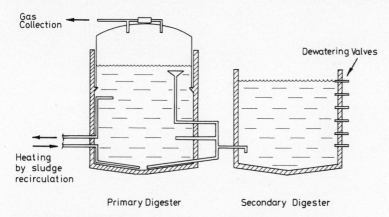

Gas Collection

Dewatering Valves

Heating by sludge recirculation

Primary Digester   Secondary Digester

Fig. 7.12. Typical arrangement of the two-stage digestion of sludge.

degree of de-watering occurs (Fig. 7.12). Most texts, when discussing the design criteria for digesters, are referring to the primary unit. The design parameters that are normally used are the solids retention time and the organic loading rate but the values which are quoted as 'standard' vary considerably. These variations depend on national boundaries and on whether a distinction is being made between high- and standard-rate digestion (see Brade & Noone, 1981). Retention times can vary from 10 to > 30 days although it has been suggested that if the retention time is less than 12 days there is a risk that the methanogens could be washed out of the digester (Institute of Water Pollution Control, 1981). The design values for the organic loading rate vary from 0.48 to 8.5 kg volatile matter m^{-3} d^{-1}, but a survey of UK digesters has shown that at rates of less than 1.71 kg m^{-3} d^{-1} temporary or persistent operational difficulties were experienced (Swanwick, Shurben & Jackson, 1969). On the basis of this type of information it is not possible to provide precise design criteria. However, a reasonable starting point might be to consider a retention time of around 20 days and an organic loading rate of about 2 kg m^{-3} d^{-1}. The tank itself should have a depth to diameter ratio of between 1:3 and 1:2 with the maximum diameter being 25 m. The floor should have a slope of between 12 and 30°. The roof of the digester can either be floating or fixed (Fig. 7.13) but whichever is used it is essential that air must be prevented from entering and forming an explosive mixture with the biogas being produced. Fixed roof digesters will however require a separate gas storage unit.

The main parameters that are used to monitor the operation of an anaerobic digester are pH, alkalinity, volatile fatty acids (VFA) and gas yield. The acceptable pH range is 7.0–7.5 and bicarbonate alkalinities should be maintained within the range of 3500–5000 mg l^{-1}. VFA

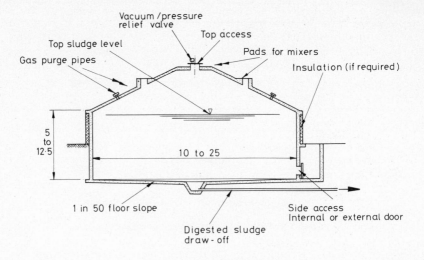

FIXED ROOF DIGESTION TANK

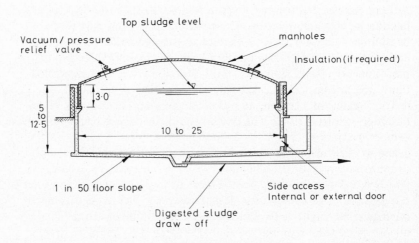

FLOATING ROOF DIGESTION TANK

Fig. 7.13. Fixed roof and floating roof digestion tanks.

concentrations are measured in terms of acetic acid and, for the digestion of sludge, need to be kept at a value below 200–500 mg l⁻¹. (This value should not be confused with the higher values that can be tolerated by some digesters treating liquid wastes; see chapter 8.) As a general rule, pH adjustment is not necessary as there is a natural buffering within the reactor due to interactions between ammonium and bicarbonate ions. Additional carbonate/bicarbonate may be provided if

Table 7.9. *Concentration of toxic material causing significant (20%) inhibition of anaerobic digestion*

Toxin	Concentration (mg kg dry solids^{-1})
Chloroform	15
Trichlorethane	20
Carbon tetrachloride	200
Nickel	2000
Cadmium	2200
Copper	2700
Zinc	3400
Anionic detergent	1.5–2.0%

From Institute of Water Pollution Control, 1981.

it is necessary to enhance this buffering capacity. If this is done it must be remembered that there is a limit for concentrations of alkali metal ions above which they become inhibitory: 3.5–5.0 g l^{-1} for sodium, 2.5–4.5 g l^{-1} for potassium. An alternative control method is to add lime. Gas production rates will vary from plant to plant. In using this parameter for monitoring the operation of a digester, therefore, it is the trend which is important rather than an absolute value.

The 'health' of a digester can also be gauged from the composition of the gas (or its calorific value); a rise in the carbon dioxide level is a distinct warning signal (Brade & Noone, 1981; Noone & Brade, 1982). These workers also provide a good appraisal of the interdependence of the various monitoring parameters. A 'sick' digester, as indicated by the VFA values and/or the gas production, can be caused by many operational aspects; for example, underloading, overloading or poor mixing. A deterioration in performance could also be caused by inhibitory or toxic material in the sludge. Heavy metal ions, detergents and chlorinated hydrocarbons are the most commonly cited toxic materials (Table 7.9). Their concentrations in sewage, and therefore in the sludge feed to digesters, can be limited by good trade effluent control (Chater 11). In attempting to control the concentrations of toxic compounds it should be recognised that their effect does appear to be additive (see Kellock, 1973 and Mosey, 1976). Remedial measures that can be taken if the performance of a digester starts to deteriorate would include reducing the rate of feeding, increasing the intensity of mixing and, in extreme cases, re-seeding the digester.

Performance data for anaerobic digesters are given in Table 7.10. The solids concentration in the sludge fed to these reactors was 3–6 per cent

Table 7.10. *Typical performance data for mesophilic anaerobic digesters*

Loading						
(kg VDS m^{-3} d^{-1})	1.0	1.7	1.4	0.79–0.88	1.27–1.36	0.97–1.39
Retention time						
(d)	19	19	23	48–56	31–33	18.5–28.1
Reduction in						
VDS (%)	54	47	48	46–52	47–50	36–47
Gas yield						
(m^3 kg $\varDelta$ VDS^{-1})	0.83	1.18	1.04	0.87–1.13	1.07–1.25	0.84–1.22
Source	IWPC, 1981			Kellock, 1973	Booker, 1981	Eves, 1981

dry solids, of which about 75 per cent was volatile matter. These data are typical of the results that could be expected from the majority of digesters operating in the UK. In comparing performances care must be taken to ensure that the performance data are based on the true working volume of the digester. Accumulations of rag and grit can cause significant reductions in the volume available for the sludge. For example, an examination of digesters at the Hogsmill Valley works near London showed that the effective volume was, in some cases, as low as 50 per cent of the total volume (Eves, 1981). A similar examination by Noone & Brade (1982) showed a 70 per cent effective volume. These results mean that actual retention times can be appreciably lower than the expected value of > 20 days, with no apparent loss in performance. This fact, coupled with the current requirements to uprate processes wherever possible, has resulted in a detailed appraisal of design and operational criteria by the Severn–Trent Water Authority (Brade & Noone, 1981, Brade *et al.*, 1982, Noone & Brade, 1982). The work has assessed methods of heating and mixing, the use of pre-fabricated structures, reduction in retention times, the use of thicker sludges and the methods of feeding primary digesters. These assessments can probably best be summarised by the recommendations that were made as interim design criteria: maximum retention time = 15 days; feed solids concentration = 4 per cent; tank height:diameter ratio = 1.0. It was also suggested that there was scope to achieve further cost savings (both capital and revenue) by using thicker sludges and direct steam heating (Noone & Brade, 1982).

Whatever the operational regime of the digester, it will produce gas. The typical rate of production is 1 m^3 kg^{-1} of volatile matter destroyed and it will contain 65–70 per cent methane. Its gross calorific value (CV) can be estimated from: $CV = 334 \times$ (methane percentage) kJ m^{-3}; in other words, 22–24 MJ m^{-3}. The problem which invariably besets engineers dealing with anaerobic digestion processes is how best to use the gas. It is all too easy to convert the energy potential to a fuel oil equivalent and assign a monetary value to it. However, using the gas will require a financial input (see Wase & Forster, 1984). For example, if it is to be considered as a fuel for vehicles it may require storage, cleansing and pressurisation; if it is to be used to produce electricity, dual fuel engines and generator equipment will be needed. The result is that, all too often, these ancillary costs are such that, whilst some of the gas is burnt to provide heating for the digesters, a significant amount is burnt uselessly in a flare. Surely, therefore, this is an area for technological innovation and improvement.

As well as producing a stable sludge, anaerobic digestion achieves a level of pathogen removal which makes the sludge acceptable, at least in the UK, for land disposal without further treatment (see §7.5; also Pike, Morris & Carrington, 1983).

7.4.2 *Aerobic digestion*

Sludges may also be stabilised by aerobic treatment, with the excess (and putrescible) organic matter being the substrate for bacterial respiration. The basic requirements therefore are good aeration, good mixing and an adequate retention time. It has been suggested that sludge stability can be defined in terms of the oxygen uptake rate (OUR). For example, Eikum & Paulsrud (1974) define stability as:

$$\text{Stability } (\%) = 118\left(1 - \left[\frac{OUR \text{ at } 18\,^{\circ}C}{\text{maximum } OUR}\right]\right).$$

The OUR values that have been suggested as being indicative of a stable aerobically digested sludge range from 1 to 5 mg oxygen g VSS^{-1} h^{-1} (Ahlberg & Giffen, 1972; Cohen, 1977). However, Mavinic & Koers (1979) have questioned the use of OUR values to define the stability of sludges that are being digested at temperatures of 10 °C or less. Instead they suggested that a mixed liquor BOD value of 0.2 kg kg VSS^{-1} was more appropriate.

Although aerobic digestion has been studied for over 25 years and although it is used considerably in North America (US Environmental Protection Agency, 1974), it is not a process which has had any real popularity in the UK. However, the development of auto-heating, thermophilic digestion appears to be changing these attitudes (Gunson & Morgan, 1982). Auto-heating, arguably the most interesting aspect of aerobic digestion, is the ability of aeration (or oxygenation) to induce a significant temperature rise in the sludge. This increase in temperature is caused by free energy being released as organic matter is converted to new cell material. The total released (ΔF, kcal l^{-1}) can be calculated from $\Delta F = 3.5E\,(\Delta COD)$, where E is the efficiency of the retention of heat and ΔCOD has units of g l^{-1}. Since the heat released, expressed as kcal l^{-1}, is approximately equal to the temperature change and since the thermal efficiency (E) is about 70 per cent (Jewell & Kabrick, 1980), the temperature rise that is achieved (ΔT) can be expressed as $\Delta T = 2.4$ (ΔCOD).

The requirements for auto-heating have been summarised by Jewell & Kabrick. They are:

(a) There should be sufficient biodegradable organics in the incoming sludge to generate between 25 and 35 kcal l^{-1}

(b) Oxygen transfer efficiencies should exceed 10 per cent (that is to say more than 10 per cent of the oxygen supplied should be used in the biochemical reactions)

(c) The reactors should be well insulated

(d) The product of temperature and sludge retention time should exceed 150 degree-days (Cohen, 1977).

Waste activated sludge, either alone or mixed with primary sludge, provides an adequate amount of biodegradable organic matter, particularly when thickened (4–5 per cent solids) sludges are used. Both air and pure oxygen have been used to achieve the oxidation. It is not at all clear, however, whether air is universally suitable. For example, Jewell & Kabrick report work which shows that air-aeration can produce auto-thermal conditions even when the ambient and raw sludge temperatures are low. Cohen (1977) on the other hand, in a comparison of aerated and oxygenated aeration, showed that significantly higher temperatures were obtained with the oxygenated systems.

In judging the success of this type of aerobic digestion there is a need to consider both primary and secondary criteria. The primary objectives are:

(a) the increase in temperature that can be achieved

(b) the reduction in volatile suspended matter (VSS)

(c) the stability of the digested sludge

(d) the retention time needed to meet these objectives.

Of secondary importance are the reduction (or removal) of pathogens by the elevated temperatures and the de-watering characteristics of the final sludge. On the basis of the performance data shown in Table 7.11, it can be seen that both oxygen and air give relatively similar results. In principle, both are capable of producing thermophilic conditions and of meeting the EPA criterion of a 40 per cent reduction in volatile suspended solids (US Environmental Protection Agency, 1974). The units, which were the source of the data in Table 7.11, operated with retention times ranging from 3 to 10 days. As has already been mentioned, the definition of stability is open to discussion. However, on the basis of the development of odours in sludge stored at 25 °C

Table 7.11. *Examples of performance data for auto-thermal aerobic digestion*

Source	Loading rate (kg VSS $m^{-3} d^{-1}$)	ΔT (°C)	ΔVSS (%)	Oxidant
Cohen, 1977	6.9–9.6	13–23	34–47	oxygen
Jewell & Kabrick, 1980	10	40	40	air
Gunson & Morgan, 1982	5.6[a]	35	48[a]	air
Anon., 1983	5	48	50	air
Matsch & Drnevich, 1977	5.1–7.4[b]	38	29–42	oxygen
	6.1–8.5[c]	36	30–45	oxygen

[a] Data based on COD; [b] Surplus activated sludge; [c] Activated and primary.

(Matsch & Drnevich, 1977), sludge which has been digested in an aerobic thermophilic reactor would remain stable for at least five weeks. Because the operational temperature of this type of digestion is usually above 50 °C, there is a high removal of pathogens (Franzen & Hakanson, 1983; Kabrick & Jewell, 1982).

The effect of auto-thermal digestion on the de-watering characteristics of sludge appears to be variable. According to the data presented by Cohen (1977), sludge from an oxygenic reactor required more conditioning than undigested sludge. Jewell & Kabrick (1980) also showed that digestion caused filterability to deteriorate. However, Matsch & Drnevich (1977) report that, in terms of vacuum filtration rates, thermophically digested sludge has de-watering characteristics which are comparable to those of activated or anaerobically digested sludge.

It can be seen, therefore, that thermophilic aerobic digestion can provide a degree of sludge stabilisation that is similar to that achieved by mesophilic anaerobic digestion. This means that there may be a need to choose between these processes. A comparison by Riegler (1982) suggests that anaerobic digestion should be the choice at large treatment works (> 50000 population) whilst aerobic digestion would be the more appropriate for smaller units. Franzen & Hakanson (1983) offer a similar suggestion. Although performance data are available for individual units, there is also a need for generalised scale-up and optimisation procedures. Some recommendations for these have been made by Vismara (1983).

7.5   Application of sludge to land
7.5.1   *General discussion*

Although it has been recommended that the most favourable method for the disposal of digested sludge was, as a slurry, to grasslands and arable land (Ministry of Housing and Local Government, 1954), the concept of returning the carbon, nitrogen and phosphorus that are present in sewage to the soil is not new. Some one hundred years ago when the treatment of sewage by land irrigation was being advocated, a report on this type of treatment stated that: 'Milch cows thrive remarkably well on this grass and it has been proven by chemical analysis that the milk is of the best quality, while the vegetables are also quite wholesome'. Certainly, even to-day when sludges are contaminated with metals and trace organics from industry, there is much to be said for utilising the nitrogen and phosphorus in what would otherwise be classified as a waste product. The concentrations of nitrogen and phosphorus in sludge shown in Table 7.3 compare well with those normally cited in the literature; that is a mean nitrogen concentration (as per cent dry residue) of 7.3 and a mean phosphorus concentration of 5.4 per cent for liquid digested sludge. Assuming an availability of 85 and 70 per cent for nitrogen and phosphorus respectively, Burley & Bayley (1977) have estimated that the gain to the farmer, at 1976 fertiliser prices, is equivalent to about £23 dry tonne^{-1}. Having said this, it must be remembered that if a dried sludge were used the benefit would be reduced, as a considerable proportion (perhaps as much as two thirds) of the nitrogen is associated with the liquid phase.

7.5.2   *Manurial value*

The benefits of using sludge on farm lands, measured in terms of crop productivity, and for land reclamation have been examined extensively (Coker *et al.*, 1982; Water Research Centre, 1979). The comparison between liquid digested sludge and conventional artificial fertiliser on the production of grass showed that, with application rates of 240 m^3 ha^{-1}, the sludge produced as great a dry weight of grass as the equivalent amount of nitrogen and potash in a conventional fertiliser (Table 7.12). The trials also showed that, if the grass were to be grazed *in situ*, there was little need to supplement the sludge with potash. However if frequent applications were being made and the grass were to be cut and used elsewhere, then supplementary potash would be needed at a rate of 34–56 kg ha^{-1} for every 101–146 kg ha^{-1} of nitrogen applied in a 67–112 m^3 ha^{-1} dressing. Trials with air-dried sludge and a sludge-straw compost have also shown that sludge application to land, particularly if the sludge is ploughed in during the autumn, can give

Table 7.12. *Results showing the effect of
digested sludge applications to ryegrass*

	Grass yield (tonnes ha^{-1})	
	No added potash	Added potash
No nitrogen	3.1	3.2
Artificial fertiliser	12.8	15.4
Liquid digested sludge	14.6	15.3
Sludge + fertiliser	17.2	18.8

From Coker, 1965.

Table 7.13. *Mean annual rates of increase in produce yield (1944–50)
from various organic manures applied at a rate of 75 tonnes ha^{-1} year^{-1}*

	Yields (tonnes ha^{-1} year^{-1})			
	Beet	Peas	Cabbage	Leeks
Artificial NPK fertiliser	0.83	1.05	0.90	1.93
Farmyard manure	1.51	1.10	1.36	1.91
Sewage sludge	1.63	0.58	1.18	2.46
Sludge-straw compost	1.10	1.43	1.46	2.21

From Mann & Barnes, 1963.

good produce yields (see Mann & Barnes, 1963, and Table 7.13). These
advantages were most marked with sandy or silty soils. In addition,
large yield increases were obtained on phosphate-deficient soils. In these
cases, it was found that as much as 100 per cent of the sludge
phosphate was made available to the crops.

7.5.3 *Metal contamination*

Unfortunately, most sludges are contaminated, to a greater or lesser
degree, by metals which can have harmful effects on crops. Fig. 7.14,
for example, shows the reductions in yield that were experienced in pot
trials when varying concentrations of copper and nickel were added to
the soil.

In addition to a yield reduction, plants do take up metals from the
soil. Fig. 7.15 shows some of the results from a plant growth-test in
which sludge, containing 1070 mg kg^{-1} of zinc, 245 mg kg^{-1} of copper
and 24 mg kg^{-1} of nickel, was applied to a coarse, sandy soil at varying

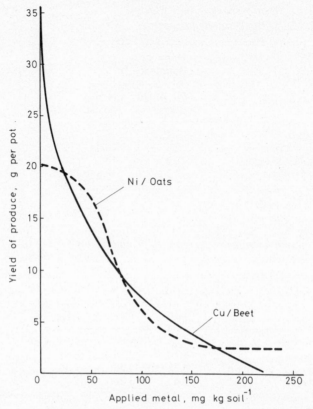

Fig. 7.14. Yields obtained with pot trials showing the effect of added metal ions. (From Webber, 1972.)

rates together with a pre-plant application of 392 kg potassium ha^{-1}. In the context of the overall effect of metals on crops it must be realised that there can be wide variations, both in yield and uptake, between crops and even between varieties of the same crop. In the UK, it is now recognised that a series of elements must be controlled whenever sludge is mixed with soil if toxic or potentially toxic effects on crops, livestock and humans are to be avoided. It has been proposed therefore that an elemental application rate should be calculated for each metal or metalloid listed in Table 7.14 and that the sludge application rate which is used should be the lowest elemental rate. The application rates for individual elements (tonnes dry solids ha^{-1} yr^{-1}) can be calculated from:

$$\text{Rate} = \frac{A - B}{C} \times \frac{1000}{D}$$

where A = suggested limit of addition, in kg ha^{-1} (from Table 7.14),

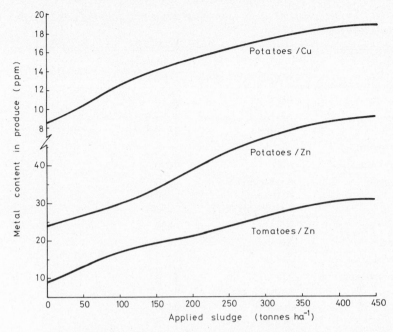

Fig. 7.15. Metal uptake by plants grown in sludge fertilised soil. (From Dowdy & Larson, 1975.)

B = concentration of available element in the soil, in kg ha^{-1} = 2.2 (concentration in mg kg^{-1} dry solids), C = total concentration of the elements in the sludge, (mg kg^{-1} dry solids), D = application period (usually 30 years). Thus, a sludge with the analysis shown in Table 7.15 being applied, over a 30-year period, to a soil which had the analysis also shown in Table 7.15 would have an application rate which was controlled by the cadmium application rather than the zinc equivalent. The application rates given by this method do assume a yearly application. In fact it is not essential that the annual increments are equal. However, the maximum annual rate should not exceed 20 per cent of the total amount that can be applied. Cadmium may well be found to be a major constraint to the use of sludge on land. Because of this, the impact of sludge cadmium on the human diet has been the subject of a detailed review (Davis & Coker, 1980). Where a metals concentration in the sludge inhibits the application to land, trade effluent controls can, and should, be used to alleviate the problem (see Chapters 11 and 12; Matthews, 1983).

When considering sludge application to land, care must be taken with sludges that have been lime-treated. The increase in soil pH which results from the addition of either a limed sludge or lime directly will, in general, reduce the availability of metals, but in the case of

Table 7.14. *Recommended 30-year limits for controlling the addition of toxic elements to soil*

Element	Receiving situation	Addition limit (kg ha^{-1})
Arsenic	All	10
Boron	Arable	3.5–5.0[a]
	Pasture	4.5–7.0[a]
Cadmium	All	5
Chromium	All	1000
Copper	Arable (pH > 7)	560[b]
	Pasture	560[b]
	Arable (pH ⩽ 7)	280[b]
Fluorine	All	600
Lead	All	1000
Mercury	All	2
Molybdenum	All	4
Nickel	Arable (pH > 7)	140[b]
	Pasture	140[b]
	Arable (pH ⩽ 7)	70[b]
Zinc (and zinc equivalent)	Arable (pH > 7)	1120[b]
	Pasture	1120[b]
	Arable (pH ⩽ 7)	560[b]

[a] Hot water soluble; annual basis. [b] EDTA extractable. From Department of the Environment, 1981.

Table 7.15. *Elemental application rates for various metal concentrations*

	Concentration in sludge (mg kg^{-1})	Concentration in soil (mg kg^{-1})	Elemental application rate (tonnes DS ha^{-1} year^{-1})
Zinc	1650	40	$\dfrac{560-(2.2\times40)}{1650}\times\dfrac{1000}{30}=9.5$
Cadmium	34	1	$\dfrac{5-(2.2\times1)}{34}\times\dfrac{1000}{30}=2.7$
Lead	150	30	$\dfrac{1000-(2.2\times30)}{150}\times\dfrac{1000}{30}=207.6$
Copper	400	15	$\dfrac{280-(2.2\times15)}{400}\times\dfrac{100}{30}=20.6$
Nickel	30	10	$\dfrac{70-(2.2\times10)}{30}\times\dfrac{1000}{30}=53.3$
'Zinc equivalent'[a]	2690	150	$\dfrac{560-(2.2\times150)}{2690}\times\dfrac{1000}{30}=2.9$

[a] 'Zinc equivalent' = $Zn+(2\times Cu)+(8\times Ni)$.

Table 7.16. *EEC recommendations for the maximum concentrations of metals in relation to the application of sludge to land*

Element	Limit in sludge (mg kg DS^{-1})		Loading limit (kg ha^{-1} yr^{-1})		Soil limit (mg kg DS^{-1})	
	R	M	R	M	R	M
Cd	20	40	0.10	0.15	1	3
Cu	1000	1500	10	12	50	100
Ni	300	400	2	3	30	50
Pb	750	1000	10	15	50	100
Zn	2500	3000	25	30	150	300
As	—	—	0.35	—	20	—
Cr	750	—	10	—	50	—
Hg	16	—	0.4	—	2	—

R = recommended; M = mandatory.

molybdenum the metal becomes more available at the higher pH and its uptake by crops is increased. Whilst molybdenum is not toxic to plants, high intakes by livestock can result in copper deficiency symptoms. Limed sludge should also not be used on soils which are likely to yield crops deficient in essential trace elements. In the future, EEC requirements will also have to be considered. The directive currently being considered suggests three methods of control:

> the maximum levels in the sludge
> the maximum loading rates over a 10-year period
> the maximum levels in agricultural soils.

As is usual with EEC directives, both mandatory and recommended values are quoted (see Table 7.16). However, as has been the case with many directives, the values and the logic behind their derivation have been questioned (see Purves, 1983).

7.5.4 Pathogen contamination

The potential biological hazards in sludge are:

(a) Human bacterial pathogens
(b) Animal or plant parasites or pathogens
(c) Viruses

The extent to which sludges are contaminated with dangerous biological components depends on the nature of sewage producing the sludge and the type of treatment it has received. The relative level of the problems associated with differently processed sludges is shown in Table 7.17; when it is considered that crude sludge has been, and frequently is, applied to land it might be expected that disease transfer to plants, livestock or man might not be uncommon.

Table 7.17. *Relative level of pathogen
contamination in sludge*

Sludge treatment	Odour	Pathogens
Raw	H	H
Raw/lime (pH = 11.5)	M	L
Raw/Cl$_2$ (pH = 2–3)	N	N
Raw/Cl$_2$ (pH = 6–7)	M	L
Digested	M	M
Digested/lime	M	L
Composted	N	N
Heat-dried	L	N

H = high; M = medium; L = low; N = negligible.

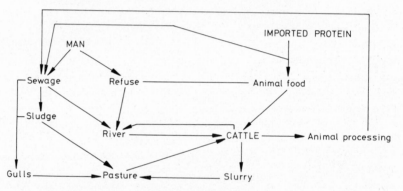

Fig. 7.16. The Salmonellosis cycle.

One of the main concerns from the point of view of animal husbandry is the transfer of *Salmonella* infections. There are many routes whereby this transfer can take place (Fig. 7.16), and although the number of incidents of Salmonellosis diagnosed by the Ministry of Agriculture veterinary centres has increased since 1960, the main increase has been caused by *S. dublin* which is a serotype that rarely infects man. This could well explain why it is that although *Salmonella* can be isolated from both raw (e.g. as many as 70 *Salmonellae* ml^{-1} of wet primary sludge) and digested sludge, the risk of spreading infection by means of sludge is thought to be marginal. The risk of disease transfer can be minimised if simple precautions are taken. Thus, raw sludges should not be used on grazing land and should only be used for those arable crops which are consumed either by animals or humans after processing. Treated sludge can be applied to pastures and grassland but an interval of at least three weeks should be allowed between application and the grazing of cattle.

In order for animals to become infected they must ingest the minimal infective dose. This will vary with the virulence of the pathogen and the health of the animal. Although most tests to determine the minimal infective dose have been done on healthy animals, it has been suggested that for *S. typhimurim* and *S. dublin* an ingested dose of 10^7–10^8 will result in fatal illness. The time interval between application and grazing is therefore to ensure that the numbers of *Salmonella* on the grass are reduced to a level well below the minimal infective dose. It is assumed that this reduction is due to the exposure of bacteria to the ultra-violet radiation in sunlight and to desiccation. In general however, after sludge is applied to soil the viability of pathogens is very variable, ranging from a few hours to several months. Spore-forming bacteria, however, can remain viable for even longer periods (Dotson, 1973; Kirkham, 1974).

The relationship between the level of pathogen contamination of a sludge and the type of treatment that sludge has received has already been mentioned, but of the treatments listed in Table 7.17 only digestion and the use of lime are common in the UK. As far as *Salmonella* removal is concerned digestion is a very unpredictable process, the removal varying between 40 and 98 per cent. Certainly there is, at the moment, insufficient knowledge about the precise mechanism of pathogen inactivation in mesophilic digestion. The use of lime on raw sludge showed that *S. typhosa* was destroyed in less than two hours when the pH was held at 11.0 or above (Doyle, 1967) and it was concluded that if lime were being used as a sludge conditioning agent the additional costs of using extra lime to achieve these high pH values would not add appreciably to the cost of sludge disposal. When de-watered sludge is stockpiled there is a certain degree of composting and the temperature within the pile does increase. Under these circumstances there is a die-off of pathogens and it has been found that the concentration of *Salmonella* reaches a base level after about three months. The choice of technique will depend on the use of the receiving farmland, the facilities (i.e. type of sludge, degree of contamination, power), the land available at the treatment works and the discounted cost of the various options. It is worth noting that under the Zoonoses Orders, 1974, all Salmonellosis cases are subjected to veterinary investigations so that the source of infection is identified and that, to date, there are no published cases of Salmonellosis resulting from the application of sludge to land (Carrington, 1980). The Waste Protein Order, 1976, on the other hand, which requires feedstuffs to satisfy a standard of 95 per cent of all samples being free of *Salmonella* and the remaining 5 per cent to contain not more than 2–4 MPN *Salmonella* 100 g^{-1}, will remove one of the primary sources of infection. This may mean that sludge may assume a greater prominence in the infection of farm animals.

Of the many known viruses to which man is a host there are

Table 7.18. *Enteric viruses and their associated diseases*

Virus group	Number of types	Common disease syndromes
Polioviruses	3	Poliomyelitis, aseptic meningitis
Coxsackieviruses A	23	Herpangina, aseptic meningitis, exanthem
Coxsackieviruses B	6	Aseptic meningitis, epidemic myalgia, myocarditis, pericarditis
Echoviruses	31	Aseptic meningitis, exanthem, gastroenteritis
Adenoviruses	31	Upper respiratory illness, pharyngitis, conjunctivitis
Reoviruses	3	Upper respiratory illness, diarrhoea, exanthem
Hepatitis A virus(es) (HAV)	1?	Viral hepatitis type A or 'infection hepatitis'
Gastroenteritis virus(es)	?	Acute infectious nonbacterial gastroenteritis

essentially eight groups which are relevant to any discussion on sewage treatment (Table 7.18). Those viruses which cause diseases of economic importance in farm animals (i.e. foot and mouth disease, swine vesicular disease) are controlled so strictly by inspection that their transmission by infected material reaching the sewerage system is extremely small. Viruses are removed from the aqueous phase quite effectively by bio-oxidation systems, mainly by adsorption processes. Activated sludge has been found to remove more than 90 per cent of the viruses present although bio-filters are not as effective (Carrington, 1980). The plant parasite which is most likely to cause problems when sludge is applied to land is the root crop eelworm (*Heterodera* spp.). There are ten species of eelworm which commonly occur in soil (Table 7.19), one of the most prevalent being the potato cyst eelworm. The cysts, which contain the eggs of the parasite, can persist in soil for a considerable time in the absence of a host plant. Indeed, once land has become infested with potato cyst eelworm a period of eight or more years when no potatoes are grown on the land may be needed to eliminate the problem. One of the main causes of heavy eelworm infestation is overcropping but, because of the very ready dispersion of the cysts whenever a contaminated soil is moved, the problem can be spread very easily. In this way cysts can enter the sewerage system in the effluents from vegetable processing factories and can accumulate in the resultant sludges. Whilst it is known that digestion can destroy the

Table 7.19. *The most common species of* Heterodera

Species	Name	Host crops
H. rostochiensis	Golden nematode, potato root eelworm	Potato, tomato, egg-plant
H. pallida	Pale potato cyst-nematode	Potato, tomato, egg-plant
H. schachtii	Beet cyst-nematode, beet eelworm	Sugar beet, fodder beet, red beet, all types of brassica, rhubarb, etc.
H. avenae	Cereal cyst-nematode, cereal root eelworm	Oats, barley, wheat, etc.
H. carotae	Carrot cyst-nematode, carrot root eelworm	Carrot
H. cruciferae	Cabbage cyst-nematode, cabbage root eelworm	All types of brassica and many other plants
H. goeltingiana	Pea cyst-nematode, pea root eelworm	Peas and beans
H. punctata	Grass cyst-nematode	Grasses
H. trifolii	Clover cyst-nematode, clover root eelworm	Clovers etc.
H. galeopsidis	Galeopsis cyst-nematode, Galeopsis root eelworm	Clovers etc.

cysts, the effect of other types of sludge treatment on cyst populations is uncertain.

Cysts can be isolated from sludge and counted using modifications to the Fenwick Can method (Linfield, 1977). It might therefore be considered possible to calculate the acceptable amount of cyst-contaminated sludge that could be applied to soil which was free from any infestation by assuming (a) that cysts will survive for eight years and (b) that the critical concentration above which yield losses are experienced is 25 cysts per 100 g of dry soil. However, the Potato Cyst Eelworm (Great Britain) Order, 1973, which complies with an EEC directive, stipulates that potatoes for export can only be produced on land that has been officially certified as cyst-free. Whilst this should gradually bring about a reduction in the number of cysts in sludge it is important that sludge disposal is never cited as the agent for re-infecting certified land.

The only other parasite which need be considered in the context of applying sludge to land is the human/beef tapeworm (*Taenia saginata*), and in particular its ova. These can remain viable for long periods: up to 23 weeks on pasture. However, although the incidence of cystercercosis is thought to be widespread amongst the human population in the UK (statistics are difficult to find as it is not a notifiable disease), the number of infected beef carcases detained at slaughter-houses is relatively low. In a survey covering 70 abattoirs between 1972 and 1974 only 666 carcases were found to be infected. This may well be due to the fact that mesophilic digestion is thought to kill the tapeworm eggs (Pike *et al.*, 1983). Nevertheless, it may be necessary in the future to monitor sludges for worm ova (as a result of EEC directives). It has therefore been suggested (Pike *et al.*, 1983) that the viability of the ova of *Ascaris suum* (the pig roundworm) might be used to monitor the effectiveness of digestion (or disinfectants). The reason for this suggestion is that *Ascaris* ova can be separated more readily than *Taenia* ova; the viability of *Ascaris* ova can be examined more easily and they are more resistant to heat. Within the UK, the public significance is low. However, in tropical countries, infection is much more prevalent and thus assumes a greater significance both in terms of community health and losses in food revenue (see, for example, Latham, Latham & Basta, 1977).

7.5.5   Application techniques

There are essentially four methods for applying sludge to land: surface spreading, trenching, irrigation and injection. Surface spreading involves the use of a vehicle directly on the land itself. In the case of de-watered sludges this would probably be a conventional manure spreader, whilst for liquid sludges either a small road tanker (e.g. 4.5–5.5 m^3 capacity) or a tractor-hauled slurry tanker (e.g. 3.6 m^3 capacity) would most probably be used. These would discharge the sludge, through air-operated valves and fishtail nozzles, in strips perhaps 4.5 m wide, the rate of application being controlled by the speed of the vehicle. The fact that the vehicle must go onto the land means that this method of application is usually limited to about 8 months of the year, i.e. April or May to October or November.

Trenching is something of a lost art but could be a satisfactory method of disposing of raw sludge if care is taken to avoid ground water contamination. In addition, it is a technique that could enable marginal land to be brought back to full agricultural production. Using trenches 0.6 m deep by 0.6 m wide at 0.6 m intervals, an application rate of about 860–1000 dry tonnes ha^{-1} is achieved. When liquid sludges are applied in this way, it can be difficult to keep the sludge in the trench during back-filling.

As far as liquid sludge is concerned, and particularly liquid digested sludge, a very useful application technique is irrigation. This is usually done with rain guns (with 15–50 mm openings) which means that a pipeline network (usually of 75–100 mm diameter aluminium pipes) and a pressurising pump are also required. There are two main problems with this method of application: the labour involved with setting and re-laying the pipe network is time consuming and it is usually a dirty and unpleasant job; and the method produces an aerosol which can be carried beyond the confines of the agricultural area causing complaints from the general public. Concern has also been expressed about the possible risk of disease transmission (i.e. virus or *Salmonella* infections) through these aerosols. If spray irrigation is to be used, very little can be done to overcome the problem of aerosol formation. However, the problems associated with the moving of pipelines can be minimised by the use of flexible hoses, mobile hosereels and winches. Probably the cleanest method of sludge application and the least objectionable from the point of view of the public is injection. This approach uses a chisel plough to inject the sludge 25–50 mm below the surface of the soil. Application rates as high as 180 tonnes ha^{-1} have been achieved at a single pass with sludge injection but at this level of application the soil was too wet to allow any further vehicle movement for 3–6 weeks.

7.6   Incineration

Although incineration is not used widely in the UK (see Table 7.1), there are situations where its use must be given careful consideration. For example, when land and sea outlets either are not available or are very limited; or when the sludge is not suitable for any other route because of biological or chemical contamination. Several types of incinerator are available; Burgess (1968) lists four whilst Thomas (1975) describes three. However, the main choice would appear to be between multiple hearth systems (Burton & Conway, 1983; Grieve, 1978) and fluidised bed incinerators (Dickens, Wallis & Arundel, 1980). Multiple hearth incinerators are operated with a counter-current flow of sludge and air, with the sludge being moved downwards from hearth to hearth by rotating arms which are air-driven. In this way, the sludge is dried, is ignited and finally the residual ash is cooled with heat transfer taking place directly between the air and the solid. One of the main features of the multiple hearth system is that there is a 'thermal jump' from 90–95 °C in the drying zone to perhaps 800 °C in the combustion zone which is claimed to minimise the risk of odour emissions. Nevertheless it is essential that gas cleaning is practised. Details of the size of units, operating temperatures and capacity have been published elsewhere (Burton & Conway, 1983; Grieve, 1978; Tench, Phillips & Swanwick, 1972; Smith, Griffin & Grahame, 1978).

Fluidised bed incinerators contain a bed of heated sand which is kept in a fluidised state by an upwards flow of air. The sand acts both as a heat reservoir and as means of breaking up the sludge into small particles. The sludge and air flow co-currently. This means that external heat exchangers are necessary together with facilities for removing the ash and fine sand particles (see Dickens *et al.*, 1980; Thomas, 1975).

Table 7.20. *Comparison of H-values with prevailing operating conditions for incinerators*

Source	Operating conditions	Calculated H-value (kJ kg H_2O^{-1})
Smith *et al.*, 1978	Autothermic	8027
Burton & Conway, 1983	Not autothermic[a]	3238[c]
	Autothermic[b]	5667[c]
Dickens *et al.*, 1980	Not autothermic	4875

[a] $d = 16\%$; [b] $d = 25\%$; [c] C assumed as 17000.

One of the central design considerations is the heat required to evaporate the water from the solids. If sufficient water has been removed by earlier processes and if there is sufficient organic matter, the sludge may be autothermic. That is to say, the energy released during combustion is greater than that required to evaporate the water. It has been suggested (Grieve, 1978) that the minimum requirements for autothermic conditions are a heat release (H) of 5400 kJ kg^{-1} of water to be evaporated, i.e.

$$H = \frac{C \times d}{100 - d} \geqslant 5400$$

where C = calorific value of sludge, in kJ kg^{-1} DS and d = dry solids (DS) concentration, %. Using the data provided in the literature already cited to calculate H-values shows that this appears to be a realistic criterion for judging the onset of autothermic conditions (Table 7.20). It has also been suggested (Jank, 1975) that the calorific value can be calculated from

$$C = 260.5V - 1535$$

where V = volatile matter percentage.

Empirical relationships for calculating calorific values, based on (a) the percentage of volatile matter and (b) the chemical oxygen demand of the sludge, have also been reported by Zanoni & Mueller (1982). Typical values for sludge calorific values are shown in Table 7.21. Obviously these values, together with the solids concentration being fed to the incinerator, have a significant impact on the performance of the process when it is measured in terms of the cost. Non-autothermal incineration requires supplementary fuel (oil or LPG). It is, therefore, better to incinerate raw sludge since digested sludge has given off some of its energy potential in the form of methane. This possible requirement for supplementary fuel could, perhaps, be linked with the question posed earlier (§7.4.1) about the usage of digester gas. Would it

Table 7.21. *Typical calorific values of sewage sludges*

Sludge type	Calorific value (kJ kg DS^{-1})	Source
Primary/humus	19 500	Dickens *et al.*, 1980
Activated	13 398	Jank, 1975
Digested	12 677	
Raw	11 268	Tench *et al.*, 1972
Raw/digested/activated	15 792	Smith *et al.*, 1978
Digested	15 400	
Raw/activated	17 200	

be possible or even realistic to envisage a large regional sludge handling centre where 'safe' sludges were digested and applied to land whilst 'difficult' sludges, which had only been partially de-watered, were incinerated with the aid of digester gas?

7.7 Sea disposal

Sludge is taken out to sea for disposal from several locations in the UK. The vessels that are used have capacities which range from 300 to 3000 tonnes and the amount of sludge dumped is 9.9×10^6 wet tonnes year^{-1} (3.4×10^5 tonnes dry matter) (see Fish, 1983; Calcutt & Moss, 1983). The disposal of sludge to sea is controlled by licences which are issued by the Ministry of Agriculture, Fisheries and Food. These licences are issued under the Dumping at Sea Act (1974) which is drafted so as to conform with two international conventions, the Oslo Convention for the North East Atlantic and the London Convention, which prohibit or limit the addition of specified dangerous compounds to the marine environment. Thus a sludge disposal licence will specify the dumping area and the quantity and the nature of the sludge being dumped. The licence is continually reviewed on the basis of ecological monitoring of the dumping zone. The UK is essentially the only European country to dispose of sludge in this way and there are increasing pressures to restrict its use (Calcutt & Moss, 1983). Are such restrictions logical? Does sea dumping constitute any serious ecological threat? The assessments of both those who dump and those who monitor would suggest that there is little logic in any proposals to restrict sea dumping. For example, McIntyre in a detailed review (1977) concluded that there was really no conclusive evidence that dumping affected the marine biota. Fish (1983) reached similar conclusions, whilst Norton (1978) reported that regular monitoring coupled with good site selection meant that any adverse effects were minimised and

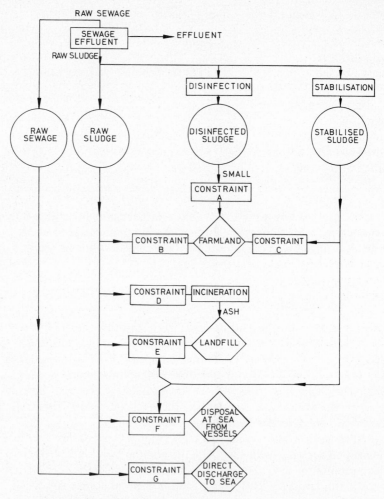

Fig. 7.17. Disposal routes for sewage sludge and the constraints that affect each option. (From Calcutt & Moss, 1983.) A DOE Guidelines – limits on metals; B A plus 6-month no-grazing limit; C As A plus 3 week no-grazing limit; D Planning permission required for incinerator construction; E Control of Pollution Act, 1974 – licence required; F Oslo Convention/Dumping at Sea Act, 1974 – licence required; G Paris Commission/Control of Pollution Act Part II – consent required. All units are in kilotonnes (DS) per year.

in most cases were insignificant. Norton, however, did state that fertilisation of the land was more logical than fertilisation of the sea. In the light of these conclusions there is a need to question whether any ban on sea dumping, which according to Calcutt & Moss would require an additional expenditure of £30 × 10⁶ per annum, can be tolerated.

7.8   Conclusions

The treatment and disposal of sludge is expensive. Currently these
operations take up about 40 per cent (£200 × 10⁶ per year) of the annual
revenue budget for sewage treatment and about 10 per cent of the total
revenue expenditure by the UK water industry. The major impact both
on these costs and on present practice is most likely to stem from
externally imposed constraints (Calcutt & Moss, 1983). The present
situation is summarised in Fig. 7.17. The most likely targets for further
constraints are likely to be (a) a restriction on sea dumping, and (b) a
requirement for all sludges to be stabilised or even disinfected. The full
significance of this has been assessed by Collinge & Bruce (1981) and by
Calcutt & Moss (1983). Both groups of authors assess the areas where
research and cost savings might be applied. These include defensive
research and monitoring, better process control and automation and
the possibilities of uprating processes. In the context of biotechnology,
mention is also made of the possibilities of utilising sludge rather than
disposing of it. For example, pyrolysis to produce oil or the recovery of
specific chemicals or class of chemical are possible. This philosophy is
not new (Forster, 1973). However, for it to be accepted, two criteria are
needed: the process must work successfully on a continuous basis and
on a large scale, and the economic climate must be conducive to their
introduction. Additional constraints on disposal routes may impose the
latter criterion; the biotechnologist must provide the former.

8   Anaerobic treatment of effluents

8.1   Introduction

Although the anaerobic treatment of wastewaters could be said to have been discovered in the middle of the last century, it is only in the last decade that serious consideration has been given to it by environmental engineers. The intensity of this consideration can be seen from the proliferation of conferences dealing with this particular process. The proceedings of these conferences are available and reference should be made to them (Conference Proceedings, 1979–1983). However, despite this high degree of research activity, there are still significant problems to be overcome. These have been defined quite rigorously by the Environmental Biotechnology Working Party of the European Federation of Biotechnology (see Sidwick, 1983). The main areas of concern are:

(a) Microbiology: biochemistry and genetic aspects of the main species still require attention

(b) Start-up procedures need to be optimised so that there is a shorter 'lag time' between the commissioning of a new reactor and its being fully operational

(c) Attention needs to be paid to the optimisation of the process engineering; in particular the ancillary equipment, small-scale reactors and the nature of the support media (where used).

In other words, this is an area of considerable scope for the biotechnologist. However, the extent of the information that is still required may help to explain why the process is not, as yet, a complete success in commercial terms. At first sight, it ought to be a highly attractive process: it produces energy, it does not require a high energy input and it does not produce large amounts of sludge; and yet the number of full-scale plants that are in operation is limited. Although this chapter will examine the various types of reactor that are available and will, where possible, provide full-scale operational data, it will not have the temerity to pass judgement on the relative merits of the various reactor designs. The reason for this is basically one of economics. The most suitable reactor at any particular site will be the most cost beneficial one and this will depend not only on the loading

236

rate that can be achieved and the rate of carbon conversion but also on:

the site conditions (i.e. the space available)
the destination of the final effluent (i.e. to sewer or to stream)
the use being envisaged for the gas (i.e. gas storage/handling costs)
(see Forster & Wase, 1984)
the nature of the waste stream (i.e. whether or not it is seasonal).

8.2   Process options

For the majority of applications, fixed biomass systems are the most commonly used. The basic reactor designs have already been discussed (§§3.4.6 and 3.5.3). However, most of the basic designs have more than one variation.

8.2.1   *Anaerobic filters*

This process, as originally described by Young & McCarty (1969), operates in an upflow mode. Under these circumstances, a significant proportion of the active biomass is present not as an attached biofilm but as an unattached growth trapped within the voids. The smaller particles move upwards through the media, grow, flocculate and then settle back through the column (Young, 1983). This movement of solids, together with the evolution of gas, affects the hydraulic regime that exists within the filter, imposing a degree of mixing upon the basic plug-flow characteristics that prevail with totally clean media. This hybrid regime is difficult both to define and to model mathematically. The importance of hydraulic definition can perhaps best be highlighted by the suggestion made by Young (1983) that a more precise definition of the hydraulics could lead to improved media design, improved performance, and reduced reactor costs.

The effect of media design has been examined by Young & Dahab (1983) and Wilkie, Reynolds & Colleran (1983). This showed that whilst different designs of packing material gave quite significant differences in performance, this was a design feature rather than one related to the specific surface area (see Fig. 8.1). The alternative mode of operation is as a downflow reactor (see van den Berg & Kennedy, 1983). In this version, the biomass is present only as an attached film as any suspended growth is flushed out of the reactor with the effluent. This means that not only is it important to develop and maintain a stable film but also that the supporting media must be designed in such a way as to minimise the potential for solids accumulation. Thus a channelled arrangement is usually employed rather than the random

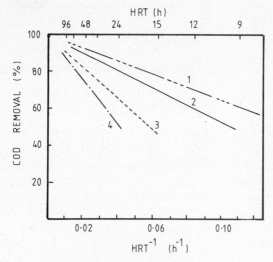

Fig. 8.1. COD removal efficiencies of anaerobic filters in relation to different types of media. (From Young & Dahab, 1982.) 1 Large modular; 2 Small modular; 3 Pall rings; 4 Spheres.

packing used in the upflow systems (Wilkie *et al.*, 1983). Because this type of filter is film-controlled, the loading rates that can be used depend on the specific surface of the packing and on its roughness.

8.2.2   *Upflow sludge blanket (USB) reactors*

Although essentially a suspended growth reactor, the USB can certainly be thought of as a fixed biomass process. The essential feature of the system is the development of a sludge blanket in which the component particles are sufficiently aggregated to withstand the hydraulic shear of the upward flowing liquid (see Fig. 3.19) without being carried upwards and out of the reactor. In addition, these shear forces must not cause the particles to break up into smaller units that could be washed out of the reactor. In other words, the sludge flocs must be structurally stable and have good settlement properties. The main point at issue is whether the particles need merely to be floccular or whether they should be granular in nature. Certainly the granular sludges have a very good settlement rate (0.012 m s^{-1}; Pette & Versprille, 1982). Thus, the typical SVI of granular sludge is 10–20 compared with a figure of 20–40 for floccular sludges (Lettinga *et al.*, 1980). The result of these settlement properties is the formation of a compact sludge bed which, for granular material, would have a solids concentration of 40–150 g l^{-1} (Lettinga *et al.*, 1980; Pette & Versprille, 1982). Nevertheless, a purely floccular bed can be operated at loading rates similar to those achieved by fully

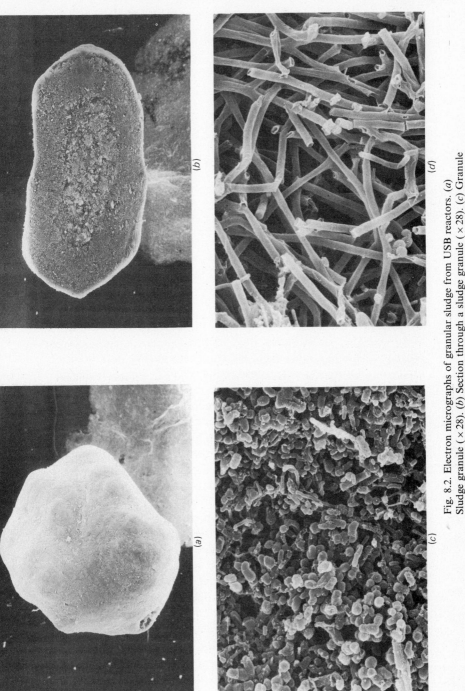

Fig. 8.2. Electron micrographs of granular sludge from USB reactors. (a) Sludge granule (×28). (b) Section through a sludge granule (×28). (c) Granule dominated by rods (×2500). (d) Granule dominated by filaments (×2500).

Table 8.1. *Elemental composition of USB granules (as measured by electron dispersive X-ray analysis)*

Concentration (%, w/w)	Source of sludge		
	1	2	3
Al	0.536	0.200	0.180
Ca	0.443	0.033	0.285
Cl	—	0.131	0.187
Cu	—	0.260	0.158
Fe	0.605	0.161	0.415
K	3.113	0.590	0.106
Mg	0.151	0.107	0.055
P	1.643	0.726	0.405
S	0.733	0.970	1.251
Si	0.764	1.120	0.762

granulated systems (i.e. up to 24 kg COD m^{-3} d^{-1}) (Alibhai & Forster, unpublished data).

The sludge granules, which can vary in size from 0.5 to 4 mm (Lettinga *et al.*, 1979), have a high volatile matter content (~ 80 per cent) and a very variable microbial composition (Fig. 8.2). Some reactors produce granules formed predominantly from rod-shaped bacteria, whilst in others filamentous forms are the predominant species (Hulshoff Pol *et al.*, 1983). Pipyn & Verstraete (1979) on the other hand have described granules with a mixed bacterial flora: rods, cocci and filaments. The floccular sludges contain a similar bacterial mixture although the large numbers of Methanothrix, which are frequently found in granular sludges, are not present. There is a sufficient similarity in the ecology of the two types of sludge to suggest that granules could be considered as 'super flocs' which have developed because of interactions with other components in the waste. In this context, calcium ions have been cited as having a significant effect (Lettinga *et al.*, 1980). However, an examination of the elemental composition of the surfaces of granular sludge from USB plants in Holland (Table 8.1) showed that calcium was not a dominant element. The significance of these results is still unclear, as is the nature of the interactions which promote granulation and the factors which determine the bacterial ecology. A more precise understanding of these points could assist in fully optimising the design, start-up and operation of this type of reactor.

The use of a gas–solids separation system in the upper part of a USB reactor is claimed to be an essential feature, whatever the settlement

Table 8.2. *Guidelines for the minimum number of inlet nozzles in a USB reactor*

Sludge type	Loading (kg COD m^{-3} d^{-1})	m^2 per nozzle
Dense flocculant (i.e. > 40 kg DS m^{-3})	< 1–2	< 1
Thin flocculant (i.e. < 40 kg DS m^{-3})	> 3	5
Granular	1–2	< 1

From Lettinga *et al.*, 1983.

characteristics of the sludge (Lettinga *et al.*, 1983). In judging whether this claim is universally true there is a need to consider the effect of loading rates (both hydraulic and organic) on the solids and the design values being used for any particular plant. An increase in the organic loading rate will result in increased gas production, a lowering of the floc density (due to occluded gas) and a greater tendency for flotation (due to attached bubbles). The net result will be a greater probability of solids carry-over. This will be exacerbated at the higher hydraulic loading rates. However, before accepting the necessity for a gas–solids separator, there is a need to judge whether this carry-out will cause an intolerable depletion of the sludge solids and to what extent solids are acceptable in the final effluent. Certainly the incorporation of a separation system will increase the capital cost of a reactor. The most logical approach is therefore that, for each specific application, an economic comparison should be made of the various options below:

Use high loading rates and install an internal separator

Design the reactor with an external solids separation system (i.e. flotation or settlement)

Operate at lower loading rates without solids separation.

The operation of a USB reactor will be affected by the degree of contacting of the sludge solids with the substrate. To a certain extent, this will be enhanced by the mixing which is induced within the bed by gas evolution. However, to maintain high loading rates without any diminution in performance, attention must be paid to the inlet distribution system. The review by Lettinga and his co-workers (1983) offers some suggestions as to the required number of feed inlet points for optimal operation (Table 8.2).

Table 8.3. *Factors of importance in the selection of the media for expanded/ fluidised bed reactors*

Microscopic pore size
Macro-pore sizes
Porosity
Specific area
Density
Durability
Cost

8.2.3   *Anaerobic expanded beds*

There are two versions of this type of reactor: the expanded bed and the fully fluidised bed. Both of them use an inert medium (e.g. sand, anthracite) which supports a film growth of the active biomass. It is important therefore that the medium be selected with a proper regard to this role. The main factors involved in media selection are summarised in Table 8.3. However, it must be recognised that the full significance of the physical properties of the media in relation to the operational characteristics is not fully understood. For example, what type of surface gives the most rapid 'start-up' and is this necessarily the type of surface to give long term stability to the film? The second critical aspect in the operation of this type of reactor is the distribution of the influent/recycle flow (Jewell, 1982). This must be arranged so as to ensure a completely even expansion of the bed. As well as being a critical aspect, this requirement for a uniformity of flow (together with the high rates of flow that are needed) is a limiting factor due to the high capital cost involved (van den Berg & Kennedy, 1983). The biofilm formed in these reactors tends to be thin and dense due to the high liquid velocities that are used. Nevertheless there is a need for media to be removed from the reactor periodically so that biomass can be separated and the clean support media can be returned to the reactor (see Sutton & Evans, 1983). Techniques for doing this have already been described (§3.4.5).

8.2.4   *Miscellaneous processes*

One of the major problems with suspended growth reactors is the solids/liquid separation stage which is necessary to ensure a sufficiently high rate of solids recycle. One way of achieving this is the use of ultrafiltration membranes to separate the treated effluent from sludge solids. In the process patented by Dorr–Oliver, the synthetic membranes are attached to polyethylene plates and used, in units of 20,

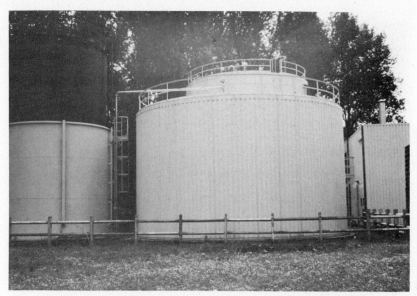

Fig. 8.3. Two-phase digestion plant (by courtesy of Dunlop Bioprocesses Ltd).

in the form of a cartridge (see Sutton & Evans, 1983). Although this concept has been evaluated at pilot-scale level, the potential, reliability and operational cost of this membrane separation system over an extended period of full-scale use have still to be determined.

The current interest in anaerobic digestion has led to the development of many other different designs of reactor. However, these designs tend to be for specific applications and, as such, are of insufficient interest to merit discussion in this very limited review of anaerobic treatment. Readers are therefore referred to the major conference proceedings of the last five years.

8.2.5 Two-phase digestion

The reactors described so far have been considered as single phase systems; that is to say, with the hydrolytic, acetogenic and methanogenic species working in the same reactor. However, anaerobic digestion can be operated in a two-phase configuration with separate reactors for acid formation and methane generation (Ghosh & Klass, 1978; Cohen, 1983) (Fig. 8.3). The logic for separating the processes is to enable each one to be operated under optimal environmental conditions thus enabling the overall through-put to be increased. Any type of anaerobic reactor (i.e. filter, expanded bed, USB) can be operated in this manner and certainly the concept has its enthusiasts. However, there are also a number of workers who would urge caution.

Van den Berg & Kennedy (1983), for example, whilst accepting that the loading rate on the methanogenic stage can be increased in this way, and the acid-forming reactor made quite compact, note that the overall loading is unlikely to be increased. In addition, they suggest that the cost of a two-phase system would be greater because of the need for additional pumps, valves and even pH control. Their conclusions are that whilst the two-phase concept offers some advantage in overall process control, its general application is likely to be limited. Similar conclusions were reached by Cohen (1983). The only real advantage of two-phase operation with soluble wastes, as seen by Lettinga *et al.* (1983), is that inhibitory compounds (e.g. SO_3^{2-}) could be eliminated in the acidogenic reactor. Nevertheless, as will be shown later, full-scale plants with this configuration are being used to treat industrial wastes.

8.3   Performance

8.3.1   *Scale-up*

To date, much of the work done on the evaluation of anaerobic reactors has used laboratory or pilot-scale systems. The transition to full-scale units requires that rational design criteria for scale-up be developed (Ross & Smollen, 1982). The dangers of using inadequate criteria can be judged from the experiences reported by Ross and his co-workers (1981) (see Table 8.4).

8.3.2   *Start-up*

The rate at which the various types of reactor can be 'started-up' varies with the design (see van den Berg & Kennedy, 1983). However, it has been suggested that the published information about start-up is less than adequate (Brunetti *et al.*, 1983). Because of this, Brunetti *et al.* have provided a review of the conditions which affect the start-up of USB reactors. Their general conclusions were that start-up could take 1–3 months and that the best criteria were those recommended by Lettinga *et al.* (1979). These are similar to the conditions suggested for the start-up of fixed film reactors (Salkinoja-Salonen *et al.*, 1983). Also, in considering start-up there is no clear consensus as to when a unit is

Table 8.4. *The effect on the volumetric loading rate of using the sludge concentration as a scale-up factor*

Reactor size (m³)	0.007	6.3	954
Loading rate (kg COD m⁻³ d⁻¹)	17.0	7.1	3.0

From Ross *et al.*, 1981.

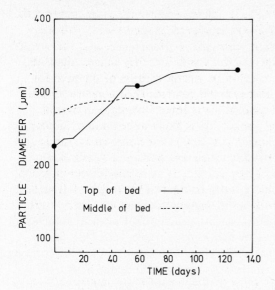

These size measurements were made

using a pre-calibrated microscope

linked to a video system. The data

are average values

Fig. 8.4. Biofilm growth at the top and middle of an expanded bed reactor.

fully 'started'. This problem can be highlighted by examining data obtained from an expanded bed reactor (Rockey & Forster, unpublished data). These show that as far as gas production and COD removal were concerned, the reactor had appeared to have reached steady-state and that start-up was complete. However, as the loading rates were gradually increased a discontinuity in the loading rate/performance curve occurred, indicating that additional biofilm could become available and achieve additional treatment. The potential for further growth can be demonstrated from the different rates of film growth at different parts of the bed (Fig. 8.4). It would seem essential therefore that 'start-up' be defined, in some way, so that realistic correlations can be made and the necessary criteria defined without ambiguity.

8.3.3 *Performance criteria*

There are several factors that can be used to assess or compare the performance of anaerobic reactors:

(a) COD removal
(b) loading rates (either in terms of the sludge, kg COD kg^{-1} VSS d^{-1}, or the reactor volume, kg COD m^{-3} d^{-1})
(c) gas yield (based on the total gas production or on methane, m^3 kg^{-1} COD removed d^{-1})
(d) hydraulic retention time.

Of these, two require comment. Loading rates require care in their definition. In the case of fixed film reactors, the sludge loading rate (kg COD kg^{-1} biomass d^{-1}) may be difficult to calculate since it is not easy to obtain a precise figure for the weight of biomass that is present. On the other hand, the volumetric loading rate (kg COD m^{-3} d^{-1}) is always easy to calculate. However, its calculation is open to ambiguity since different volumes may be used. For example, with USB and expanded bed reactors, should the volume be taken as the total working volume of the digester or as the volume occupied by the active biomass? As yet no agreement has been reached as to which is the more correct, and although a recent attempt to standardise analytical methods and operational parameters, such as rates (Colin *et al.*, 1983), has specified that rates should be expressed 'per unit working volume', no suggestions were offered as to what constituted the 'working volume'. Until this is done, anomalous loading rates will continue to be reported. Comparisons must therefore be made with care.

Although gas yields are reported in terms of either the methane or the total gas, it can be argued that the former is the more appropriate. This is because when the total gas production is used, there must always be some uncertainty as to how much carbon dioxide has not been measured due to absorption. According to the composition of the waste being treated, this absorption can be as high as 100 per cent (Godwin, Wase & Forster, 1982). Gas yields based on methane should be judged against the theoretical yield of 0.35 m^3 of methane per kg of COD removed.

8.3.4   *Operational performance*

Although there is a large amount of data available in the literature (see Conference Proceedings, 1979–1983) describing the performance of laboratory and pilot-scale plants, the data for full-scale is very limited. Indeed, there are conflicting opinions as to the number of plants in operation. Verrier, Moletta & Albagnac (1983) report that within the European Community there are only 39 reactors treating food/food processing wastes. On a world-wide basis, 29–39 USB plants have been reported (BV Machinefabriek Spaans; Esmil; personal communications). Filter systems do not appear to be a popular option;

Table 8.5. *Performance data for full-scale anaerobic reactors*

Process	Loading rate (kg COD m^{-3} d^{-1})	Gas yield (m^3 kg^{-1} ΔCOD)	Retention time (h)	COD removal (%)	Volume (m^3)
Anaerobic filter					
Witt *et al.*, 1979	7.53	0.38	30	60.3	1020[a]
Badger Co. Inc.	9.50	0.37	33	85	5700
Taylor & Burm, 1973	9.52	—	22	63.8	453[a]
Bedogni *et al.*, 1983	22.2	> 0.27	22	> 55	1500[a]
Szendrey, 1983	3.79	0.33	199	71	13254
USB					
Pette & Versprille, 1982	⎧ 12.0	0.38	4	70	800
	⎪ 12.0	0.33	4.8	75	1300
	⎨ 16.5	0.30	5.7	75	1425
	⎩ 5.0	0.33	20	75	500
Maaskant & Zeevalkink, 1983	7.5	—	6	88	400
B.V. Machinefabriek Spaans	8.2	0.32	9	93	750
Contact digesters					
Seyfried *et al.*, 1983	1.65	0.25	175	88	3500
Parker & Lyons, 1983	11.3	0.27	166	70	1200
	8.4	0.31	120	75	1200
Morfaux *et al.*, 1982	3.2	0.27	161	95	5000
	3.0	0.26	127	95	5000

[a] Void volume.

Table 8.6. *Performance data for full-scale USB reactors*

Plant	Gottem[a]	Naveau[a]	Steenhuffel[c]
Loading rate (kg m^{-3} d^{-1})	15–34	17–20	10–15[d]
Reactor volume (m^3)	12[b]	360[b]	320[d]
Influent COD (mg l^{-1})	6000–9500	4000–5000	5000
Effluent COD (mg l^{-1})	900–1300	290–600	500
Average removal (%)	86	90	90
Gas production (m^3 d^{-1})	125–280	2160–3600	1300–2000
Methane content (%)	65–75	80–85	—

[a] By courtesy of Biotim SA.
[b] 'Active' volume.
[c] By courtesy of Dunlop Bioprocesses.
[d] Based on the second stage methanogenic reactor.

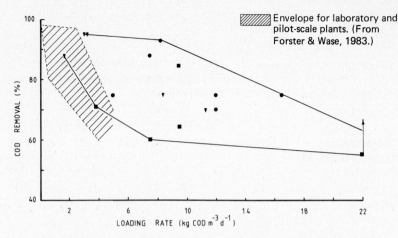

Fig. 8.5. COD removal efficiencies of full-scale plants in relation to the organic loading rate.

Young (1983) lists only six although others are being designed or constructed (Hall, 1983). Expanded bed systems are either small (1–3 m³) or merely at the design/construction stage. However, a report by Nyns, Naveau & Demuynck (1983) suggests that the digester capacity available in industry within Switzerland and the European Community is 174000 m³, equivalent to a significantly higher number of reactors than suggested by other reports.

The data that are presented in Tables 8.5 and 8.6 are typical of the performances that can be achieved by the various designs of anaerobic reactor. These show that:

(a) the amount of methane gas that is produced is usually close to the theoretical volume. This is something which frequently is not demonstrated with laboratory and pilot-scale plants (see Forster & Wase, 1983). It must also be noted that the yields which appear to exceed the theoretical figure do so because average values have been taken for the components used in calculating the yield figures (*cave media*).

(b) the modern anaerobic reactor is capable of high COD removal efficiencies often at high loading rates and short retention times.

(c) the performance envelope for removal efficiency/loading rate (Fig. 8.5) is similar in shape to that reported for laboratory and pilot-plants (Forster & Wase, 1983). However, the full-scale data extend over a much wider range of loading rates. This is a further emphasis of the need to develop sound scale-up procedures.

8.3.5   *Process stability*

The stability of these anaerobic processes can be considered in terms of the way in which the chemical environment influences the microbial flora. In other words, in terms of the balance and availability of nutrients and the effect of toxic compounds.

The chemicals which are normally considered in assessing the nutritional balance are carbon, nitrogen and phosphorus. As far as these elements are concerned, anaerobic processes are less demanding than their aerobic counterparts. Huss (1977) quotes a BOD:N:P ratio of 100:0.5:0.1 whilst Henze & Harremoës (1983) show that the COD:N:P can vary from 42:0.7:0.1 (at the higher loading rates) to about 150:0.7:0.1. Thus, the need for (and cost of) supplementing the feedstocks is much less. Some trace elements are also necessary, for example the divalent ions of iron, nickel, magnesium, cobalt and barium (see Henze & Harremoës, 1983). The only other element which has been reported as having any significant effect on process stability is calcium, the role of which in promoting sludge pelletisation in USB reactors has already been discussed.

The effect of toxic substances has been examined by a number of researchers, the work of whom has been reviewed by Speece & Parkin (1983) and by Henze & Harremoës (1983). Apart from the obvious and more usual toxic agents (e.g. chlorinated hydrocarbons, heavy metals, cyanides), two compounds can cause a serious reduction in gas production. These are sulphide and ammonia. Both of these compounds can either be present in the feedstock or, as is more often the case, be formed by the anaerobic reactions. However, in both cases the concentrations which have been reported as starting to cause inhibition vary quite widely. This appears to depend on the degree to which the microbial flora are acclimatised, the pH at which the reactor is operating and even the rate at which gas is evolved from the liquors. The minimum inhibitory concentrations cited are: ammonia – 0.4–14 g l^{-1}; sulphide – 50 mg l^{-1} – 1 g l^{-1}.

Reactors can recover from this type of inhibition once the toxic agent is removed or reduced in concentration although the rate of recovery does depend on the concentration of the inhibitor that was originally present. One industrial concern would appear to have overcome the problem of sulphide generation/inhibition during the treatment of sulphate-rich wastes (Anderson, Donnelly & McKeown, 1984). As described, the process uses a 'microbial association' which 'maximises the formation of methane in the presence of sulphate'. However, the same report mentions a 'control' procedure (details of which were not disclosed) which suggests that something other than microbial manipulation is being used. Until these details are made public,

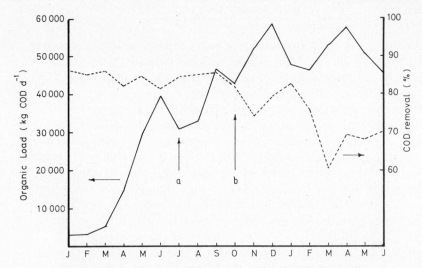

Fig. 8.6. Performance characteristics of the Bacardi Corporation filter. (From Szendrey, 1983.) (*a*) Distillery shut-down for three weeks. (*b*) Distillery shut-down for two weeks.

sulphide poisoning will have to be controlled by the more conventional techniques of:

> sulphide stripping from the gas
> dilution of the feedstock
> *in situ* precipitation of metal sulphides.

Process stability can also be considered in terms of the ability of a reactor to re-start rapidly after a period of shut-down. This is a facility that has always been claimed for anaerobic digesters. The data provided by the Bacardi filter (Szendrey, 1983; Fig. 8.6) show just how true this claim is.

8.4   Post-digestion processes

Although anaerobic reactors can remove carbonaceous pollutants very efficiently, the residual BOD (or COD) will be appreciable because of the high concentrations in the original feed-stock. If the effluent is being discharged to sewer the level of this residue may be unimportant. However, the discharge consent conditions (be they to sewer or stream) may require that even more BOD is removed. This is an aspect of treatment that is not often considered. There would appear to be no reason why this residual organic matter cannot be degraded by conventional aerobic reactors (see Chapter 3) and indeed anaerobic and aerobic systems have been combined in the Anamet process (Fig. 8.7).

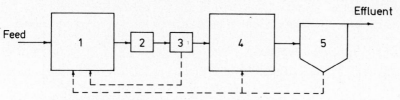

Fig. 8.7. Schematic diagram of the Anamet process.

Table 8.7. *Performance of an Anamet plant*

	1979	1980
Design flow (m³ d⁻¹)		2160
Design load (kg BOD d⁻¹)		9800
COD reduction (%)		
Anaerobic stage	79	92
Aerobic stage	83	65
Overall	97	97
Final COD (mg l⁻¹)	230	216
Final BOD (mg l⁻¹)	122	21

From Huss, 1982.

Since 1972, some 25 plants based on this principle have been built or are under construction, the largest operational one having a capacity of 38 tons BOD d^{-1} (Huss, 1982). The effectiveness of the Anamet combination can be seen from the data obtained for the treatment of wastewater from the processing of sugar beet during the three month campaign period (Huss, 1982) (Table 8.7). The anaerobic reactor is a well-mixed contact digester and can be operated as an acidogenic/methanogenic system or merely as a methanogenic process. In the latter case, acidification is achieved in an anaerobic storage lagoon (Shore, Broughton & Bumstead, 1984).

Anaerobic processes convert the majority of the organic nitrogenous material in the feed to ammonia (or ammonium ions). In many cases, this will also have to be removed or oxidised. The techniques that are envisaged for this include biological nitrification (and de-nitrification if necessary) and stripping (using either air or steam) (Berends, 1983). In the latter case, the ammonia can then be recovered by absorption, using sulphuric acid, nitric acid or urea.

8.5 Utilisation of solid substrates

Solid substrates can be used to produce biogas just as effectively as a feed-stock which is predominantly soluble. The solids which have been used in this way can be considered in three categories: agricultural wastes; land-fill material; and biomass grown for this specific purpose.

8.5.1   *Agricultural wastes*

Agricultural wastes (usually animal excreta in the form of a slurry) have received most attention (see Hobson, Bousfield & Summers, 1981). The use of this type of digestion is not new. However, the development of intensive farming techniques, coupled with an increased awareness of environmental pollution and energy costs, has resulted in considerable attention being focussed on digestion processes. The degree of this interest can be seen from the fact that within Switzerland and the countries of the European Community, 95000 m³ of digester capacity was installed between 1978 and 1983 for the treatment of farm wastes (Nyns *et al.*, 1983), and in Italy alone there are more than 60 plants treating animal wastes. Commercialisation of this aspect of anaerobic digestion is also taking place in North America (Hashimoto, 1983).

The type of reactor most suited for the digestion of farm wastes is the simple stirred tank system (Hobson, 1984), although anaerobic filters have been used for pig slurries (Colleran *et al.*, 1983). For the contact digesters, plug-flow is the preferred regime (Stafford & Etheridge, 1982). The retention times that are necessary depend on the nature of the waste being treated, but typically they would range from 14–20 days with the corresponding loading rates ranging from 4–7 kg VS m⁻³ d⁻¹ (Hashimoto, 1983). Apart from possible difficulties with solids handling (i.e. the delivery of feed to the digester, mixing the digester contents and the removal of the digested material), one of the main problems is the potential for ammonia toxicity (particularly with pig slurry).

For the concept of digestion to succeed in the farming industry, the process must be cost beneficial. The assessment of costs and benefits is an exercise fraught with potential hazards. For example, if the biogas is being used to generate electricity what value should be given to that electricity – the present value or a projected value? In addition, factors such as the savings in slurry handling costs and the fertiliser value of the digested material must be considered (see Stafford & Etheridge, 1982; Hashimoto, 1983). In other words, each case must be considered as a unique situation and costed as such.

8.5.2   *Biogas from land-fill sites*

The biological processes necessary for the stabilisation of the organic matter in a land-fill site generate methane. One estimate of the amount of gas that could be recovered from these sources, if *all* the sites in the UK were suitable, was 8×10^8 m³ year⁻¹ (equivalent to some 2000 tonnes of coal per day) (Campbell, 1983). However, it must be recognised that many sites are either too small, contain (or receive) unsuitable wastes, or are too remote. Nevertheless, the exploitation of land-fill gas is a definite possibility and in the UK, North America and Europe demonstration and feasibility studies are being undertaken. The major challenges in this area relate to site management so that the gas yields can be maximised. This could involve adopting new philosophies about choosing the site, filling the site, and selecting (and even supplementing) the material placed in the site. In other words moving from a dumping philosophy (land-fill) to one of reclamation (biofill) (Richards, 1983).

8.5.3 *Biogas crops*

Methane can also be produced from crops grown specifically for this purpose or from crop residuals. The latter category includes unwanted leaves and stalks (e.g. from root vegetables or peas and beans) and possibly even pulverised timber residues. The crops grown specifically for conversion range from the water hyacinth to algae. The main criterion for success is that the energy expended in their growth, harvesting and preparation should not exceed the energy recovered in the form of biogas (Stewart, Badger & Bogue, 1982).

8.6 **Gas utilisation**

Until relatively recently, biogas has invariably been thought of as an asset, and has been costed as such in economic appraisals without much thought of the cost entailed in realising the energy potential. The biogas generated by anaerobic reactors, which typically will have a calorific value of around 24 MJ m^{-3}, can:

> be burnt to produce heat
> be burnt to generate electricity
> fuel vehicles
> supply energy to a National Grid (either as gas or electricity).

However, each of these possible routes can require some intermediate processing. At the very least, storage is required, whilst the most sophisticated treatment requires cleaning and even compression. The cost of these processes must also be considered and readers are therefore referred to specialist reports for specific applications, techniques and costing methods (e.g. Hashimoto & Chen, 1980; Sullivan, Petters & Ostrovski, 1981; Stewart *et al.*, 1982; Meynell, 1983; ADAS, 1982; Henrich & Phillips, 1983).

8.7   Conclusions

Anaerobic digestion is now an established process both for reducing pollution and producing energy. However, its commercial application is currently restricted to a limited number of countries. Some of the reasons for this have been discussed by Hashimoto (1983) and by Nyns and his co-workers (1983). Other points have been discussed in this chapter (e.g. the need for a better understanding of some of the biochemistry and of the physico-chemical interactions which govern attachment, flocculation and thus reactor design and operation). It could thus be argued that the full commercial realisation of the potential of anaerobic digestion is the biggest challenge currently facing the biotechnologist involved in wastewater treatment and environmental control. However, it must be remembered that, because of the explosive nature of methane/air mixtures, this challenge must be answered within the confines of strict safety limits (Anon., 1982).

9 Disinfection

9.1 Introduction

In considering any form of disinfection it must be realised that absolute sterility is only approached asymptotically, as microbial inactivation is dependent not only on the disinfection techniques being used but also on the number of microbes which are present in the system. Thus, the number of microbes which remain after any given time (N_t) is usually determined by:

$$N_t = N_0 \, e^{-kt}$$

where $N_0 = $ initial number, $t = $ contact time; $k = $ rate constant. However, in the case of the chlorination of effluents, the empirical relationship

$$N_{t_2} = N_{t_1} \left[\frac{t_2}{t_1} \right]^m$$

(where m is a constant) has been found to be more applicable (White, 1972). This means therefore that in practice, dilution and dispersion by the receiving waters, in addition to the action of the disinfectant, must be relied upon to achieve the low microbial concentrations required by the standards outlined in §9.3.4.

There are, at present, essentially only two biocidal agents that are widely used for the treatment of either raw or treated sewage (e.g. Venosa, 1983). These are chlorine (or sodium hypochlorite) and ozone, the former being the more commonly used chemical. Both chemicals rely on their oxidising properties (Table 9.1) to effect sterilisation, a comparative assessment of which is shown in Table 9.2. Chlorine is thought to act on the sulphydryl groups of one of the bacterial enzymes, triose phosphate dehydrogenase; however the mechanism of disinfection by ozone, despite intensive investigations, is still open to question (Venosa, 1972). The mode of attack on viruses, for both agents, has been summarised by Sproul, Pfister & Kim, 1982.

Table 9.1. *Oxidative properties of sterilising agents measured in terms of their oxidation–reduction potential*

Sterilant	Oxidation potential (volts)
O_3	-2.07
HOCl	-1.49
Cl_2	-1.36
NH_2Cl	-0.75

From Kinman, 1972.

Table 9.2. *Concentrations ($mg\ l^{-1}$) of disinfectant required to inactivate 99% of the listed organisms within 10 minutes*

Disinfectant	Enteric bacteria	Viruses	Bacterial spores
O_3	0.001	0.10	0.2
HOCl	0.02	0.40	10
OCl^-	2	> 20	> 1000
NH_2Cl	5	100	400
Free Cl_2 (pH 7.5)	0.04	0.8	20

9.2   Use of ozone

9.2.1   *General description*

Ozone, which is an allotropic form of oxygen, is produced when air or oxygen is subjected to either an electrical discharge or ultra-violet irradiation. It is important that the feed gases for either technique should be dry (i.e. dew-point less than $-50\ °C$), since water vapour reduces the ozone yield. The basic components of an ozonolysis unit are shown in Figs. 9.1 and 9.2 and the basic operating parameters in Table 9.3. One of the main problems with the use of ozone is the dosing technique. Dissolution of the gas is difficult and it is usual therefore to form what amounts to a gas/water emulsion by creating a large number of very small bubbles either by using porous ceramic diffusers, venturi injectors or by injecting the ozone-rich air through a propellor set just below the surface of the water to be treated. In this way, the maximum mass transfer across the gas/water interface is obtained. The most commonly used modes of operation are (a) diffusers which usually operate on a counter current flow basis with a liquid depth of 4.5–6 m and a contact time of 5–15 minutes, (b) 'partial injection' in which a high pressure flow of some of the liquid is used to

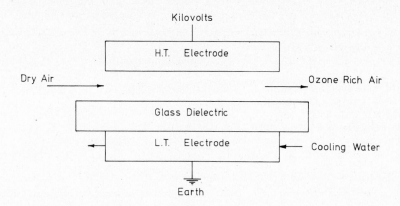

Factors affecting ozone production

Dryness of air   Electrical power & frequency
Rate of flow of air   Electrode dimensions
Pressure of air   Width of discharge gap
         Temperature

Fig. 9.1. Schematic diagram of an ozonolysis unit.

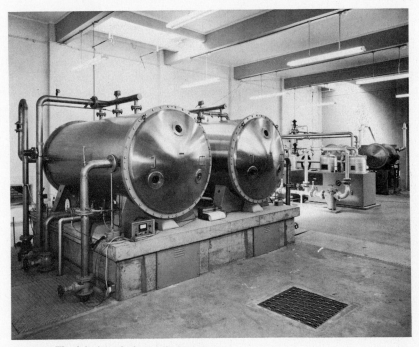

Fig. 9.2. A typical ozonolysis system.

Table 9.3. *Typical operation parameters for an ozonolysis unit*

Operating power (kv)	5–25
Electrode material	Aluminium or stainless steel
Dielectric material	Borosilicate glass
Yield (g O_3 m^{-3} air used)	15–25
Output (g O_3 h^{-1})	20–45
Power utilisation (Wh g O_3^{-1})	15–18

Table 9.4. *Ozone dosages for sewage treatment*

Type of wastewater	Objective	Dose (mg l^{-1})	Contact time (min)
Secondary effluent	Virus destruction	15	5
Secondary effluent	1000 coliforms 100 ml^{-1}	5	1
Tertiary effluent	Complete bacterial disinfection	5	1.6
Primary wastewater ⎱ Storm water overflow ⎰	Treatment	> 50	Not reported

From McCarthy & Smith, 1974.

produce an ozone-rich 'solution' which is then mixed with the rest of the liquid to be treated, and (c) 'total injection' in which all of the liquid flow is passed through the injector. In all cases the vented gases which still contain some ozone can be recycled through the ozoniser. However, if this is done, the gases must be dried before further treatment.

9.2.2 *Operational data*

The role of ozone in the disinfection of domestic wastewater has been reviewed recently by Rice, Evison & Robson (1981). In the UK, the main attention for the use of ozone has been focussed on tertiary treatments. In this type of usage not only is the microbial population decreased, but also there have been reductions both in BOD and COD (e.g. Majumdar & Sproul, 1974). In the case of effluents containing phenols and cyanides, reduction in the concentration of both these constituents has also been found (e.g. Ogden, 1970; Joshi & Shambaugh, 1982). In general however, ozone could be applied to wastewater at any stage of its treatment, although this would of course affect the dosages required (Table 9.4). Nebel *et al.* (1972) found that the following ozone dosages were required: (a) 10–100 mg l^{-1} for the treatment of raw sewage and storm water overflows, and (b) about

Table 9.5. *A comparison of the costs and performances of disinfectants used for the control of* Salmonella *in a poultry processing effluent*

| Disinfectant | Costs (Canadian $ m^{-3}, 1977 basis) | | Dose (mg l^{-1}) | Time (min) | Control effect (% of time) |
	Capital	Operating			
Chlorination/de-chlorination	9.43	0.008	10	45	100
Ozone	57.02	0.014	30	60	30

From Hrudey, 1984.

50 mg l^{-1} to convert secondary effluents to water of a potable quality. Majumdar, Ceckler & Sproul (1973) found that both the time of contact and the concentrations of the ozone were important factors in determining the rate at which polio viruses were inactivated. As a result of their work, two relationships were suggested:

$$Ct = 0.10\,(S)^{-1.12} \quad \text{when } C < 1.0 \text{ mg l}^{-1}$$
$$Ct = 0.13\,(S)^{-0.36} \quad \text{when } C > 1.0 \text{ mg l}^{-1}$$

where, C = concentration of ozone, in mg l^{-1}, t = time of contact, in minutes, and S = surviving fraction of virus particles.

One of the strongest criticisms against the use of ozone is its operational cost. The cost data obtained during a North American study have been summarised by Hrudey (1984) and are shown in Table 9.5. However, it has been claimed (Ogden, 1970) that the cost of chlorination is not expected to be reduced significantly in the foreseeable future, whereas many ozone equipment manufacturers predict that the overall cost of ozonolysis can be reduced. If these predictions are correct, an increased use of ozone as a disinfectant for untreated domestic effluents may well be seen.

The effectiveness of ozone for reducing bacterial numbers can be seen from an examination of data from both pilot and full-scale plants. However, direct comparisons between the data are not possible because (a) different targets were used for the ultimate bacterial concentrations, and (b) in some cases the ozone concentrations used were discussed as the applied dosage and in others as the absorbed dose. Nevertheless, the data do show that ozone can reduce bacterial numbers significantly using only short contact times. For example, Rakness & Hegg (1980) describe the use of ozone for the tertiary treatment of effluent from a works whose design flow-rate was 5680 m^3 d^{-1}. The ozonolysis unit was designed to use air at a dew-point of -51 °C and a pressure of 41–103 kN m^{-2}. the air flow-rate being 118 m^3 h^{-1}. This gave a maximum rate of ozone production of 1.08 kg h^{-1}. The contact tank was 3.66 m deep and was baffled to give a serpentine flow pattern and a retention time of 14 minutes at the design flow. Ozone was diffused into the wastewater through porous stone diffusors at the bottom of the tank. Although a number of commissioning problems occurred, Rakness & Hegg report that the target concentration of less than 200 faecal coliforms per 100 ml was achieved, on average, using applied ozone dosages of 7 mg ml^{-1}. The data reported by Stover & Jarnis (1981) for a 216 m^3 d^{-1} pilot-study show an even better performance, with a concentration of 70 total coliforms per 100 ml being achieved with an absorbed dose of 3 mg ozone l^{-1}. However, both Leeuwen & Prinsloo (1980) and Legeron (1982) report performance figures which are more comparable with those of Rakness & Hegg.

9.3.   Use of chlorine
9.3.1   *General description*

The chemistry of the disinfectant action of chlorine, which is the more commonly used gas, is more complex than that of ozone. This is further complicated by the reactions which can occur between chlorine and some of the components (particularly nitrogenous compounds) of sewage. Three distinct phases, all of which are well documented, can be recognised (Culp, 1974; Irving & Solbe, 1980):

(a) The formation of hypochlorous acid
(b) The dissociation of hypochlorous acid
(c) The formation of chloramines.

All the end products from these reactions have biocidal properties. Therefore, depending on the characteristics of the water being treated (i.e. pH, amount and form of nitrogen compounds), the rate and the degree of disinfection as well as the basic mechanism of inactivation can vary. For example, Whitlock (1953) has reported that 25 times more chloramine than free chlorine was required to obtain a 100 per cent kill of the test bacterium *Eberthella typhosa* in the same exposure time, indicating that hypochlorous acid was the predominant sterilising agent. However, White (1974a) states that the formation of chloramines precedes any reaction with bacteria and that the transient presence of hypochlorous acid is of no significance. Whatever the outcome of this argument, chlorine is used widely and effectively and, as a result, the design of chlorination equipment (i.e. flow regulation, materials of construction) is well established (e.g. White, 1972). However, there are several criteria which must be met to optimise this effectiveness. These have been well described by White (1974b) and more recently by Geisser, Garver & Murphy (1979) and Longley, Moore & Sorber (1982). The main points are summarised in Table 9.6. This shows that

Table 9.6. *Operational parameters that affect chlorination*

pH	No major effect but in some cases sterilisation improves with acidity since more dichloramine is formed
Mixing	Good mixing is essential if excessive chlorine doses are to be avoided. Turbulence represented by a Reynolds Number of 10^4 is suggested
Contact time	In most cases the contact time should be at least 30 minutes, at peak dry weather flow
Contact chamber	Should be designed for easy cleaning to prevent an excessive build-up of solids
Chlorine residue	The maintenance of a chlorine residue of 3–4 mg l^{-1} is the best control parameter although this figure may have to be increased if high chlorine demand trade wastes are present

From White, 1974*b*.

the main features that affect the efficiency of chlorination are mixing and contact time, whilst the best parameter for controlling the overall performance is the chlorine residue. The fact that mixing is so critical can be seen from the mathematical model which was developed by Collins, Selleck & White (1971) and relates the initial coliform concentration to the chlorine residue and the contact time. This is:

$$N_t = N_0 (1 + 0.23 \ Ct)^{-3}$$

where C = total chlorine residue and t = contact time, in minutes.

It can be seen from this that when the initial microbial count is high it is essential that the mixing of the chlorine solution and the liquid to be treated be very good, particularly when miscellaneous debris can be expected to act as a screen for the bacteria. The hydraulic regime that optimises the effectiveness of the chlorine, and the cost of the operation, is one which approximates to plug-flow conditions (Hart & Vogiatzis, 1982; Sepp, 1981).

9.3.2 *Operational data*

Chlorine can be taken from storage containers either as a gas or a liquid. The liquid phase is used when the rate of utilisation is such that gas phase operation is impractical (e.g. the maximum rate of gas withdrawal from ton cylinders is approximately 180 kg d^{-1}). The use of liquid chlorine means that an evaporator must be incorporated into the system before the chlorinator (Fig. 9.3). This enables an accurate and safe metering of the gas to be made since the metering is done under the vacuum which is created by the injector system producing the chlorine solution. The details of all these pieces of equipment are well

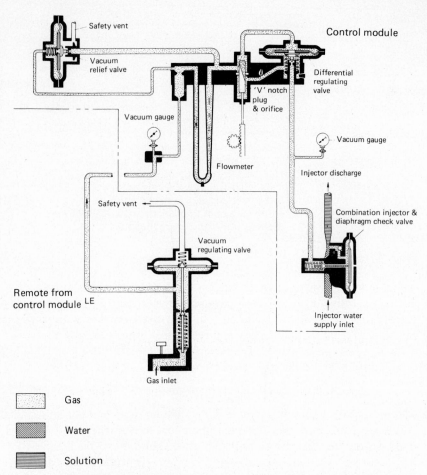

Fig. 9.3. Typical flow diagram for a chlorine injector (by courtesy of Wallace & Tiernan Ltd).

documented (e.g. White, 1972). The maximum concentration of chlorine in the solution produced by the injector is 3500 mg l⁻¹. This solution must then be mixed with the wastewater and a variety of mixing devices have been described previously (Benzina, Lin & Wang, 1974; Hart & Vogiatzis, 1982). These range from mechanical mixing devices fitted with baffles to the use of the hydraulic jump (Fig. 9.4). One disadvantage of the latter system is that there can be a longitudinal shift of the jump and also a variation in the submergence of the diffuser. White (1974a) has assessed the power requirements for both these systems and has estimated that they are comparable up to flows of about 10⁵ m³ day⁻¹. With flows in excess of this figure more energy will be required for mechanical mixing.

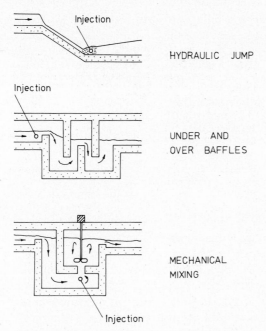

Fig. 9.4. Systems for mixing chlorine solutions and sewage.

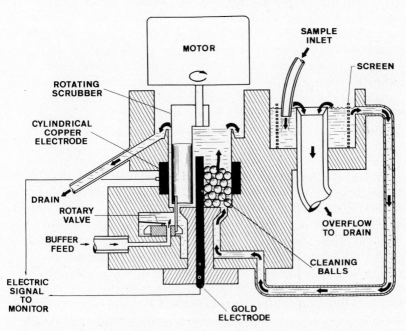

Fig. 9.5. Electrode system for measuring chlorine residuals (by courtesy of Capital Controls Ltd).

Table 9.7. *Typical chlorine dosages for various types of wastewater*

Source	Type of treatment	Chlorine dose (mg l^{-1})	Contact time (mins)
White, 1974*b*	Primary	8–10	30
White, 1974*b*	Activated sludge	13–15	30
White, 1974*b*	High-rate biofilter	8–10	30
Bradley, 1973	Raw sewage	6–24	15
Bradley, 1973	Settled sewage	3–18	15
Bradley, 1973	Activated sludge	3–9	15
Whitlock, 1953	Raw sewage	10–13	30

The use of chlorine residual as the most effective control system has already been mentioned. In wastewater plants the technique which is most commonly used for measuring the chlorine residual is amperometric. A typical cell (Fig. 9.5) consists of two electrodes mounted coaxially, a reference electrode of platinum or gold and a measuring electrode of copper. Free chlorine is measured directly but the measurement of combined chlorine requires the addition of potassium iodide. This produces free iodine quantitatively. The presence of either halogen in the flow-through cell produces a small current which is proportional to the halogen concentrations. Fouling of the electrode surfaces is prevented by the circulation of an abrasive and the pH is controlled, by the addition of a buffer solution, between 4 and 4.5. Temperature compensation can also be provided. There are essentially two variations which can be used: one in which the analyser system provides control for both the change in flow rate and the chlorine demand, or one in which the control apparatus receives independent signals from the flow measuring device and the residual analyser. This latter system is preferable because it can deal more effectively with sudden changes in flow. For optimal operation of a control system the sample for the analyser should be taken down-stream of the chloride mixing device within 30 seconds of the chloride application under average flow conditions. The level at which the control is set will depend on the nature of the effluent but the optimum value is quoted as being between 3 and 4 mg l^{-1} with a contact time of 30 minutes (White, 1974*b*). Values of the chlorine dosages which have been used in practice are shown in Table 9.7.

9.3.3   *Electrolytic generation*

In the majority of cases where chlorine is used to sterilise raw or final effluents, it is brought to the site. However, it is possible in the case of coastal discharges to generate chlorine by the electrolysis of sea water

(Marson, 1967; Wei & Heinke, 1974; Poon & Brueckner, 1975).
Although the electrolysis of sewage was first reported in 1880, most of
the early plants were abandoned by 1930. However, pilot-scale studies
have been re-examining this concept both in North America and in
Europe since the middle 1950s as attention has focussed increasingly on
physico-chemical treatment. Nevertheless, very few full-scale plants
have been built. Present studies are examining not only the disinfective
action of the chlorine but also the removal of nutrients and suspended
solids by the combination of flocculation and flotation which occurs in
the electrolysis cell. Whether this more complete treatment is being
attempted or not, the electrode systems can be divided into two classes:
those in which the anode is constructed from a dissolvable metal such
as iron, stainless steel or aluminium, and those in which an inert
material such as platinum, lead dioxide or platinised titanium is used.
In the former system the metal that dissolves during electrolysis can act
as the flocculating agent.

There is considerable variation in the operating parameters of the
plants that have been described in the literature. The sewage:sea water
ratio varies from 3:1 to 20:1, the retention time from less than one
minute to about an hour, and the power requirements from
0.45–2.11 kWh m^{-3}. Despite this, a high removal (i.e. about a 99 per
cent reduction) of coliforms is usually claimed. Electrolytic generation
of chlorine from a sodium chloride solution has also been described
(Bennett, 1974), although its application was primarily intended for
potable water. The operating costs for this unit were found to be lowest
when 8–10 gm l^{-1} available chlorine were being produced. At lower
concentrations the salt utilisation was poor, whilst at higher
concentrations there was a loss in current efficiency which made the
operation economically unattractive. Cells of this type which are
capable of producing up to 450 kg day^{-1} of chlorine are now
commercially available in America.

9.3.4   *Design problems*

The chlorination of effluents is an established process in many countries
and as such is considered as being an essential public health measure.
Indeed, in some countries this type of disinfection is mandatory and
sound designs are available (e.g. Thalhamer, 1981). However, in the
UK chlorination either of sewage effluents or raw sewage is the
exception rather than the rule. As a result, data on its use and its effect
on UK systems are somewhat limited. If, because of the EEC directive,
it is necessary to provide some form of disinfection for an existing sea
outfall discharging crude sewage, the outfall pipe itself may have to be
used as the contact chamber. There is, however, an inherent difficulty in
using the outfall for this purpose and that is the indeterminate nature

of the contact time. For example, consider the pipeline at low water during a spring tide cycle when the flow of sewage is insufficient to cause the pumps to operate. Under these conditions the pipe would be empty. As the tide began to rise the pipeline would begin to fill with sea water, top water level being equal to sea level. When the pumps cut in, the sewage that was discharged would flow down the pipeline until it reached the sea water. Assuming that the sewage had the lower density, it would then float on the sea water and since, under dry weather flow conditions, the rate of inundation of the pipeline by the sea would exceed the rate of discharge from the pumps, the sewage would be conveyed back up the pipe by the rising tide. Eventually, the upper part of the pipeline would be filled with sewage as a discrete body and beyond the sewage/sea water interface the remainder of the pipeline would be filled with sea water. Up to this point, which might be 30 to 40 per cent of a tide cycle, it is unlikely that any appreciable dilution of the sewage would take place, and an adequate contact time would be achieved. Thus, provided that sufficient chlorine has been added, disinfection should be satisfactory.

Conditions over the remainder of the tide cycle cannot be predicted in this way. Little is known about the behaviour of miscible liquids of differing densities conveyed together in the same pipeline. Stratification might take place, with the sewage travelling seawards in the upper part of the pipeline and the sea water remaining static in the lower part. If this occurred, the velocity of travel of the sewage would be increased, as it would only occupy a proportion of the pipe depth, reducing the contact time. If complete mixing of the two liquids, which has been observed, occurred in the outfall, contact time would be further reduced. The effects of chlorination with pumped discharges should therefore be monitored carefully and if unsatisfactory results are obtained, tests with discharges at specific points of the tidal cycle should be carried out. To match chlorine supply with demand, a compound loop residual control system would have to be employed. Using this system, chlorine supply would be related to both the quantity of sewage discharged and the chlorine demand per unit volume of sewage by monitoring the free chlorine residual some time, say two minutes, after chlorine application. It then remains for the operational chlorine residue and the type of chlorination to be chosen. The decision on which form of chlorination to employ may well rest on safety considerations; pumping stations for sea outfalls are not infrequently near to populated areas. Sodium hypochlorite solution is 2–4 times more expensive than chlorine gas, per unit weight of chlorine supplied, but a leakage of gas would be potentially more hazardous than a leakage of hypochlorite solution. If gas is used, the injector should be located as near to the application point as possible, since it is safer to run a chlorine gas line through a pumping station than a hypochlorous acid line. This is because the injector sets up a partial vacuum in the gas line and chlorine is therefore sucked into the injector, whereas the hypochlorous acid line is at a pressure both greater than atmospheric and greater than the head supplied by the sewage pumps. Therefore a minor leak in the gas line ought to result in air being sucked into it (thus preventing the escape of gaseous chlorine) whereas a leak in the hypochlorous acid line would cause the solution to be pumped out and chlorine to be liberated into the atmosphere. Chlorine leak detectors linked to an alarm system should also be installed so that the supply would be cut automatically in the event of any escape of gas. Chlorine storage and control equipment should be housed outside the pumping station in order to further reduce the risks of leakage within the station. The transfer of chlorine into the sewage also has implications for the choice of system. Injectors are easily blocked which means that it may not be possible to use raw sewage for dissolution of the chlorine without installing filtration equipment. However, the cost of this must be compared with the alternative of using mains water (unless there is an adjacent water course from which an abstraction can be made). An advantage of the sodium hypochlorite solution is that additional water is not essential although mixing with the sewage is improved by dilution.

The results of sewage chlorination in relation to marine disposal have been discussed in general terms by Irving & Solbe (1980) and by Irving (1980), and for a specific application by Toms, Saunders & Hodges (1981). The latter report describes the use of chlorine to reduce the number of bacteria in the sewage being discharged by means of a short sea outfall. The objective was to bring the water in the adjoining bay within the limits demanded by the EEC directive for bathing waters:

total coliforms not greater than 10 000 per 100 ml
faecal coliforms not greater than 2000 per 100 ml.

The results of the investigation show that although the sewer system is a complicated one, involving three pumping stations, and although the arrangement of the pumps at the main pumping station was such that chlorine could only be injected into dry weather flows and the first flush of storm sewage, a 95 per cent compliance with the EEC limits was achieved when chlorination was taking place (Fig. 9.6). This achievement has an even greater significance when it is realised that the natural 90 per cent die-off time of coliforms in the bay (T90) was 29–39 hours. This was the result of high turbidity reducing the penetration of ultra-violet light. By comparison, the T90 values in clear sea water (e.g. the English Channel) were 2–4 hours. The level of chlorination which achieved this performance was 15 mg l^{-1} and the contact time in the

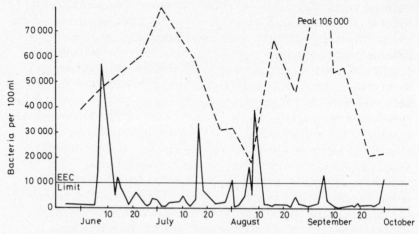

Fig. 9.6. The effect of the chlorination of a sea discharge on bacterial numbers. (From Toms *et al.*, 1981.) —— with chlorination, – – – – without.

outfall pipe was 30–60 minutes. Both these figures relate to the main pumping station. The overall operating costs (including an element for mains water which had to be purchased for use as the solvent for the chlorine) over the four-month bathing season (June–September) amounted to 0.74p m⁻³ of treated sewage, or about 15p per head of summer population. The total capital cost of the equipment was less than 0.5 per cent of the cost of constructing a new long sea outfall. Biological surveys did not detect any short term (i.e. over the four years of the investigation) effects within the bay.

Although the results show the effectiveness of this method of using chlorine, Toms and his co-workers stress that it ought not to be considered as a permanent means of controlling bacterial pollution. Rather, it should be used as a temporary measure which would be discontinued when a properly sited long sea outfall was constructed.

9.4   Other disinfectants

9.4.1   *Ecological considerations*

Whilst there is no doubt as to the efficiency of chlorination in reducing the level of microbes to one which will satisfy the increasingly stringent requirements for the discharge of wastewater, there are doubts as to the effect that this practice, and the resultant addition of toxic materials, will have on the aquatic environment. Free chlorine residues can obviously be toxic to aquatic life but their effect is of limited duration. Bound residual chlorine in the form of chloramines, however, is more of a problem as the toxicity of these materials both towards fish and the populations which make up the micro-ecology of the receiving water system is maintained for a longer period. Chloramines are particularly toxic to bacterial predators so that food chains could be disrupted, and 'unnatural' populations could then become dominant. In addition, when wastewater is chlorinated other toxic compounds such as cyanogen chloride may also be formed, and concern has also been expressed that by-products (e.g. chlorinated hydrocarbons) of the chlorination process may be carcinogenic (Ward, 1974). Whilst this is a problem which is specifically relevant to drinking water, there is at the moment no way of knowing what effects this may have within the various aquatic food chains. It is known that certain chlorinated hydrocarbons (e.g. PCBs) do accumulate in the organs of certain species. Therefore, it may well be that the excessive use of chlorine may be producing a 'biological time-bomb'; at the moment we do not know the answer to this. However, the present practice of effluent treatment in the UK does not utilise chlorine on a wide scale. The main concern must therefore be on the acute rather than the chronic toxicological effects. Thus if an effluent, which had been chlorinated so that it had a residual chlorine level of 4.0 mg l^{-1}, were to be discharged through a sea outfall designed to avoid slick formation (i.e. an initial dilution of at least 100), the maximum concentration of chlorine residuals would be less than the level at which a serious disturbance of biological species is thought to occur. Therefore, unless the design of the outfall was such that (a) poor dilution occurred or (b) inadequate dispersion of the effluent resulted in a build-up of chlorine levels, the use of chlorination ought not be expected to produce any short term adverse effects in the marine eco-system. Nevertheless, in assessing the use of chlorination, both the potential long term effects and the cumulative effect of multiple discharges must be considered. Thus, if a number of outfalls were to be contemplated within a confined area, it might be necessary to consider the use of de-chlorination techniques. This could be done with sulphur dioxide (White, 1974c), which could reduce the residual chlorine levels to around 0.1 mg l^{-1}, using a feed-forward control system based on the measurement of the chlorine residual:

$$SO_2 + NH_2Cl + 2H_2O = NH_4HSO_4 + HCl$$

However, this could increase the cost of the overall treatment process. The combined process of chlorination–de-chlorination–post-aeration has been quoted (Ward, 1974) as being 2.0 cents m^{-3} and it is claimed that this is starting to compare unfavourably with the cost of ozone treatment (see Table 9.5).

9.4.2   *Chlorine dioxide*

Chlorine dioxide is an explosive gas and therefore when it is being used as a disinfectant for water systems it is normally generated in the aqueous phase by the reaction of a chlorine solution with a solution of sodium chlorite:

$$2NaClO_2 + Cl_2 = 2ClO_2 + 2NaCl$$

The biocidal properties of chlorine dioxide result from its powerful oxidising capacity, although the precise method by which microbial inactivation occurs is not known. Critical comparisons of chlorine dioxide with other disinfectants suggest that it is more effective than chlorine (Longley *et al.*, 1980), and in some cases may have a greater efficiency than ozone. For example, in a test (Roberts & Vanjdic, 1974) using sterile sewage effluent to which a known cell density of *E. coli* had been added, chlorine (5 mg l^{-1}) achieved a 90 per cent kill in 5 minutes compared with a 100 per cent kill by chlorine dioxide (2 mg l^{-1}) in 30 seconds. However, the efficiency of chlorine dioxide is pH dependent, greater effect being achieved at values higher than neutral. An important advantage of chlorine dioxide is that it is claimed not to react with ammonia or other nitrogenous compounds so that there is no chloramine formation. This means that there are no known toxic residues formed when chlorine dioxide is used. However, the possibility of unknown side-reactions with waste organic compounds to form trace amounts of refractory toxins must not be ignored. If these can be elucidated and the by-products shown to be ecologically safe then chlorine dioxide could become a useful tool for the disinfection of sewage. However, its potential will depend on its cost effectiveness and this has been questioned (Geisser *et al.*, 1979). For a more complete appraisal of chlorine dioxide, readers are referred to the report by Roberts *et al.* (1981).

9.4.3   *Ultra-violet irradiation*

Ultra-violet radiation, because of the action on cellular nucleic acids, has a bactericidal effect which is greatest at a wavelength of 265 nm. Low-pressure mercury arc lamps produce a radiation with a wavelength of around 254 nm and therefore have a significant potential for use in the disinfection of wastewater. However, the electromagnetic waves must be absorbed by the bacteria and both the turbidity and colour of raw sewage act as shields. To overcome this problem it is necessary to pass the sewage through small diameter irradiated tubes or in a thin film over irradiated plates, and even under these conditions some shielding would take place. Such systems are liable to blockage by sewage solids and require further head to be supplied by the pumps.

For these reasons it is unlikely that this method would be appropriate for treating raw sewage, although it has been suggested that it might have an application in the treatment of a polished final effluent. A state-of-the-art survey by Venosa (1983) reports that, using thin (< 5 mm) film irradiation, the total coliforms in a tertiary effluent could be reduced to less than 70 per 100 ml as long as the turbidity was below 11 JTU. The same report describes the results of both pilot-scale (flow $= 3$ l s^{-1}) and full-scale (maximum flow $= 4.4$ m^3 s^{-1}) evaluations. These show that ultra-violet radiation can consistently produce effluents with faecal coliform counts of better than 200 per 100 ml. They also suggest that the cost is comparable with chlorination/de-chlorination. Finally, Venosa highlights the questions which must be answered if ultra-violet radiation facilities are to be designed so as to optimise both cost and efficiency.

9.4.4 *Sludge disinfection*

As has already been discussed, much of the sludge produced in the treatment of sewage is used in agriculture. In the UK, this is done on the basis of the requirements laid down by the Department of the Environment (DoE) guidelines and, in the future, by the EEC (see Chapter 7). However, in other parts of the world there are even more stringent requirements for the reduction of pathogens (Hansen & Tjell, 1979). The US EPA, for example, identifies two categories of treatment to reduce pathogens: category A, the initial step, should achieve a 'significant' reduction, whilst the subsequent category B should effect a 'further' reduction. The processes falling into category A include digestion, liming, and composting and therefore produce a sludge which is analogous to that required by the DoE. Category B processes are more intensive (and more expensive) and include pasteurisation and irradiation (Osborn & Hattingh, 1978; Yeager & O'Brien, 1983; Bruce, Havelaar & L'Hermite, 1982; Homann, Hartwigsen & Zak, 1982).

Radiation can kill microbes in one of two ways. In a dilute environment, the energy of the gamma photon can modify molecules in the surrounding medium so that they become toxic to microbes. In sludge, the photon energy damages molecules within the cell, the target usually being DNA. The application of gamma radiation, using cobalt-60 and caesium-137, has been examined both in North America and Europe (Roberts & Vanjdic, 1974; Englmann & Wizigmann, 1979; Suss, 1980; US Department of Energy, 1981; Yeager & O'Brien, 1983). These studies have shown that it is the total radiation dose absorbed by the effluent which determines the microbial kill, and the susceptibility of the target organisms is usually defined as the D_{10} value. This is the absorbed dose of radiation (krad) necessary to reduce the population by 90 per cent; a high value is thus indicative of a resistant species.

Typical values for specific bacteria irradiated in de-watered sludge (42–57 per cent solids) are (Yeager & O'Brien, 1983):

$$\left.\begin{array}{lr} \textit{Salmonella typhimurium} & < 60 \\ \textit{Streptococcus faecalis} & 130 \\ \textit{Escherichia coli} & 22 \end{array}\right\} \text{krad.}$$

The work described by Yeager & O'Brien also examined the irradiation of parasites (*Ascaris* ova) and fungal spores (*Aspergillus fumigatus*) and found that their susceptibility was similar to that of vegetative bacteria. However, viruses were found to have much higher D_{10} values (~ 500 krad). The irradiation of *Ascaris* ova has also been examined by Melmed & Comninos (1979). These workers showed that although gamma radiation (Co-60) did reduce the number of infective larvae developing, the larvated ova were more resistant than segmented eggs.

Radiation therefore would appear to have considerable potential as an agent for the disinfection of sludge. However, whether or not this potential is realised will depend on more detailed evaluations of full-scale plant, particularly in terms of cost. It will also depend on whether high degrees of pathogen removal are really necessary. At the present time this is not thought to be the case in the UK.

9.5   Conclusions

The disinfection of wastewater can now be achieved commercially by a number of chemical means. However, none of what might be described as 'new' disinfectants (i.e. ozone, chlorine dioxide, ultra-violet) appears to show sufficient advantages over chlorine to replace it as the most common method. The main problem is cost. Admittedly the use of chlorine does pose a question of ecological acceptability but as yet this fact cannot be included in a cost–benefit analysis.

10 Wastewater treatment in developing countries

10.1 Introduction

It is now fully accepted that the majority of the processes that have been described in earlier chapters are in the main unsuitable for use in the developing countries. As a result there has been a growth, in recent years, in the development of new processes and the study of not so new systems that are applicable in the Third World. These processes are often termed 'appropriate technology'. However, before discussing individual technologies, it is important to ask: appropriate to what? The answer must really be appropriate to the particular community or area being dealt with at that particular time. This should therefore be thought of as a unique situation. In other words, the technology that is applicable at one site may well be totally inappropriate elsewhere. This is particularly true of Western concepts, designs and operational procedures. Perhaps this is best illustrated by two examples.

A windmill is a well-tried unit for pumping water and a compact, purpose built one was offered to an Indian village. Its cost was small in Western eyes – £150 – but as this was considerably beyond the resources of the village it was a totally inappropriate technology. The second example relates to operational technique, as noted by a Western visitor, at the only substantial sewage treatment plant in an African country. The plant was a stabilisation pond and had been well designed. However, no flow was entering the pond at the time of the visit. Following the sewer up-stream led to the discovery of a large hole in the sewer-pipe. The entire flow, including waste from a hospital, was pouring through the hole into a ditch. On making enquiries, it transpired that the accident had occurred sometime before, but no one had bothered to do anything about it. It is, therefore, all too easy to assume that something will be done or be suitable, particularly if one has been trained by Europeans or European-trained personnel. Western concepts of treatment and perhaps more importantly of appropriate technology have a role to play in developing countries but it is also necessary, at times, to forget those ideas and learn from the client.

10.2   Waste stabilisation ponds

Except for the larger urban areas in developing countries, conventional western technology is usually inappropriate for the treatment of sewage. What is required are simpler techniques which require low capital investment and only minimal operational attention. In tropical countries, stabilisation ponds are frequently the most suitable method of treatment. These are shallow lagoons, which are usually rectangular, designed and constructed so that the wastes are degraded by a variety of microbial processes. These processes are allowed to develop and to proceed with fewer constraints than those imposed by man on, for example, the activated sludge process. In addition to being a cheap process to operate, stabilisation ponds can achieve a very effective removal of pathogens: a removal which is claimed to be superior to that of chlorination. Four types of stabilisation pond can be considered:

> anaerobic ponds
> facultative ponds
> maturation ponds
> high-rate, aerated ponds.

High-rate ponds will be considered separately. The other three are frequently used in sequence and therefore will essentially be examined together.

10.2.1   *Anaerobic ponds*

These are used for high-strength, high solids wastes or as the initial step in a sequence of ponds. Under the quiescent conditions prevailing in the pond, solids settle out and are gradually digested. The overall result is a significant reduction in BOD. At temperatures above 20 °C one could expect the following amounts of BOD removal:

Retention time (days)	BOD reduction (%)
1	50
2	60
5	70

At temperatures of 15–20 °C, 20 per cent less than these figures should be allowed. Typical design criteria would be:

> Surface loading, 1000–6000 kg BOD $ha^{-1} d^{-1}$
> Volumetric loading, 0.19–0.24 kg BOD $m^{-3} d^{-1}$
> Retention time, 5 d
> Depth, 3–5 m.

The effluent quality, in terms of BOD, can either be estimated on the basis of retention time, using the table above, or can be calculated from:

$$L_e = \frac{L_i}{k \left[\dfrac{L_e}{L_i}\right]^n [R+1]}$$

where L_e = effluent BOD, L_i = influent BOD, k = rate constant = 6 at 20 °C (see Lumbers, 1979), n = constant = 4.8 at 20 °C (see Lumbers, 1979), R = retention time (days). Obviously there is a gradual accumulation of solids in such a pond and therefore some de-sludging will be necessary. However, in most cases this need only be done at 3–5 year intervals.

10.2.2 *Facultative ponds*

These depend on a symbiotic relation between algae and bacteria and a balance between aerobic and anaerobic processes. Thus, in the surface layers, the dominant populations are algae and aerobic bacteria whilst in the bottom layers and in the sediment, anaerobic populations predominate. If the balance is disturbed, such that there is a reduction in the aerobic zone, the degree of stabilisation is reduced. One way in which the balance can be disturbed is if thermal stratification occurs. Under these conditions, when the non-motile algae sink, they remain at the bottom, receive little or no light and thus exert an oxygen demand rather than producing oxygen. Motile algal species also move from the immediate surface, where the temperature may be so great as to be inhibitory, and usually form a dense band just above the thermocline (0.3–0.5 m below TWL). This results in significant amounts of self-shading and therefore a reduction in oxygen output. Thus, the overall effect of thermal stratification is a reduction in the oxygen transfer to the aerobic zone with the resultant reduction in aerobic bacterial activity, which in turn affects the BOD removal. Mixing is therefore very important to the efficient operation of facultative ponds. Wind-induced mixing is an effective means of ensuring that stratification is minimised. Therefore in siting a facultative pond, the designer should ensure that the best use of the wind is achieved. Ideally, a wind rose should be obtained before the orientation of the pond is finalised. Also, wherever possible a clear distance of some 100 m should be provided around the pond to eliminate the effect of obstruction. The efficiency of wind mixing will depend on the fetch and for a typical pond depth of 1.5 m, 100 m has been found suitable. If these conditions cannot be met, or if wind speeds are less than 20 km h^{-1}, artificial mixing (circulating pumps, bubble guns etc.,) may be necessary. Diurnal mixing will often occur as a result of thermal stratification, with turn-over occurring during the night. However, this should not be thought of as at all adequate, as the day-time stratification will still result in a diminished oxygen concentration and pond efficiency.

The role of the facultative pond is primarily BOD removal. Design is therefore based on first order kinetics:

$$\frac{L_e}{L_i} = \frac{1}{1+kt}$$

Where L_i = influent BOD, L_e = effluent BOD, k = rate constant, T = mean temperature of coldest month, °C, t = retention time, days. Two methods have been suggested for the calculation of the rate constant:

$$k = 0.3\,(1.05)^{T-20} \qquad \text{(Mara, 1976)}$$
$$k = 1.2\,(1.085)^{T-35} \qquad \text{(Lumbers, 1979)}.$$

The area (A) required for the pond is given by

$$A = \frac{Qt}{D},$$

where Q = volumetric flow rate, in $m^3\,d^{-1}$, t = retention time, in d, D = mid-point depth (i.e. the depth the pond would have if the walls were vertical), in m. Substituting for t gives:

$$A = \left[\frac{Q}{D}\right]\left[\frac{L_i-L_e}{L_e}\right]\left[\frac{1}{0.3(1.05)^{T-20}}\right]$$

The surface loading rate (λ_s) is also important in the design of facultative ponds and is given by:

$$\lambda_s = \frac{10\,L_i Q}{A} \text{ kg BOD ha}^{-1}\,d^{-1}.$$

If the surface loading rate is too high, the pond will not operate satisfactorily. The limiting loading rate (λ_s^*) may be determined from an equation developed by McGarry & Pescod (1970) from a survey of operational ponds:

$$\lambda_s^* = 11.2(1.054)^\theta$$

where θ = mean monthly temperature, in °F. This can be given a safety margin for operational purposes by incorporating a factor of 1.5; thus $\lambda_s = 7.5(1.054)^\theta$. The data used by McGarry & Pescod can also be interpreted as following the simpler relationship when temperatures are between 15 and 20 °C: $\lambda_s = 20T - 120$ where T = mean monthly temperature, in °C.

Volumetric loadings, which are often used in the design of 'conventional' plant, are also used, although merely as a guide to the nature of stabilisation ponds. Thus, if the volumetric load, calculated as

$$\lambda_v = \frac{L_i Q}{AD} \equiv \frac{L_i}{t},$$

Table 10.1. *Relationships for predicting the BOD removal efficiency (BE, %)*

Primary lagoon	$BE_1 = 0.61 \lambda_{s1} + 13$
Secondary lagoon	$BE_2 = 0.49 \lambda_{s2} - 16$
Overall	$BE_{(1+2)} = 0.8 \lambda_{s1} - 9$

From Bradley, 1983.

is in the range 100–400 g m^{-3} d^{-1}, the pond should be operated as an anaerobic unit. For facultative ponds, λ_v is usually in the range 15–30 g m^{-3} d^{-1}. The data examined by McGarry & Pescod have also been used to develop a regression relationship between λ_s and the removal rate per unit area (λ_R). Thus:

$$\lambda_R = (0.725 \lambda_s + 10.75) \text{ kg BOD removed ha}^{-1} \text{ d}^{-1}.$$

A survey made by one firm of consultants (Lumbers, 1979) has concluded that this is the best technique for design purposes, as the method based on first order kinetics can give an overestimate of BOD reduction due to the fact that the first order formula assumes complete mixing in the reactor, a condition far from that found in practice.

Having completed the basic design calculations the actual pond dimensions need to be determined. Usually a depth of 1.5 m would be used and, to minimise short-circuiting, a length to breadth ratio of 2–3:1 would be provided. Wherever possible, two parallel streams should be used. This eases the problems of maintenance and gives greater flexibility of operation, particularly during low-flow periods. Evaporative losses can reduce retention times significantly and can cause such an increase in the concentration of pollutants that operational difficulties can be experienced. It is important therefore that this is allowed for at the design stage. If necessary and if possible, re-circulation can be considered to ease operational problems (e.g. anaerobiosis, malodours).

Facultative lagoons can also be operated in series. Under these circumstances, the total lagoon volume is considerably less than that required for a single facultative lagoon which was achieving the same degree of treatment (Bradley, 1983). The design criteria that have been provided earlier are not applicable for the design of lagoons in series. The BOD removal rates can be predicted from the equations given in Table 10.1 and the maximum efficiency can be achieved by having the ratio of primary lagoon surface area:secondary lagoon surface area less than unity and maximising the load on each lagoon.

10.2.3   *Maturation ponds*

The object of these ponds, which are fully aerobic systems, is to remove pathogenic bacteria and viruses. As such, they are designed on the basis of first order bacterial die-off:

$$N_e = \frac{N_i}{(1 + k_b\, t)^n}$$

where N_e and N_i = faecal coliforms per 100 ml in the final effluent and influent, t = mean hydraulic retention time, n = the total number of ponds used in the sequence, and k_b = faecal coliform rate constant at $T\,°C$. This rate constant is very temperature dependent and is calculated from: $k_b = 2.6\,(1.19)^{T-20}$.

In a way, therefore, maturation ponds can be thought of as a tertiary treatment to be used after a sequence of other systems, i.e. anaerobic, facultative or a combination of the two. As far as possible, each of the maturation ponds used in the treatment sequence should have an equal retention time. This would be between 3 and 7 days. The normal design depth is 1–1.5 m but it has been found desirable to increase this at the take-off point to enable the effluent to be withdrawn with the minimum algal concentration. In operating a maturation pond, it must also be remembered that bacteria die at different rates, with some pathogens dying more slowly than faecal coliforms; e.g. k_b for *Salmonella* spp. = 0.8 d^{-1}, while k_b for *E. coli* = 2.0 d^{-1}. Also, bacterial die-off is greater when a large variety of algae are present. Design formulae are not available for BOD removal in maturation ponds. However, it has been found that as long as the BOD of the liquors entering the pond is less than 75 mg l^{-1}, the final effluent from two maturation ponds in series ($t = 7$ days) should be less than 25 mg l^{-1}.

The final point that needs to be considered is that of dissolved solids (salts and toxic compounds) in the final effluent. This should be of concern when effluent re-use for agriculture is being contemplated, particularly in arid zones.

10.2.4   *Lagoon performance*

Ponds of the type discussed so far are used because of their simplicity and low cost. Their simplicity should be obvious; their low cost can be seen from the data in Fig. 10.1 (Gunn, 1976).

The performance of lagoon systems will obviously depend on the degree of attention paid to them during their operation. The amount of attention that is needed can be reduced by ensuring that a degree of common sense is applied during their construction. Some of the points to be remembered are:

Location – To avoid nuisance (i.e. odours, flies) they should be located at least 0.8 km from city limits

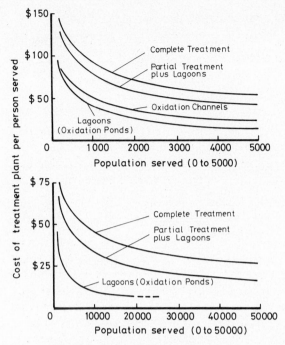

Fig. 10.1. Costs (1976 basis) of wastewater treatment plants in New Zealand. (The cost of land, inlet and outfall sewers is excluded.) (From Gunn, 1976.)

Ground – Loose, sandy or fissured limestone should be avoided as seepage losses are too high.

Pond base – Should be as impermeable as is reasonably possible. It should be sealed if the seepage rate is greater than 10 per cent of inflow. This is expensive and another site should be considered. Sealing can be clay, bitumen, or asphalt plastic.

Embankments – Usual slope 1 in 3 with a crest width of 3–5 m. Unnecessary weed growth around banks can encourage mosquitoes. Concrete slabs at and below TWL can prevent growth. They also reduce erosion by waves.

Inlet – Should be submerged to minimise scum. If possible multiple inlets should be used. Discharge away from banks (> 25 m) with the protection of coarse screens. If possible, measure influent flow (i.e. venturi or Parshall flume).

Outlet – Protect outlet (pipe or weir) by scum board. Consider multiple depth take-off to reduce algal concentrations.

Assuming a correct design and a sensible construction the performance of lagoon systems is more than satisfactory, as is shown in Tables 10.2, 10.3 (CPHERI, 1972) and 10.4.

The results reported by Bradley (1983) not only show that lagoons

Table 10.2. *Performance of an anaerobic pond (38 × 38 × 2.1 m)*

	Range	Average
Temperature (°C)	25–33	28.5
Influent solids (mg l^{-1})	290–720	530
Influent BOD (mg l^{-1})	276–560	352
Retention time (d)	4–5	4.4
Loading (kg BOD ha^{-1} d^{-1})	970–1480	1160
Effluent solids (mg l^{-1})	50–170	110
Effluent BOD (mg l^{-1})	70–156	100

Table 10.3. *Performance of a facultative pond*

	Four-year averages	
	Influent	Effluent
BOD	121	34
Suspended solids	100	64
Amm. N.	4.2	0.46
MPN 100 ml^{-1}	—	325
Retention (d)	2.7	
Temp. (°C)	27.30	
Loading (kg ha^{-1} d^{-1})	252.405	

operated in series can produce an effluent of a very reasonable standard (BOD/SS better than 35/84) but they also enable performance relationships to be developed. These relationships question whether existing design procedures (§10.2.2) are suitable for 'in series' treatment since they do not take account of the reduced BOD removal in the secondary lagoon.

10.3   Aerated lagoons

Aerated lagoons are a natural design extension of stabilisation ponds in the sense that mechanical aeration (see Chapter 4) is a logical means of providing additional oxygen in those cases where oxygen from algae is insufficient (i.e. in temperate climates). However, it was found that the use of aerators led to the disappearance of the algae and the formation of microbial flocs similar to those found in an activated sludge plant. Aerated lagoons must therefore be considered as a separate process with distinct differences from other lagoon or aeration tank systems. For convenience the process may be thought of as an extended aeration activated sludge system without sludge recycle.

Table 10.4. *Typical performance data for lagoon systems*

Lagoon type	Facultative[a]		Anaerobic and facultative	
	(Bradley, 1983[b])	(Bradley, 1983[c])	(Bradley & da Silva, 1977)	
Flow ($m^3 d^{-1}$)	1799	1324	—	—
Retention (d)	4.1+4.1	6.1+7.3	6+10	23+39
Primary				
Feed BOD ($mg l^{-1}$)	163	124	325	517
Effluent BOD ($mg l^{-1}$)	57	33	163	109
Load ($kg ha^{-1} d^{-1}$)	514	304	1050	661
Secondary				
Effluent BOD ($mg l^{-1}$)	35	29	46	56
Load ($kg ha^{-1} d^{-1}$)	180	68	84	31
Overall removal (%)	79	77	86	89

[a] Two lagoons in series.
[b] Six year average.
[c] Two year average.

These lagoons are normally operated with a hydraulic retention time of between 2 and 6 days, and under these conditions a BOD removal of 85–90 per cent would be achieved. The mixed liquor solids concentration would be about 200–400 mg l^{-1} and these solids would have to be removed from the effluent before it could be discharged to any watercourse. The simplest way of doing this would be to use a series of maturation ponds. The first would provide the necessary settlement whilst the others would remove faecal bacteria. This is necessary as aerated lagoons do not have very high removal efficiencies for coliforms. An alternative method is to use a conventional settlement tank.

Aerated lagoons are built in a very similar way to any other lagoon system. However, they are usually deeper (3–5 m) and both the embankments and the lagoon bottom must be protected from any scouring caused by turbulence generated by the aerators. This can be achieved by lining (e.g. with butyl rubber) and the use of a more steeply sloped (1 in 2) embankment.

In attempting to quantify the design of aerated lagoons both the growth of bacteria and the BOD removal rates need to be considered. Microbial growth can be calculated from:

$$\frac{dx}{dt} = y\frac{dS}{dt}$$

where x = cell concentration in lagoon, in mg l^{-1}, y = yield coefficient (0.6–0.7), S = soluble BOD. If the lagoon has a volume V and a hydraulic retention time t_r, this equation can be re-written as:

$$\frac{xV}{t_r} = \frac{y(L_i - S_e)V}{t_r}$$

where L_i = total BOD entering the lagoon, S_e = soluble BOD in the effluent. Under steady state conditions, the amount of cell growth will be balanced by the amount of cells lost in the final effluent and by death. Cell death depends on the number of cells present (i.e. the concentration and the volume) and the autolysis rate constant, b. A typical value for this constant would be 0.07 d^{-1}. Thus:

$$\frac{y(L_i - S_e)V}{t_r} = bxV + Qx$$

This can be rearranged, with $t_r = \dfrac{V}{Q}$, to give

$$x = \frac{y(L_i - S_e)}{1 + bt_r}$$

The value of S_e can be calculated by assuming that BOD removal in an aerated lagoon will follow first order kinetics:

$$S_e = \frac{L_i}{1 + kt_r}.$$

It should be remembered that this type of rate constant is temperature dependent and, assuming a value of 5 d^{-1} at 20 °C, is given by:

$$k_T = 5(1.035)^{T-20}$$

It is possible therefore, to calculate the concentrations of both the soluble BOD and biological solids in the effluent (i.e. effluent solids = lagoon solids). It has been suggested that it is possible to 'convert' the solids concentration into a concentration of BOD by using a chemical formula ($C_5H_7NO_2$) for a 'typical' cell. If this is done and it is assumed that the 5-day BOD = $\frac{2}{3}$ (ultimate BOD), then it can be said that the BOD per unit weight of cells is 0.95 and hence a *total* effluent BOD can be calculated:

$$L_e = S_e + 0.95x.$$

However, many other chemical formulae have been suggested as being appropriate to describe microbial cells and it is therefore possible that this equation may not be altogether suitable.

The design of the aerators for lagoons is no different from the design of aerators for any other type of activated sludge system in so far as the oxygen transfer is concerned (See Chapter 4). However, the aerators must also mix the lagoon contents and this will require a power input of 5–20 W m^{-3}. The types of aerator used for lagoons will have an oxygen transfer efficiency (in clean water) of 1.2–2.4 kg O$_2$ kWh^{-1}. It is also important that aerators are not placed too close to one another. The object of this is to prevent eddy interference. The suggested minimum spacing for, for example, a 75 kW aerator would be about 20 m^2.

A typical aerated lagoon system is that used in Lagos. Night-soil from 14 000 households is screened, macerated and diluted before being fed to the lagoons. Two lagoons (300 m^2 × 3 m) are used and each lagoon has four 56 kW (75 h.p.) aerators.

10.4 Biogas systems

The use of anaerobic digesters is just as applicable in developing countries as in the Western world. Indeed many factors favour biogas production in developing countries:

Biogas digesters are relatively easy to build
The digesters can be built with locally available material
The digesters can be built in different sizes according to need
Methane fermentation is favoured by a warm climate
In many developing countries the supply of biomass (organic waste + energy crops) is abundant
The waste material (e.g. human excreta) is made biologically safe (i.e. pathogens are removed)
The digester effluent is rich in nutrients, e.g. N, P and K, and can replace commercial fertiliser
The operation of a biogas digester is relatively simple and not very time-consuming
The biogas produced can be used for cooking, lighting and pumping
Building of digesters can initiate a local industry and create new jobs for biogas technicians
Biogas replaces other sources of energy (e.g. wood) and consequently diminishes the risk for erosion and drought brought about by deforestation
It is more efficient (in terms of energy) to digest manure to biogas and burn the gas, than to burn the dried manure directly.

It must be recognised, however, that, despite the obvious advantages, there are constraints to general acceptance. These can be either

284

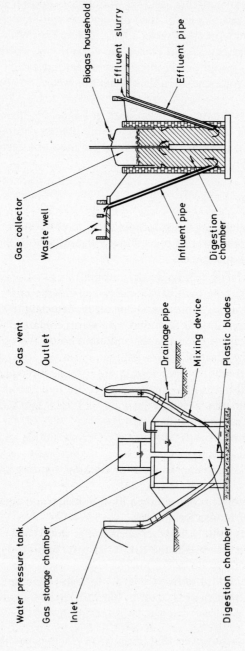

Fig. 10.2. Schematic diagrams of biogas reactors. A Polprasert, 1979; B McGarry, 1977.

Table 10.5. *An estimate of the numbers of biogas installations*

Country	Estimated number of reactors
China	7.2×10^6
India	10000–70000
Korea	29000
Taiwan	7000

economic or social. Nevertheless there are a large number of biogas reactors being used, particularly in Asia (Table 10.5). Although there are a wide variety of different designs, essentially there are two major types: the fixed cover (Chinese type) and the movable cover (Indian type) (Fig. 10.2). Whichever type, or type modification, is used, the main aim should be to achieve a system that is simple to operate and can be built at a low cost (using readily available materials, e.g. bamboo tubes, and local labour).

As can be seen from Fig. 10.2, a typical reactor consists of a digestion chamber built into the ground, an inlet and outlet and a gas collection system. As far as operation is concerned, the main requirements are that the inlet and outlet should not become blocked, that, if possible, some mixing of the tank contents should take place, and that the feed to the digester should be balanced nutritionally. An approximate guide to the nutriment balance is the carbon:nitrogen ratio, the optimum value of which is about 30:1. Cattle dung is high in carbon ($C:N \simeq 58:1$) whilst human excreta, particularly that including urine, contains more nitrogen ($C:N \simeq 15:1$). Thus biogas production can be enhanced by using a feed-stock containing both cattle and human excreta (or some other urine-rich waste, e.g. from pig pens). The increase in gas production is significant (0.19 to 0.44 m^3 kg dry solids^{-1}). Furthermore, the gas itself is likely to contain more methane. The requirements of preventing blockages and obtaining mixing can both be achieved quite simply by the use of a rope and paddle system (Fig. 10.2) which requires the input of only a little human energy. In an ideal situation, the organic loading rate would also be controlled, probably at 4 kg volatile solids m^{-3} d^{-1}. This would result in a retention time of about 10 days. However, in rural plants, loading rates tend to be below 2.4 kg m^{-3} d^{-1} with correspondingly longer retention times. Under these conditions, with a feed-stock of animal manure (pig:poultry = 6.5:3.5), the gas production rate has been found to be relatively constant at about 1.32 l h^{-1} with a methane content of 65–70 per cent. This corresponds to a yield of 0.29 l gas g VS^{-1} d^{-1}. Gas yields and other operational criteria of digesters are, of course, temperature dependent. In developed countries, the temperatures at which the large sludge digesters operate are carefully controlled. In a Third World village little can be done to control temperature of operation, so ambient temperatures must suffice. Thus, digesters operate usually over the range 18–30 °C, but also run the risk of temperatures falling below 18 °C with the resultant significant fall-off of gas production.

Gas of this composition will have a calorific value of around 20 MJ m^{-3} and would, most commonly, be used directly for household purposes (cooking and lighting). However, when used in conventional (propane) burners the energy utilisation is poor (35 per cent). This is due to the design of the burners and if these are modified specifically for the use of biogas, greater efficiency (60 per cent) can be achieved.

Irrespective of energy balance sheets there are a number of additional benefits to be obtained from using digesters. The first of these is that the slurry produced by the digestion process is rich in readily available plant nutriments. This is the result of the degradation of large molecules and the loss of carbon as gas. It is therefore a better fertiliser than the original wastes. Secondly, pathogens, particularly those bacteria and helminths of human origin, are reduced in number by passage through a digester. The production of biogas, therefore, would be expected to reduce the incidence of disease within a community as compared with one in which night-soil was applied directly to land.

Obviously one must ask, what does this process cost to install and what are the costs of the benefits? The construction costs will, of course, depend on the size of the digesters, a 60 l digester costing £12 while a 3000 l one costing £63. Data from China suggest that the biogas from a 10 m^3 digester (yielding 0.15–0.20 m^3 gas m^{-3} digester volume d^{-1}) is normally sufficient to cook three meals for a family of five and boil 15 l of water each day. The pay-back period for such a system has been estimated as being one year. Other estimates from Asia have suggested that the manure from 3–4 cattle would be enough to provide the heating and lighting needs for a family of five to six people. Furthermore, when compared with the existing methods of collecting, drying and burning cattle dung a greater efficiency of energy conversion can be achieved (36 per cent as opposed to 11 per cent). Biogas development in the Third World is very promising and hopefully will be pursued vigorously. A dialogue between the developing and the industrialised countries could promote this programme even more. Fruitful areas of co-operation could be digester design and development of efficient and economic devices for heating and stirring of the digester contents.

Digestion schemes in the future may well be based on villages rather than on individual families. Under these circumstances it might be necessary for some additional benefits to accrue to those families with cattle. One suggestion has been that whilst all families would receive light, heat and pumped water, only those families with cattle would receive slurry fertiliser.

The final assessment of the value of the biogas digesters will probably rest with the people who are required to use them. Apathy and fear of technical advances may inhibit this unless there is a positive decision taken by Central Government to support their large-scale use with financial assistance. This type of decision is seldom taken without the backing of a fully quantified cost–benefit analysis and unfortunately not all the benefits can be adequately quantified. For example, what price can be put on health improvements or reduced rates of deforestation caused by the use of gas instead of firewood? There is still a real danger that the biogas prodigy may be still-born.

10.5 Oxidation ditches

Developed countries, according to the WHO definition, are the USA, Canada, Europe, Israel, South Africa, Japan, Australia and New Zealand. However, when considering sewage treatment facilities, it must be recognised that some developing countries have an extensive

Table 10.6. *Extent of sewage treatment based on (i) percentage of the population served by sewerage and (ii) percentage of sewage receiving secondary treatment*

	Population served (%)	Sewage treated (%)
UK	93	80
Sweden	83	78
New Zealand[a]	79	62[b]
USA	73	51
Italy	57	6
Urban Brazil	50	50
Latin America	39	4[b]
Belgium	30	5
India	7	1[b]
Kenya[c]	4.6	4.0[b]
Uganda[c]	1.7	1.4[b]

[a] Gunn, 1976.
[b] Percentage of population.
[c] Pineo & Subrahmanyan, 1975.
From Simpson & Bradley, 1978.

Table 10.7. *Criteria used for the design of ditches in temperate and tropical climates*

	India[a]	New Zealand[b]	Europe
Sludge loading (kg BOD kg MLSS^{-1})	0.1–0.3	0.05	0.05
Volumetric loading (kg BOD m^3 of ditch^{-1})	0.4–1.2	—	0.2
Oxygen requirement (kg O$_2$ kg BOD^{-1})	1.5–2.0	2.35	2.0
Sludge production (g *capita*$^{-1}$ d^{-1})	5–10	—	25–30
Land requirement (m^2 *capita*$^{-1}$)	0.123	—	0.93–1.86

[a] Arceivala & Alagarsamy, 1972.
[b] Gunn, 1976.

investment in treatment whilst some developed countries have poor facilities (Table 10.6). It must also be recognised that developing countries do not always accept that water-borne sewage disposal is desirable. For example, in Japan there is a well-developed and effective practice of collecting night-soil for centralised treatment. Similarly, in rural areas of developing countries, local practices and behavioural patterns often mean that Western technologies are inappropriate. In those areas where water-borne sewage schemes are practical, the treatment options that are normally considered are lagoons, stabilisation ponds and oxidation ditches. These options are usually considered in preference to biological filtration and conventional activated sludge purely on cost grounds. In tropical countries, oxidation ditches can be operated at higher loadings than those used in European and other temperate countries (Table 10.7). This means that more compact plants can be designed. Ditch construction in developing countries is frequently less sophisticated than elsewhere. This, together with the more compact nature of the process that can be used, means that construction costs are significantly different from those prevailing in developed countries (Table 10.8).

A survey of the relative costs of various treatment options in India (Arceivala, Bhalerao & Alagarsamy, 1972) showed that stabilisation ponds were undoubtedly the cheapest method and that 'conventional' treatment the most expensive. Oxidation ditches and aerated lagoons were of a comparable cost. A different situation was shown to exist in Thailand (Suwanarat, 1972). There, the price of land played such a significant role that the least cost option changed from being

Table 10.8. *Construction costs in £ for ditches* (*indexed to 1980*)

Population served	N. America[a]	UK	New Zealand[b]	India[c]
1000	187	121	53	—
3000	94	84	29	—
5000	69	71	25	4.5

[a] Ettlich, 1978.
[b] Gunn, 1976 (does not include land costs).
[c] Arceivala *et al.*, 1972.

conventional treatment, in urban areas, to oxidation ditches, in rural locations. The performance of oxidation ditches in tropical conditions is comparable to that found in temperate zones – for example, BOD reductions of 95 to 99 per cent, concentrations of suspended solids in the final effluent of 20 to 57 mg l^{-1} and SVI values of 33–50 (Handa, 1972). A high-rate version of the ditch process, the BOD Moderator, has also been used in India to treat industrial wastes as well as domestic sewage. In the former case, complex organic effluents having BOD values as high as 3000 mg l^{-1} could be treated sufficiently to comply with the standard limits for industrial discharges to sewers (500 mg l^{-1}) recommended by the Indian Standards Institute (Antani, 1972).

In assessing the design of oxidation ditches on the basis of BOD loading, one final point needs to be made, which is in fact applicable to any bio-oxidation plant. The strength of raw sewage depends on the daily *per capita* BOD contribution and the daily *per capita* effluent flow. In Europe, a value of about 55–60 g per person per day is commonly used as a design value for the BOD contribution. This is almost certainly too high for use in hot climates, especially tropical developing countries. Some values which have been measured are:

Zambia	36 g
Kenya (Nairobi housing estate)	23 g
SE Asia	43 g
India	30–45 g
Brazil (São Paulo)	50 g
France (rural areas)	24–34 g
UK	50–59 g
USA	45–78 g.

Thus it would appear that as urban communities develop, the BOD contribution increases (40 per cent of the USA figure of 78 g was due to sink-installed garbage grinders); in rural areas lower values are found presumably because some wastes are not discharged into sewers. In the absence of local data, 40 g would seem to be a suitable design value for the daily *per capita* BOD contribution in urban areas of developing countries.

10.6   Conclusions

The subject of selecting and designing wastewater treatment systems for Third World countries is of sufficient size to fill an entire book and indeed this has been done. This chapter can do little more than highlight certain limited aspects of the subject. Readers are therefore directed to the bibliography that is provided.

11 Industrial effluent control

11.1 Introduction

One of the statutory responsibilities of all water authorities is the well-being of their rivers and to this end they have powers to control discharges to them, whether the discharge is from a sewage treatment works or directly from a trader's factory. Because discharges to sewers can affect the ability of the sewage treatment processes to produce an acceptable final effluent, it is necessary for the control requirements to embrace every trade effluent which discharges into the sewers. Trade effluents are often of such volume and composition that the provision of increased treatment capacity is required, involving abnormally high capital investment. The effluents may also contain constituents which are toxic or inhibitory and this can make the treatment process difficult, expensive or even impossible. Even after treatment, residues may be harmful to the river ecology or, in some cases, make the treatment of abstracted water difficult. Similarly, the sewage sludge may be too contaminated to be disposed of economically (i.e. to land or to sea).

The prime purpose of trade effluent control is therefore to protect both the sewerage system and the sewage treatment plant and processes, including sludge disposal. It is also essential that the personnel maintaining and operating them are protected. It must be borne in mind that even where a sewerage system is too small for a man to enter, there are still areas where vapours and gases can collect (e.g. pumping stations, manholes) and create a potential hazard. Trade effluent control is often said to be the first stage of sewage treatment. As such there is a responsibility upon every member of a trade effluent control team to be thoroughly conversant with all sewage treatment processes. Bearing these points in mind, whenever a trade effluent discharge to sewer is being assessed, the following questions need to be asked *for each constituent* in the effluent:

(a) Is the effluent likely to affect the treatment of sewage and the disposal of the resultant sludge in any prejudicial manner?
(b) Is the effluent likely to damage the sewer?
(c) Is the effluent, either alone or in combination with the contents of the sewer, dangerous, the cause of a nuisance or likely to be

291

Table 11.1. *The effect of trade effluent components on personnel, sewers and treatment processes*

Factor	Effect on personnel	Effect on sewerage system	Effect on sewerage treatment works
Volumetric flow-rate	(1) Sudden large discharges dangerous to men in sewers	Hydraulic overloading of sewers due to sudden large discharges can cause: (1) surcharging leading to flooding (2) operation of storm sewage overflows leading to discharges of crude sewage to watercourses	Sudden flushes can lead to: (1) strong sewage entering storm tanks (2) interference with treatment Hydraulic overloading can cause: (1) overloading of sedimentation tanks giving decreased retention times leading to stronger effluent for biological oxidation treatment (2) deterioration in final effluent quality
Acidity/alkalinity	(1) Skin or eye contact with strong acids or alkalis is an obvious danger (2) Strong acids in combination with other sewage constituents may lead to the production of toxic gases, e.g. hydrogen sulphide and hydrogen cyanide.	(1) Strong acids can attack and weaken sewer fabric leading to collapse in extreme cases (2) Strong alkalis may precipitate scale in hard water areas leading ultimately to blockages	(1) Inhibition of biological oxidation processes which operate at optimum pH of 6.0–8.0 can be caused by excessive variation in pH of sewage
Suspended solids	Heavy solids may induce silting of sewers leading to reduced flows and septicity leading to hydrogen sulphide production	(1) High levels of suspended solids of heavy or inorganic nature lead to progressive silting of sewers and ultimately a blockage	High solids lead to: (1) Increase in the amount of screenings and sludge requiring more plant such as digesters, sludge presses, etc.

		(2) Blockages due to fibrous solids, e.g. hair, wool, etc.
		(2) Occupation of valuable space in sludge digesters by non-degradable solids, e.g. cellulose fibres from paper making
Organic matter (High oxygen demand)	Wastes from food and fermentation industries may cause: (1) septicity (2) odour nuisances	(1) septicity (2) possible acid attack on sewer fabric (1) Fermentable wastes may lead to septicity and gassing in primary sedimentation tanks leading to rising sludge and odour problems (2) High oxygen demand may mean excessive loading of biological oxidation treatment leading to deterioration in final effluent (3) Effluent with dissolved organic matter may lead to excessive secondary sludge production (4) High volumes of carbonaceous waste may lead to imbalance of nutrients in sewage leading to 'sludge bulking' activated sludge plant
High temperature	Discharge of steam or very hot liquids produces obvious danger of scalding	(1) High temperature leads to increased rate of corrosion of sewers (2) High temperature may lead to odour nuisances (3) Thermal stress

Table 11.1. (*cont.*)

Factor	Effect on personnel	Effect on sewerage system	Effect on sewerage treatment works
Sulphate	Anaerobic condition may lead to production of hydrogen sulphide by the reduction of sulphate	Sulphate in excess of 100 mg l^{-1} can attack concrete and weaken it	Sulphate attack on concrete structures if present to excess
Oil and grease	Could cause hazardous condition if excessive	Oil and grease can combine with solid matter to cause blockages. Oil may also foul up the float gear of pumps and seriously affect pumping sequences	Excessive oil and grease can cause clogging of screens and percolating filters. Oil reduces the efficiency of oxygen uptake in activated sludge plants Excessive grease can cause difficulties in sludge pressing due to 'blinding' of the filter cloths
Injurious and Toxic Materials I *Cyanide*	Obvious danger to sewer-men particularly when mixed with acidic wastes		
II *Metals* Those found in trade effluent include: Chromium and chromate Copper Nickel Cadmium Zinc			(1) biological treatment – percolating filters and activated sludge – may be poisoned by shock loads although a degree of tolerance to low levels may be built up All are toxic in varying degrees to biological oxidation and anaerobic sludge digestion. These metals generally concentrate in the sludge and can affect sludge disposal policies (both to land and to

III *Sulphides*	Danger to sewer-men from production of hydrogen sulphide gas at low pH	Corrosive to concrete due to bacteriological oxidation to sulphate. This occurs particularly in turbulent zones and at the water level/air interface	
IV *Flammable and toxic solvents*	Danger to sewer-men from fire and explosion, and also gassing by such materials as carbon tetrachloride, trichlorethylene, etc.	Danger to sewer structure from explosion. Petroleum spirit is forbidden in sewers – Public Health Act, 1936, Section 27.	Chorinated solvents such as carbon tetrachloride, trichlorethylene used for de-greasing and dry cleaning can inhibit anaerobic sludge digestion
V *Radioactivity*		Radioactive effluents are discharged from hospitals and research laboratories in accordance with Radioactive Substances Act, 1960. The Government Radio-chemical Inspectorate controls all discharges of radioactive effluents	
VI *Others*			A large variety of industrial chemicals may cause problems to various aspects of sewage treatment e.g. phenols, pesticides, biocides, algicides, fungicides, etc. Dye-wastes may cause colour problems in the receiving watercourse

injurious to the health of persons entering the sewer? In this context, particular regard must be paid to the Health and Safety at Work Act, 1974.

(d) Will the effluent affect the river system (including fish and vegetation) adversely when discharged from the works?

Conditions should then be set to as to minimise damage at the most sensitive stage.

11.2   Components requiring control

These are summarised in Table 11.1 and typical sets of consent conditions are shown in Tables 11.2 and 11.3.

11.2.1   *Solvents*

This term covers a wide range of chemicals which can cause problems at several stages. Some, such as the chlorinated hydrocarbons, are very volatile with low flash points and can cause a serious danger of explosion in the sewers (e.g. 1,1-dichloroethylene, 1,2-dichloroethane). Some accumulate in deposits within sewers and, if disturbed by sewer workers, may produce dangerous atmospheres which can result in

Table 11.2. *Typical concentration limits for trade effluent components in discharge to sewers*

Trade effluent component	Limit concentration (mg 1^{-1})
Calcium carbide	⎱
Solvents	⎰ Nil
Petroleum	
Tar and tar oils	20
Grease, oil, fats	100
Sulphates (as SO_4^{2-})	1000
Cyanides (as CN)	5
Sulphides (as S)	10
Suspended solids	500
Copper	5–10
Nickel	5–10
Tin	5–10
Lead	5–10
Cadmium	2–5
Chromium	5–10
Mercury	0.1
Total non-ferrous metals	30
Total soluble non-ferrous metals	10
Temperature (°C)	40
pH	6–10

Table 11.3. *Acceptance standards for discharge to major sewerage systems in Australia and Germany*

Parameter	Maximum permissible concentration (mg l^{-1})				
	Germany[a]	Sydney[b]	Hunter Valley[b]	Brisbane[b]	Melbourne[b]
pH	6.5–10	6.8–10	6.8–10	7–9.5	6–10
Temperature (°C)	35	37	—	38	38
Suspended solids	—	600	350	600	10000[c]
BOD	—	600	350	600	4000[c]
Oil and grease	250	200	100	200	1000
Cyanide (as CN)	20	7	7	2.7	10
Sulphate (as SO$_4$)	600	—	500	1000	150
Sulphide (as S)	3	10	10	1.8	1
Phenols	100	—	—	20	100
Formaldehyde (as HCHO)	—	—	—	100	200
Cadmium	0.5	30	30	4	10
Chromium	0.5	100	100	20	10
Copper	2	5	5	10	10
Lead	2	10	10	100	10
Mercury	0.05	NIL	0.001	NIL	2
Nickel	4	100	100	20	10
Zinc	—	30	30	100	10
Silver	—	—	—	5	2
Tin	5	—	—	20	10

[a] ATV, 1980. [b] D. Barnes, personal communication. [c] For discharges after 1.10.79.

unconsciousness and subsequent drowning (e.g. carbon tetrachloride). Many solvents tend to be absorbed onto sludge solids and as such can be extremely toxic to the anaerobic sludge digestion process (e.g. 15 mg kg^{-1} dry solids of chloroform or 20 mg kg^{-1} dry solids of trichloroethane can produce 20 per cent inhibition of digestion) (Water Pollution Research Laboratory, 1971). Nitrification in aerobic processes is also very sensitive to inhibition by some solvents (e.g. 75 per cent inhibition of nitrification in unacclimatised activated sludge was obtained with 18 mg l^{-1} chloroform or 35 mg l^{-1} carbon disulphide) (Jackson & Brown, 1970).

Volatile flammable substances are usually prohibited. However, as far as trade effluent control is concerned, some difficulty can arise in properly defining the term 'flammable solvent' in such a way that it can be used in general terms to exclude those materials which create problems and yet allow the discharge of those which can be safely conveyed and treated. The simplest course is to exclude all organic solvents from public sewers. This will present some problems in that some contamination of water by water-soluble solvents and small spillages may be unavoidable, but, with careful attention in factories to ensure that solvent-containing waste and accidental spillages of solvent cannot pass to the sewers, these effects can be minimised. The alternative course is to consider each case and each solvent on its merits and thus specify individual solvents in the consent. Those which cause no problems in the sewers and can be successfully treated in biological systems can be identified through the Water Research Centre, Stevenage, INSTAB service or by testing in pilot-scale treatment systems. This approach is obviously more time consuming but may be considered justified in certain cases.

11.2.2   *Petroleum products*

Legally (Public Health Act, 1936), petroleum is defined in terms of the Petroleum (Consolidation) Act 1928:

> '"Petroleum" includes crude petroleum, oil made from petroleum or coal, shale, peat and other bituminous substances and other products of petroleum. "Petroleum spirit" means such petroleum as when tested in the manner prescribed in part II of the second schedule of this Act gives off an inflammable vapour at a temperature of less than 22.7 °C.'

Petroleum and petroleum spirit by these definitions are legally prohibited from discharge to sewers because of the danger of explosion. However, dissolved solids or mixtures of two or more solvents may increase the flash point and remove liquids from the scope of petroleum spirit definition. This should not necessarily result in their being allowed into the sewers.

11.2.3   *Tar and tar oils*

As with the term 'solvents' this category includes a heterogeneous collection of substances having a variety of effects on sewers and treatment processes. The term includes tar, tar acids and tar bases. The effect of tar is a physical one. It acts as a binding agent with other material causing blockage of sewers. Partial blockage of the sewer by tar-bound masses can allow increased growth of slimes by protecting them from the hydraulic scouring action. In these growths sulphide can be biologically oxidised to sulphuric acid which can seriously damage concrete sewers (Simpson, 1970).

Tar acids are very corrosive; they are difficult to treat biologically and can reduce the efficiency of the treatment system. They also have surfactant properties and can cause foaming. Where tar acids are produced in any quantity, it is best to treat them chemically before discharge. It has been suggested that tar acids and tar bases should be limited to 3 mg l^{-1} although the usual limit for tar not dissolved in aqueous phase is 60 mg l^{-1} (Burgess, 1957). The main problem with tar however usually arises from accidental or surreptitious discharges, although the latter can be traced and stopped.

11.2.4 *Calcium carbide*

Discharge of calcium carbide to sewers is completely forbidden by Section 27(1)(c) of the Public Health Act, 1936 due to the dangers of accumulation of acetylene in the sewers.

11.2.5 *Grease, oils and fats*

In discharge consents these are usually grouped with hydrocarbon oils (e.g. lubricating oil and industrial oils). The solids and heavy oils and fats cause physical blockages in sewers, pumps, screens and filter distributor arms, all of which increase maintenance costs. The materials are mainly of biological origin although in some cases heavy lubricating oils can have the same effect. Lighter oils can accumulate in wet wells of pumping stations, fouling electrodes or float systems so that pump controls fail to operate. Flammable oils may also cause an explosion hazard. Layers of fat can be adsorbed to activated sludge flocs or biological filter media reducing treatment efficiency, and floating oil may be passed to rivers with the final effluent.

The consent limits imposed by various sewage authorities have ranged from nil to 500 mg l^{-1} (Mattock, 1969). The consent conditions depend on the volume of the effluent in relation to the sewage works capacity. For a relatively small discharge, 400 mg l^{-1} for total grease and oil is a common condition. It has been suggested however, that a properly maintained, adequate oil interceptor should be able to achieve a standard of 100 mg l^{-1}. The usual method of measurement is as ether extractable material (EEM). Values of around 100 mg l^{-1} are found in domestic sewage. No differentiation has been made between 'free' or immiscible EEM and emulsified EEM in consent conditions and it has been suggested that separate limits should be set. However, emulsifying agents are frequently biodegradable, thus releasing the oil in the biological system with the consequent adsorption to the activated sludge flocs or filter media. These conditions would result in inhibition of the treatment processes or the appearance of floating grease balls in the effluent.

When considering the conditions relating to fats, oil and grease for discharge to a sewer, it is worth remembering that the discharge from the receiving sewage works may be restricted by the consent conditions of 'no visible oil' or alternatively a permitted range of 5–10 mg l^{-1}.

11.2.6   *Sulphates*

Sulphate discharges are controlled because of their potentially damaging action on cement sewers, the effect increasing with the cation combined in the order $Ca < Mg < Na < NH_4$. However, pipes of ordinary Portland cement are not likely to suffer serious damage over a 15–20 year period from concentrations of 1000 mg l^{-1}. If sulphate in an effluent is precipitated as calcium sulphate, the residual concentration of sulphate is likely to be about 1500 mg l^{-1} and this is considered reasonable as long as there is adequate dilution available to reduce it to below 1000 mg l^{-1} on discharge to the sewer. If concentrations of 1500 mg l^{-1} are likely for more than 1 h d^{-1} then sulphate-resisting cement sewers should be used. For concentrations of greater than 2000 mg l^{-1} sulphate, super-sulphate or high alumina cement should be used. These two cements should also be used if the pH is other than neutral or slightly alkaline. Therefore the usual limit for sulphate to ordinary sewers is 1000 mg l^{-1}, with the proviso that 1500 mg l^{-1} may be allowed where adequate dilution is available. In this latter case one of the sulphate-resisting cements should be used for the trade sewer which leads to the public sewer.

11.2.7   *Cyanide*

Cyanides and cyanide-producing substances can produce toxic atmospheres in sewers and have a deleterious effect on biological treatment processes. Experiments in London have shown that sewage should not contain more than 10 mg l^{-1} where men have to work for several hours, if toxic atmospheres are to be avoided (Lockett, 1952).

The biological processes are also sensitive to cyanide inhibition. The rate of formation of activated sludge of high activity has been found to be retarded by 1 mg l^{-1} and 2 mg l^{-1} can reduce effluent quality (Burgess, 1957). Also, 0.65 mg l^{-1} when fed to unacclimatised activated sludge produced 75 per cent inhibition of nitrification (Jackson & Brown, 1970). Cyanide can be oxidised by biological processes and filters have been acclimatised to 15 mg l^{-1} cyanide with very little appearing in the effluent, although the general quality of the effluent was reduced (Burgess, 1957). The usual standard for sewage works discharges to rivers is 0.1 mg l^{-1}. Therefore trade effluent limits are usually set to ensure that less than 1 mg l^{-1} is present in the mixed sewage arriving at the works. Frequently, only 1 mg l^{-1} is allowed in the trade waste, although some large sewage works will allow 10 mg l^{-1} and even 20 mg l^{-1} for small discharges which are quickly diluted. Most consents are less than 10 mg l^{-1} for cyanide and materials producing cyanide on acidification. Some consents differentiate between simple soluble cyanide, cyanide complexes (excluding ferrocyanide) and ferrocyanide.

Cyanide is fairly easily oxidised by free chlorine and a concentration of 0.1 mg l^{-1} is as easy to achieve as 10 mg l^{-1} once treatment equipment is installed, as long as complexes such as ferrocyanide and nickelocyanide are not present (see Chapter 12). For this reason, cyanide from metal-plating processes should be treated before being mixed with iron- and nickel-containing wastes which are also produced by plating factories.

11.2.8 *Sulphides*

Sulphides should be restricted because they can cause fatal atmospheres of hydrogen sulphide and can cause damage to the fabric of the sewer if they are oxidised microbially to sulphuric acid (see Chapter 6). Typical consents specify less than 10 mg l^{-1} of sulphide and substances which produce hydrogen sulphide on acidification (e.g. hydrosulphides and polysulphides), although up to 50 mg l^{-1} is often allowed for small discharges which are quickly diluted to below 10 mg l^{-1}. Sulphide differs from most other toxic constituents of sewage in that it can be formed in the sewer from domestic sewage which has become anaerobic (Chapter 6).

Where sewage septicity is a problem in a sewerage system, further additions of sulphide in trade effluents will aggravate the potential for corrosion and such discharges should be prevented. However, if the formation of sulphide is only slight, some addition in trade effluent discharges may be allowed. The pH of the sewage also plays a part, in that being a weak acid in solution, the proportion of hydrogen sulphide in the molecular form depends on the pH (pH 6 – 83 per cent; pH 7 – 37 per cent; pH 8 – 5 per cent). Therefore alkaline sewages will be less likely to produce corrosion from this cause. Since any sulphuric acid production will occur in slimes on the wall, the faster the sewage travels, the greater the scouring action and the less slime there is; velocities of greater than 0.7 m s^{-1} are considered adequate to minimise the problem. Therefore, the limits to be set for sulphide in any particular discharge will depend on factors such as the volume of discharge, the dilution available in the sewer, the gradient of the sewer and the frequency of rising mains and whether the sewage is liable to become septic.

11.2.9 *Suspended solids*

Suspended solids concentrations need to be controlled to prevent the possibility of blocking of sewers, solid deposits in sewers and, in some cases, the overloading of sludge handling facilities at the sewage works.

Any limit that is imposed must consider the nature of the solids, the volume of effluent, the dilution available in the sewerage system, the velocity of the sewage in the sewers and the capacity of the works. Total suspended solids by filtration is the normal method for measuring this constituent.

The limit should be set so that problems will not be caused at the point of minimum flow velocity in the system. For solids of high density (i.e. mineral matter), 200 mg l^{-1} is a recommended maximum where reasonable velocities of flow are maintained in the system; for flocculent suspended matter, in good flow conditions, 800–1000 mg l^{-1} could be allowed. Higher levels can be set if the sewers and solids are suitable and the sewage works has the capacity.

Some suspended solids (e.g. colloidal material) can be a problem at sewage works, as they can reduce settleability and reduce sludge de-waterability. However this type of material is difficult to remove by pretreatment. In general, it is better, where possible, to accept solids into the sewerage system if it is considered that they will not cause problems and the capacity is available, as they are more effectively dealt with at the sewage works and the extra cost can be charged to the manufacturer under the charging formula (see Section 11.4).

11.2.10   *Biochemical oxygen demand*

In general, restrictions on BOD are only applied where there is a danger of overloading the sewage works and then they should be calculated in terms of the total load on the sewage works (i.e. taking into account volume, strength, treatment capacity of works and limits imposed on the final effluent). Carbohydrates in industrial wastes may be limited in certain cases as they are usually readily biodegradable and readily cause septic conditions in the sewers, producing H_2S and foul smells. They may also ferment in primary settling tanks producing anaerobic conditions and rising sludge. In secondary treatment systems, they can cause excess slime growth in filters producing ponding, or bulking of activated sludge. For these reasons, the discharge of readily biodegradable carbohydrate material is sometimes controlled. Where such discharges form only a small part of the total sewage flow to a sewage works they can be successfully treated and may even benefit the treatment system by correcting any excesses of nitrogenous material. Problems arise in small works, particularly where such loads arrive as 'slug' loads from the emptying of process tanks (e.g. yeast fermentation wastes from pharmaceutical factories, or milk waste). To avoid problems in the sewers such wastes may be transported by tanker direct to larger sewage works where the addition can be controlled. If adequate dilution with sewage, to produce a balanced nutrient load to the biological system, is not available, or where the high BOD of the waste could overload the sewage works capacity, some pretreatment would be necessary before discharge to the sewer. This can readily be performed either by chemical means or with a biological 'roughing' filter using plastic media. The limit most commonly applied is 1000 mg l^{-1} as glucose. Wastes likely to present a problem are usually from food processing, drink manufacturing and yeast fermentation industries.

11.2.11 *Phenols*

Phenols are not now a common constituent of trade wastes. The principal source was gas liquor and with the introduction of natural gas this source is decreasing. They are also commercially valuable and are recovered wherever economically possible. Consents usually quote a concentration of less than 500 mg l^{-1} and acclimatised biological systems have treated up to 2000 mg l^{-1} fairly successfully (see Catchpole & Stafford, 1977; Luthy, 1981). Nitrophenols are resistant to treatment and satisfactory effluents are difficult to obtain so these should be restricted. A limit of 10 mg l^{-1} on polyhydric phenols has also been suggested to avoid inhibition of biological processes.

Although treatment of high concentrations of phenol has been successful, the addition of sewage containing 5.6 mg l^{-1} of phenol to unacclimatised activated sludge produced 75 per cent inhibition of nitrification (Jackson & Brown, 1970). The higher concentrations of phenol recommended by most consent standards may therefore be too high for unacclimatised biological processes, particularly if a nitrified effluent is required. Lower limits have been set elsewhere; in Auckland (New Zealand) a maximum of 5 mg l^{-1} is permitted and in Germany zero phenols in a petrochemical plant effluent has been demanded (Fassbender, 1967).

11.2.12 *Toxic metals*

The metals commonly considered in this category are chromium, cadmium, lead, zinc, tin, nickel and copper. Many of these are common in industrial effluents, particularly metal-plating wastewaters. A lot of consideration and research has been devoted to the effects of these metals on biological treatment systems and on watercourses after treatment.

In general, the hexavalent form of chromium is more toxic to biological systems than the trivalent form. From the results of a number of experiments on pilot-scale and municipal treatment plants it has been concluded that the activated sludge process could tolerate continuously a total concentration of 10 mg l^{-1} of hexavalent chromium alone, although this concentration as a shock load would slightly reduce the treatment efficiency and completely inhibit nitrification

(Moore *et al.*, 1961; Barth *et al.*, 1965). Much of the chromium (28–45 per cent) is removed in the primary sludge. The chromium is concentrated in the sludge and is fairly rapidly reduced to the trivalent form. The maximum concentration in the sludge before inhibition of digestion occurs depends both on the retention time in the digester and on the solids concentration in the digester. For example 300 mg l^{-1} in wet sludge did not affect digestion when the mean retention time was 21 days, but when the retention time was only 14 days, 50 mg l^{-1} had a significant effect on gas yield (Jackson & Brown, 1970). Surveys show that, overall, sewage works remove 70–80 per cent of the chromium present in the influent so that 20 per cent is discharged with the effluent – the majority associated with the suspended solids (Lawson & Fearn, 1970). With a continuous discharge, this could have an appreciable effect on the river ecology.

Cadmium is fairly toxic in biological systems, being more toxic than nickel, zinc, chromium, tin and lead, but less so than mercury, copper and silver. More than 1 mg l^{-1} in settled sewage has been shown to inhibit aerobic treatment processes. Cadmium is inhibitory to anaerobic digestion but, like most other metals, this effect is reduced at higher pH values and toxicity is prevented by sulphide. It has been recommended that the concentration of sulphide ions be monitored to detect incipient inhibition. Addition of ferrous sulphate to digesters increases the concentration of sulphide and prevents inhibition (Mosey, Swanwick & Hughes, 1971). Only about 90 per cent of cadmium is removed in sewage treatment processes, 1.0 and 2.1 mg l^{-1} in sewage giving 0.07 and 0.3 mg l^{-1} respectively in the effluent. Cadmium is also concentrated in the sludge, which may cause toxic effects on crops if the sludge is disposed of on agricultural land. It is this and the effect of cadmium-containing effluents on watercourses which are the more important effects of cadmium, although cadmium contamination can also result in restrictions being placed on the sea disposal of sludge.

Lead in solution is fairly toxic, 1 mg l^{-1} significantly affecting aerobic treatment and 0.5 mg l^{-1} being toxic to protozoa and inhibiting nitrification (Stones, 1960). It readily forms insoluble salts however, and is largely removed in the sludge. Fairly high concentrations in settled sludge are needed to inhibit digestion (200 mg l^{-1} gives 33 per cent inhibition of gas production) and this can be prevented by ferrous sulphate addition as with cadmium. High concentrations in sewage sludge will increase the problem of disposal to land.

Zinc is one of the commonest metals found in trade wastes. It is also present in domestic sewage and 10 mg l^{-1} has been shown to produce a measurable deterioration of BOD removal and a reduction of gas production during anaerobic sludge digestion. This level of zinc in sewage also produces a sludge containing over 1 per cent dry weight of zinc which is rather high if it is to be spread on agricultural land. A survey of sewage works showed that the removal of zinc between incoming sewage and final effluent is between 60 and 100 per cent with a median of 86 per cent (Jackson & Brown, 1970).

Tin is one of the least toxic of the metals usually present in trade wastes. No deleterious effects on sewage treatment, aerobic or anaerobic, have been observed at concentrations as high as 20 mg l^{-1} in sewage (Burrows, 1969).

BOD removal in biological processes shows inhibition when the incoming sewage contains 2.5–5 mg l^{-1} nickel, although nitrification is inhibited at concentrations of less than 1 mg l^{-1} (Burgess, 1957; Sherrard, 1983). Anaerobic processes are affected at around 2000 mg kg dry solids^{-1}, which gave 20 per cent inhibition of gas production. Nickel is less strongly absorbed than most other metals and in consequence far less is removed by sewage treatment processes. A survey of a number of sewage works showed 30–40 per cent removal (median 31 per cent), so most nickel appears in the effluent. The nickel retained with the sludge solids produces problems when disposed of to agricultural land, as weight for weight it is approximately eight times more toxic to crops than zinc.

Because copper is strongly complexed by organic material, fairly high levels (25 mg l^{-1}) can be tolerated in sewage before the oxidation of organic material is affected. Protozoa and nitrifying bacteria are more susceptible and 1 mg l^{-1} in incoming sewage reduces nitrification considerably and increases the turbidity of the effluent by killing protozoa. It has also been shown that concentrations of 1–3.5 mg l^{-1} will cause the microbial population to decrease in diversity (Hunter, Painter & Eckenfelder, 1983). Copper inhibition of treatment processes shows a synergistic effect with nickel and zinc. Inhibition of anaerobic treatment depends on the concentration of free copper which is inversely proportional to the sludge concentration, sulphide concentration and pH. In one case the maximum concentration of soluble copper in a digester before gas production was inhibited was 0.7 mg l^{-1}, although the total copper concentration was several thousand mg l^{-1} (McDermott *et al.*, 1963). The toxicity in rivers depends on the amount of organic matter present. Most of the copper discharged by sewage works in the final effluent is complexed with the organic material.

Obviously with toxic, conservative pollutants like the heavy metals it would be best to exclude them as far as possible from the sewage system. The problem is that removal from wastes is expensive. Settling tanks prior to discharge to sewers can reduce the level considerably, but where discharge standards are high, this method is not reliable, especially if the metal is in solution. Metals may be precipitated as metal hydroxides, and since this is considerably more effective with high pH values, pH control may be necessary. Even with polishing filters, where there is a mixture of metals, this method cannot give reliable results much better than 10 mg l^{-1} metals. Improvements in the effluent discharged to sewers may also be affected by some modification of the production processes or the treatment of metal-containing wastes before they are diluted by other liquors. It has been suggested that differentiation in consents should be made between dissolved and total metals, allowing 10 mg l^{-1} dissolved and 20–30 mg l^{-1} total metals as fairly readily achievable limits for industrialists (Mattock, 1968). Alternatively, consents should be based on the total daily weight of individual metals arriving at a works. If this were maintained at a level equivalent to a concentration of less than 1 mg l^{-1}, treatment processes should not be significantly affected and nitrification should not be inhibited. However, as metals are concentrated by the sludge and further concentrated by digestion, consideration must be given to the effect of metals on the sludge disposal techniques – particularly land disposal. If one particular metal is restricting disposal (see Chapter 7) then further restriction of its discharge to sewer must be contemplated.

The average removal of metals in sewage works rarely exceeds 80 per cent and therefore considerable amounts will pass out in the effluent. It has been estimated that metal toxicity accounts for the fish-less state of a number of Midland rivers (Jackson & Brown, 1970). It is recommended that the concentration in final effluents should not exceed 0.1 mg l^{-1}. In connection with this, it is beneficial to set separate limits for each metal, since toxicities and removal in sewage works vary. Cadmium, for instance, is, on average, 90 per cent removed in sewage works but is extremely toxic to fish, 10 mg l^{-1} being the three-week LC50 for rainbow trout. The chronic sub-lethal effects of low concentrations of metals on fish are for the most part unknown, but initial work at the Water Research Centre, Stevenage indicates that significant deleterious effects may occur at concentrations considerably below the short term lethal concentrations.

11.2.13 *Temperature*

The Public Health Act 1936 prohibited the discharge to sewers of waste waters above 44.3 °C (112 °F) although higher temperatures may be authorised under the 1937 Act. At higher temperatures there is a danger of damage to sewers due to uneven expansion and contraction of the sewer walls. Higher temperatures also accelerate the development of anaerobic conditions in the sewer leading to increased rates of sewer-wall corrosion and odour nuisances. The limit which is often used is 40 °C.

11.2.14 *pH*

Acidic conditions in the sewer release hydrogen sulphide from sulphide, hydrosulphides and polysulphides, and hydrogen cyanide from cyanides. As well as causing toxic atmospheres, the hydrogen sulphide can be oxidised to sulphate which corrodes the sewer (see Chapter 6). Acid wastes may also react with the other contents of the sewer; in one incident a carpet manufacturer discharged an acid dye waste and a latex waste, with the result that the acid precipitated the latex and the sewer was blocked. Alkaline wastes can also cause problems. The commonest is carbonate precipitation where alkaline waste combines with hard water waste or milk waste and carbonate is precipitated. This process can be extremely rapid. In one incident a 305 mm diameter sewer was reduced to 51 mm in three weeks. The usual limits set by most authorities are pH 6–10. The sewage should be between 6 and 8 at the sewage works. Where there is a large flow to a small works, limits of 6–8 may be appropriate; for a small flow to a large works the limits could be extended to 5–10. In all cases consideration should be given to possible reactions with other contents of the sewer.

11.2.15 *Miscellaneous problems*

Boiler and cooling waters should be discharged to surface water drains and not to foul sewers. However, these waters frequently contain additions which make them unsuitable for discharge direct to a watercourse. Care needs to be taken in assessing how to deal with this problem.

Organophosphorus and organochlorine pesticides may well be present in some trade effluents. These compounds accumulate in biological systems and many are not affected by the normal treatment processes, passing into the receiving watercourse with the final effluent with a deleterious effect on the stream ecology. Compounds of this type should be excluded wherever possible.

Detergents can affect both treatment processes and the receiving stream. In the latter case they can produce foams, be toxic to fish and reduce the re-oxygenation capacity of the river. To minimise these effects, the Standing Committee on Synthetic Detergents has recommended a maximum limit of 0.5 mg l^{-1} in the river. In the works itself, excessive amounts of detergent can produce foaming in activated sludge tanks together with a reduction in the oxygen transfer capacity of the aerator and, perhaps a more important point, it can cause inhibition of anaerobic digesters. The control of discharges to sewers must therefore be made with these points in mind, but as a general rule, the use of non-biodegradable anionic detergents should be discouraged or even banned and the increasing use of non-ionic detergents should be carefully monitored.

Radioactive wastes may be discharged to sewers under the provisions of the Radioactive Substances Act, 1960. This Act is enforced (in England) by the Secretary of State for the Environment, not the regional water authority. The radiochemical inspectorate consider risks to sewer workers when setting limits.

11.2.16   *Volume of discharge*

The rate of effluent discharged from trade premises must be regulated for a number of reasons: to ensure that there are no sudden large discharges that could be a danger to personnel working in the sewer; to prevent surcharging which could either cause flooding or the improper operation of storm water overflows; to prevent hydraulic overloading at the treatment works and to ensure that large 'plugs' of strong industrial liquor do not disrupt the bio-oxidation stages. In other words, the maximum daily flow and the maximum hourly rate of discharge may need to be specified. This may mean that balancing tanks will be required to ensure either a smoothed flow-rate or a discharge limited to certain times of the day.

11.3   Sampling and metering

A regular inspection programme of all trade premises is necessary both to ensure that the consent conditions are being complied with and to provide data on which charges can be based.

11.3.1   *Sampling*

A suitable, accessible sampling point should be provided by the trader, the minimum dimensions of which should be preferably not more than 1000 mm and the cover should be easily removable. In assessing a new sampling chamber, the points to bear in mind are mainly those related to safety – e.g. suitability of steps/ladder into the chamber, sufficient ventilation, accessibility of the sampling point. In addition it must be remembered that sample points are often sited in remote parts of the trade premises, which are convenient for storage of drums, carboys and barrels, and that in the event of a spillage or leakage from these containers, chemicals could find their way into the sewerage system. This danger should be pointed out to the trader, and the area kept free of such containers.

The importance of samples of trade discharges cannot be over-emphasised. The basis of the charging scheme is the strength of effluent to strength of sewage ratio. As soon as traders realise that the strength of the trade effluent, as shown by an analytical result, is almost directly convertible into cash terms there will be a most searching inquiry into the sampling programme and if there are any flaws in the scheme these will be found and exploited.

The basis of any sampling programme should be statistical analysis of each discharge, and hence an assessment of the number of samples required to achieve 90–95 percentile confidence. However, in the absence of statistical data or the facilities to carry out such a programme, a rough and ready rule of thumb could be applied. However, this must be regarded as an absolute minimum (a statistical basis of sampling is of the order of 13 samples per half year charging period):

> For discharges of 4.5 m³ (1000 gal) per day or less – 2 samples per charging period
> For discharges of 114 m³ (25080 gal) per day or less – 4 samples per charging period
> For discharges of 114.1 m³ (25107 gal) per day or more – 6 samples per charging period.

Even these guide-lines need to be interpreted with care. For example in the case of a car-wash, where a daily flow of perhaps 90 m³ is discharged, four samples per charging period is clearly excessive. Conversely, an abattoir discharging 4.5 m³ per day (or less) needs more attention than two samples per charging period. Some attention also needs to be paid to the use of snap samples and composite samples. This will again depend on the type of effluent being discharged.

As a general rule however, composite samples should be used for determining charging data except where a discharge is known to be so constant in its quality that a snap sample is genuinely representative. In all other cases snap samples should be used purely for policing purposes. In the event of a repeated lack of compliance with the consent conditions or a single flagrant breach a formal sample should be taken in accordance with the procedure prescribed in Section 10 of the Public Health (Drainage of Trade Premises) Act, 1937.

11.3.2 *Flow measurement*

Every trade effluent discharge line passing 4.5 m³ d⁻¹ or more should have a suitable means of directly measuring the flow of effluent from the premises. Clearly, where water supply input figures are easily related to effluent volume, they may be acceptable as an alternative. However, no authority should be expected to enter into complex calculations, especially where some tenuous relationships exist, to calculate effluent flow. It must also be remembered that not only are data about the total flow required, but also information on peak flows. Consideration must therefore be given to the installation of a continuous chart recorder. These meters should be inspected at least twice a year.

11.4   Charging
11.4.1   *General policies*

Traders are generally required to pay for discharging their effluents to public sewers (Dart, 1977). This charge takes into account the expenditure involved by a water authority in providing, operating and maintaining the foul sewers as well as the treatment plant (including the disposal of residual solids). Thus the standard charge (C) in pence per m³ is calculated from

$$C = R + V + \left[\frac{O_t}{O_s}\right] B + \left[\frac{S_t}{S_s}\right] S$$

where C = Total charge per cubic metre of trade effluent (in pence),
   R = Reception and conveyance charge per cubic metre,
   V = Volumetric and primary treatment cost per cubic metre,
   O_t = The COD (in mg l^{-1}) of the trade effluent after one hour quiescent settlement at pH 7,
   O_s = The COD (in mg l^{-1}) of settled sewage,
   B = Biological oxidation cost per cubic metre of, settled sewage,
   S_t = The total suspended solids (in mg l^{-1}) of the trade effluent at pH 7,
   S_s = The total suspended solids (in mg l^{-1}) of crude sewage,
   S = Treatment and disposal costs of primary sludges per cubic metre of sewage.

The unit cost per item R (reception and conveyance) should be calculated by taking an agreed proportion of the net annual revenue expenditure (including financing charges on capital) on all sewers and pumping stations in an authority's area other than those used solely for surface water and those pumping stations with rising mains discharging directly to sewage treatment works.

The unit cost for the term V (volumetric and primary treatment) should be derived from the net annual revenue expenditure including financing charges on capital on:

   (a) all pumping stations with rising mains discharging directly to sewage treatment works
   (b) all inlet works, including screenings, comminution, grit removal and pre-aeration
   (c) all primary settlement units other than storm treatment works
   (d) tertiary treatment for reduction of the concentration of residual suspended solids
   (e) all outfalls for treated sewage.

The biological treatment term B should be calculated so as to include expenditure on:

(a) the biological filtration units and humus tanks, including re-circulation and ADF, as well as pumping of humus sludge
(b) the activated sludge plant and final settling tanks, including return sludge pumping
(c) the proportion of total sludge treatment and disposal costs associated with secondary sludge treatment and disposal.

The sludge treatment and disposal costs (S) should include that portion of the annual expenditure (i.e. pumping, conveying, de-watering, treatment and disposal) which is related to primary sludge treatment. It has been suggested that the proportioning of the *total* sludge costs should be one-third to secondary sludge (and therefore to the B factor) and two-thirds to primary sludge.

Charges are usually levied on the basis of the processes available at the treatment works. Therefore, if a sewerage system drains to a pumping station and sea outfall, only reception and conveyancing charges would be levied on traders connected to that particular sewer.

An industrialist can reduce his annual charges in two ways: by making a capital contribution (if the water authority agrees) towards the extensions to the treatment works necessitated by the industrial discharge; or by a simple good housekeeping within the factory aimed either at reducing the volume of the discharge or its strength. The organic strength of both the settled sewage (O_s) and the trade effluent (O_t) will, in the majority of cases, be measured as the dichromate chemical oxygen demand. Most water authorities will provide data on the standard sewage strengths (O_s and S_s) which are used within their region and these are the targets at which the cost-conscious industrialist should aim (Dart, 1977).

12 Industrial effluent treatment

12.1 The scope of the problem

In general, industrial effluents pose a number of very similar problems irrespective of their source. They are (a) highly polluting, and (b) subject to daily, and often seasonal, variation in both flow and strength. In addition, they may well contain toxic materials or be nutritionally unbalanced. This means that, whether the effluent is discharged directly to sewer or is treated on site prior to discharge, the treatment processes will require a more rigorous consideration, at the design stage, than would be necessary for a plant treating a purely domestic sewage.

Industrial effluents constitute a significant proportion of the polluted water generated by any developed country. A significant amount of this is discharged to inland streams; not all of it in a satisfactory manner (Tinker, 1975). The options open to any industrialist faced with the problem of disposing of process water are:

(a) discharge directly to a municipal sewer and pay the appropriate charge (see Chapter 11);
(b) achieve a degree of treatment on site and then discharge to sewer. Under these circumstances a reduced trade effluent charge would be levied but there would be capital and operating costs associated with the treatment process;
(c) achieve full treatment of the effluent (with increased capital and operating costs) and discharge to river.

These various costs need to be examined very carefully so as to determine the least cost option. However, it may not always be possible to calculate the various costs so as to achieve a clear minimum; this is due to uncertainties over the variations in sewer charges, labour costs or interest rates over the life-time of any plant likely to be installed.

The type of treatment plant will depend on the nature of the pollutants in the waste water. Although the range of these is extremely wide, they can, in general, be classified as:

(a) readily degradable organics (e.g. from the food industry)
(b) complex organics (e.g. from the organochemical industries)
(c) reactable inorganics (e.g. heavy industry and plating)

312

(d) inert inorganics (e.g. coal mining and quarrying)
(e) thermal pollution (e.g. cooling water).

Each of these general types tends to require its own type of treatment.

12.2 Readily degradable organic wastes

Although the treatment of this type of waste might, at first sight, appear to have few significant differences from the treatment of domestic sewage, each waste has specific characteristics which require that specific processes, or modifications to processes, be used. Some of the major differences between this type of waste and domestic sewage are the strength of the polluting matter, the balance of nutriments (industrial wastes often contain an excess of carbon) and, quite often, the seasonal nature of the discharge. These problems and their solution are best considered by examining specific cases.

12.2.1 *Dairy effluents*

Effluents produced by the dairy industry are characterised by the presence of milk solids. Their actual quantity and thus their polluting load will depend on the degree of processing and the variety of products. However, since whole milk has a high BOD ($c.$ 110000 mg l^{-1}), they invariably constitute a significant potential for de-oxygenation (see Table 12.1 and Marshall & Harper, 1984). The data in Table 12.1 show that the ranges for any one determinand are very wide; however, the majority of plants have a BOD of between 500 and 4000 mg l^{-1} and a COD of about 4000 mg l^{-1}. This strength coupled with the readily degradable nature of the carbonaceous matter (BOD rate constant = 0.31; Brown & Pico, 1980) means that biological activity, either in the bio-oxidation unit or prior to it, can cause rapid de-oxygenation. If this occurs and anaerobicity results, the lactose can be degraded to lactic acid and the pH will drop. It may therefore be

Table 12.1. *Typical characteristics for dairy effluents (mg l^{-1})*

	USA	NZ
BOD	40–48000	90–12400
COD	80–95000	180–23000
Suspended solids	24–4500	7–7200
Nitrogen	1–180	1–70
Phosphorus	9–240	4–150
Fat	35–500	0–2100

From Marshall & Harper, 1984.

necessary to incorporate pH adjustment in the treatment sequence. This will also control any pH fluctuations resulting from the use of alkaline detergents in cleaning cycles. Although the milk residues in dairy effluents are readily degradable, the overall effluent can frequently be deficient in nitrogen. Therefore, if a high removal efficiency is required, nitrogen must be added. This will add to the cost of treatment.

The hydraulic load from a milk processing plant can be expected to vary significantly both throughout the day and seasonally. Indeed it is not uncommon, in some countries, for plant to be shut down for two to three months during the winter or for plants to be operated for five days a week. Within these variations the main factor affecting the waste-water volume is the on-site management. If this is good then low (*c.* 0.5) waste coefficients (m^3 of water or kg BOD per m^3 milk) can be achieved; if not the waste coefficients can be expected to be high (both > 3.0). The first essential in any waste treatment proposal is therefore to reduce waste. The methods for doing this are well documented (e.g. Chambers, 1980; Galpin & Parkin, 1981) and well proven. For example, effective control measures at one plant reduced the BOD load from 5500 to 2800 kg d^{-1}.

Although measures such as this can greatly reduce the polluting load, and therefore the cost of treatment, there will always be a significant amount of carbonaceous material that will require treatment. There are a range of methods that can be used; however, it would appear that the preferred method varies geographically. For example, in New Zealand the dominant technique is spray irrigation; in Europe extended aeration is preferred; whilst in the United Kingdom the use of bio-filtration (either ADF or with plastic media) is the most widely used. Nevertheless, there are a number of processes which, by way of pretreatment, are common to all these methods. Flow-balancing is nearly always essential, but when this is used it is important to provide sufficient aeration capacity to ensure that no anaerobicity (with the resultant drop in pH and increase in potential odour nuisance) occurs. The flow-balancing stage can also be used for the adjustment of pH and, if necessary, the addition of nutriments. The removal of fat is another essential process which is common to most of the bio-oxidative methods. This is best done at an acid pH to ensure that as little of the fat as possible is present in an emulsified state. Fat traps may be used to effect the removal but in the more modern plants dissolved air flotation tends to be preferred.

The irrigation of agricultural land with dairy effluent offers a very low cost treatment option. It is also a method which can result in beneficial effects for the farming communities in that it stimulates both microbial and earthworm activity and adds trace elements to the soil. An example of the benefits is illustrated in Fig. 12.1 which shows the

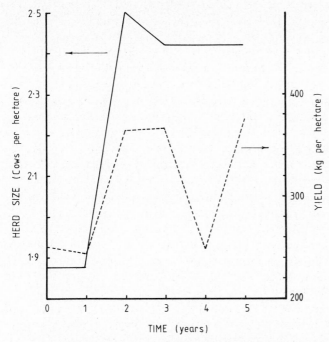

Fig. 12.1. Variation in the annual milkfat yield (kg ha^{-1}) and the farm capacity (cows ha^{-1}) resulting from irrigation with dairy effluent. (From Marshall & Harper, 1984.)

variation in the cattle numbers per hectare and annual milk yield per hectare over a five-year period of application (Marshall & Harper, 1984).

The techniques used for irrigation are well documented (e.g. Harper, Blaisdell & Grosskopf, 1971; Parkin & Marshall, 1976). However, it is important to ensure that (a) the irrigation rate does not exceed the infiltration rate of the soil; (b) there is a suitable rest period between applications; and (c) the removal of fats and solids has been adequate to ensure that the soil pores do not become blocked. In New Zealand, the average dose is about 450 m^3 ha^{-1}, at a rate of < 8 mm h^{-1}, and the rest period is 14–21 days.

Practically all the conventional types of process based on bio-oxidation (see Chapter 3) can be used to treat dairy effluents. The only possible exception is the activated sludge process unless it is operated in the extended aeration mode. This is due to the fact that even with good flow-balancing facilities, careful pH control and adequately sized aerators, filamentous bacteria can all too readily dominate the sludge flora and cause severe sludge settlement problems. Extended aeration, with its very low organic loading rates

Table 12.2. *Typical performance data for the treatment of dairy effluents by oxidation ditches*

Ditch volume (m³)	675	3300	496
Flow rate (m³ d⁻¹)	59–225	400	160–180
Sludge load			
(kg BOD kg MLSS⁻¹ d⁻¹)	0.11	0.02	0.08
Retention time (d)	4.8	8.0	3.1
Mean influent BOD			
(mg l⁻¹)	2850	950	950
Mean BOD reduction (%)	99.5	99.0	99.3

From Forster, 1983.

Table 12.3. *Typical performance data for high-rate (plastic) filters treating milk effluents*

BOD$_{in}$ (mg l⁻¹)	1660	1500	1500	1200
Load				
(kg BOD m⁻³ d⁻¹)	2.4	2.97	3.0	2.97
Efficiency (%)	60	66	66	60
Polishing				
system	Aeration	ADF	ADF	Municipal

(< 0.1 kg BOD kg⁻¹ MLSS) coupled with the aeration phase where endogenous respiration is dominant, provides an environment more favourable to non-filamentous species. It is for this reason that extended aeration and in particular the oxidation ditch is preferred in Europe (Scheltinga, 1972). Typical performance data of ditches treating dairy wastes are shown in Table 12.2.

Although the biological filter is generally a more stable process than activated sludge, the regular shock loads produced by dairies can cause ponding. It is for this reason that ADF (see Chapter 3) is the more popular mode of bio-filtration for this type of waste if a Royal Commission effluent is required. Alternatively, high-rate filtration with plastic media can be used to reduce the polluting load by $\frac{2}{3}$–$\frac{3}{4}$. The effluent can then be discharged to sewer or 'polished' by any of the conventional biological processes (see Table 12.3). The applied load will determine the degree of removal that can be effected during the 'roughing' process (see Fig. 3.8).

Any of the four main types of lagoon (aerobic, aerated, facultative or anaerobic; see Chapter 10) can be used to treat dairy wastes in those areas where land costs are low. Typical operating characteristics for lagoon systems are shown in Table 12.4. In general terms, the performance of lagoons would seem to be variable, and in addition,

Table 12.4. *Typical operating characteristics for lagoons*

	Aerobic	Aerated	Facultative	Anaerobic
Depth (m)	0.18–0.3[a] < 1.0[b]	1.8–4.6[a] 3.7[c]	0.6–1.5[a]	2.4–3.0[a]
Retention time (d)	2–6[a] 10–40[b]	2–10[a] 45–80[c]	7–30[a]	30–50[a]
BOD loading (kg ha^{-1} d^{-1})	20–40[a] ≯ 70[b]	— 342[c]	4–9[a]	55–90[a]

[a] Harper *et al.*, 1971.
[b] An Foras Taluntais, 1974.
[c] US EPA, 1974.

they are systems which have a very high potential for nuisance (odours and insects). Their use therefore is limited to sites where this would have only a minimal effect.

Although dairy wastes are readily degradable and contain no toxic matter other than cleaning agents, the cost of treating them is relatively high (see Marshall & Harper, 1984). Nevertheless they can be treated and high quality effluents can be produced if necessary. However, whichever method is used it is essential that good on-site management is practised to ensure that there are no wastages that would add unnecessary costs to the treatment budget.

12.2.2 *Other food industry effluents*

The majority of the problems associated with dairy wastes are typical of those which occur with other food industry effluents. Because of this, only the more significant processes used in the treatment of other food industry wastes will be discussed. These are usually processes which are exclusive to a particular waste and a particular problem.

The effluents from the fruit and vegetable processing industry can pose a number of problems in that not only are there seasonal variations but also there is a wide variety of products and, therefore, of waste streams. In addition it is becoming increasingly common for some pretreatment to be made before the produce reaches the factory so that both processors and growers have effluent problems. In the raw state the organic matter in fruit and vegetables is not readily soluble in cold water but as soon as heat or mechanical action damages the tissues, the organics start to pass into solution. The BOD of the effluent from any process will therefore depend on where that process is situated in the production line and the time of contact between the water and the food material. It is therefore clear that no overall

Table 12.5. *Loading rates for the treatment of fruit and vegetable effluents*

Effluent	Process	Loading rate $(kg\ m^{-3}\ d^{-1})$
Fruit cannery	Trickling filters + re-circulation	0.049
Fruit processing	Activated sludge	2.000
Cannery	High-rate bio-filtration (86%)	4.950
Fruit/vegetable washings	High-rate bio-filtration (93%)	3.120
Potato processing	Activated sludge	4.200
Potato processing	High-rate bio-filtration (90%)	1.110

From Forster, 1974.

generalisations can be made about these effluents. Each factory must be examined and its effluent must be considered as a unique case. What can be said however is that the effluents contain organic matter, which is biodegradable, in concentrations high enough to give BOD values up to 8000 mg l^{-1}. The majority of this BOD is present as soluble matter: 80 and 87 per cent from peach and tomato processing respectively. It is also relatively common for the effluents to be deficient in nitrogen.

Because of the fairly readily degradable nature of effluents, bio-oxidative systems can be used for their treatment. The main problems lie in maintaining a steady loading, both organic and hydraulic, on that system, particularly since storage for any length of time can result in a rapid drop in pH. The various treatment processes have been reviewed by Holdsworth (1970) and the treatment of specific wastes by specific techniques has also been described (e.g. Chipperfield, 1968; Lunt & Hemming, 1979). Some of the loading rates for various treatments are shown in Table 12.5. However, with these wastes solids can also be a significant problem. These can be present either as silt (from the washing of vegetables) or as the skins, and other unwanted debris, of fruits. The removal of these from the waste streams and their subsequent disposal are therefore of considerable importance. The techniques for doing this have been reviewed by Harrison, Licht & Peterson (1984). They highlight the use of screens, silt ponds and primary settlement and discuss the advantages and disadvantages both of these methods and the options for solids concentration and disposal. In addition, they indicate how some of these solid residues can be used as by-products.

Solids can also be a major problem in the effluents produced by the meat and poultry processing industry. Since at any one site a variety of processes may be used (e.g. slaughtering, bone de-greasing, rendering), the characteristics of the effluent will vary quite widely. Table 12.6 gives

Table 12.6. *Effluent characteristics (mg l⁻¹) of meat processing wastes*

	BOD	SS	FOG
Complex slaughterhouse[a]	1477	1300	800
Bone de-greasing[b]	11300	5170	—
Packing houses[a]	1286	840	720
Chicken processing[a]	500	350	213
Turkey processing[a]	350	220	60

[a] Hrudey, 1984.
[b] Ashworth & Tristram, 1973.

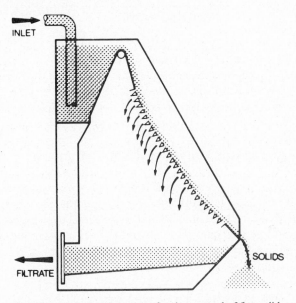

Fig. 12.2. Typical wedge screen for the removal of fine solids.

typical values both for individual processes and for overall combinations. This shows not only the high solids concentrations that can be expected but also that another problem area is fats, oils and grease (FOG). The origin of the FOG is obvious and its high specific BOD (> 2 g BOD g lipid⁻¹) means that its removal will not only ease operational problems within the treatment plant by elminating the risk of blockages, but will also reduce the polluting load quite considerably. The solids, which can be bone, feathers, hair, flesh residues and even paunch manure (partially digested food), are best removed from the wastewaters by screening. The type of screen which has found one of the widest applications is the tangential or wedge wire screen. As is

Table 12.7. *Dissolved air flotation performance data*

Plant type	Load ($m^3\ m^{-2}\ d^{-1}$)	Coagulant dose ($mg\ l^{-1}$)	Removal (%)	
			BOD	FOG
Red meat	46	—	55	90
Pigs	63	—	33	62
Pigs	88	Ferric sulphate = 100 Polymer = 10	41	95
Poultry	160	Alum = 75 Soda ash = 75 Polymer = 2	74–98	97–99

From Hrudey, 1984.

shown in Fig. 12.2 these are curved screens constructed of wedge-shaped wires (or bars) placed at 90° to the downward flow of effluent. The 'liquid' fraction passes through the screen whilst solids slide down it and are collected at the bottom. Most applications of this type of screen in the meat and poultry industry use wire spacings of 0.25–1.5 mm (Hrudey, 1984).

Grease traps can be used to remove FOG but it is probably more common to use gravity clarification or dissolved air flotation (DAF). If clarifiers are used they can serve a dual function, i.e. the removal of settleable solids as well as floatable FOG. Assuming that flow balancing is being practised, a retention time of 1–2 hours at the average daily flow should ensure good separation, and surface scrapers should be used to remove the separated FOG. The loading rates for a DAF system usually range from 30–60 $m^3\ m^{-2}\ d^{-1}$. Chemicals can be used to improve the efficiency of the process but their use will result in a lower quality tallow being produced if the recovered material is used to manufacture by-products (Hrudey, 1984; Table 12.7).

Another essential part of the waste treatment stream is the segregation and recovery of blood for use either as an animal feed supplement or as fertiliser. In addition to producing a valuable by-product, blood recovery helps to reduce the polluting load in the waste stream. Material segregation of this type is an essential part of the on-site management that should be encouraged to ensure that treatment costs are kept to a minimum. This may necessitate the use of separate sewers so that low impurity effluents can by-pass specific treatment units thus ensuring that they are designed only for those flows which genuinely require treatment.

The effluent that is produced by these preliminary processes (i.e. flow equalisation, solids removal, settlement and DAF) will still contain

Table 12.8. *Performance characteristics for secondary biological systems treating meat and poultry effluents*

Effluent source	Process	Flow (m³ d⁻¹)	BOD loading rates (kg m⁻³ d⁻¹)	BOD loading rates (kg kg⁻¹ MLSS d⁻¹)	BOD reduction (%)
Poultry	Plastic filter	545	1.48	—	74
Poultry	Plastic filter	431	2.36	—	60–66
Abattoir	Plastic filter	1130	8.25	—	50
Meat[a]	Activated sludge	1800	3.00	0.6	97
Meat[a]	Activated sludge	—	—	0.25	84
Poultry[a]	Activated sludge	—	0.24	0.05	> 94
Meat packing[b]	Activated sludge	3709	—	0.26	95

[a] Hrudey, 1984.
[b] Forster, 1983.

soluble and colloidal carbonaceous material. However, the majority of this is biodegradable and can be treated with almost any of the standard biological processes. These have been discussed in detail by Hrudey (1984). This discussion not only details loading rates and performances but also provides information about the costs of treatment. Some of these data are summarised in Table 12.8.

Because of the nature of the raw material used in this industry there is a risk of pathogens being present in the effluent. These will, in the main, be bacterial (*Salmonella, Brucella, Campylobacter*) although other species may be present in the effluents from specific plants. If the presence of pathogens is either suspected or proven, then the treatment stream should include disinfection. Chlorine or ozone are the disinfectants normally considered for this purpose (see Chapter 9). However, the data derived by Dearbourn (1978) during a study into the treatment of poultry processing effluent (4560 m³ d⁻¹) suggest that, on the basis of both cost and performance, chlorine ought to be preferred (Table 9.5).

The industries which come within the scope of this section are many and varied. They include distilleries and breweries, cider and vinegar making, yeast production and the processing of yeast (i.e. extraction), and at the periphery (at least in terms of the food industry), antibiotic production. As a general rule, the effluents produced by these industries contain a strong organic load (Table 12.9). However, provided that proper attention is paid to the nutrient balance, in particular nitrogen, and pH control the organic matter can be treated by the normal bio-oxidation routes (see Table 12.10).

Table 12.9. *Strength of effluents for the fermentation industry*

	BOD (mg l⁻¹)
Distillery	2000–30000
Brewery	800–1450
Cider making	600
Yeast production	4000–10000
Yeast extraction	6500
Antibiotics	3500–30000

Table 12.10. *Performance data for bio-oxidation plants treating effluents from the fermentation industry*

Source of effluent	Treatment process	BOD loading rate ($kg\ m^{-3}\ d^{-1}$)	($kg\ kg^{-1}$ MLSS d^{-1})	Removal (%)
Brewery	Activated sludge	0.97	—	96
Brewery	Plastic filter	2.41	—	84
Winery	Activated sludge	0.2	0.05	98
Maltings	Plastic filter	2.43	—	52
Maltings	Oxidation ditch	0.36	0.05	99
Distillery (condensate)	Activated sludge	0.29	—	91.5
Distillery (steep water)	Plastic filter	1.72	—	66
Distillery (pot ale)	Plastic filter	4.29	—	45
	(3-stage)	2.36	—	60
		0.94	—	73

The possible exception to this are distillery wastes. Considerable difficulty has been reported (Sheehan & Greenfield, 1980) in using activated sludge treatments for the very high strength wastes that can be produced by some distilleries (e.g. pot ale). In their review, these workers report that, even with careful balancing of the flows and pH adjustment to 7.2–7.5, only a mediocre (33 per cent) reduction of COD could be achieved. In addition, difficulties in maintaining a satisfactory sludge and in controlling foam have been reported. Pot ale can often be evaporated to recover material for addition to animal feeds. As far as the activated sludge process is concerned, the condensate from this evaporation (BOD = 500–2000 mg l⁻¹) is more suitable as a feed-stock than are high strength distillery effluents. High-rate biological filtration using plastic media, on the other hand, would appear to be applicable to the entire range of distillery effluents (see Table 12.10), although to achieve high removal rates multi-stage filtration is necessary. However, it is worth echoing the note of caution put forward by Sheehan & Greenfield (1980). Distillery wastes can be very variable both in strength and composition; their treatability is therefore also variable. These workers also suggested that this variability could well be compounded by the increasing interest in producing fuel ethanol from biomass.

Anaerobic treatment processes and their potential for treating strong readily degradable organic wastes have already been discussed (see Chapter 8). However, the effluents that have been discussed in these preceding sections are of the type most suited to anaerobic treatment. They are strong and frequently are produced at a temperature well above ambient. It is therefore worth considering these processes. It must be remembered however that they are very unlikely to produce a final effluent capable of being discharged to an inland stream. Their application should therefore be limited to:

(a) pretreatment for sewer discharge
(b) roughing treatment prior to polishing by an aerobic process, and, possibly,
(c) treatment before discharge to coastal or estuarine waters.

12.3   Complex organics

Not all the organic material which is discharged in chemical effluents is as biodegradable as that present in food industry effluents. In some cases the material is present in a sufficiently high concentration to be toxic to the microbial flora, in other cases the compounds are structurally so complex that any degradation takes an excessively long time. Phenol is a typical example of the former whilst the latter is typified by highly substituted aromatics or polynuclear aromatics.

Nevertheless, it is possible to use biological processes to treat these effluents provided that both adequate dilution and aeration time are provided. The process can be assisted by designing the pretreatment stage so that there is an appreciable removal of those constituents likely to interfere with the bio-oxidation. These points are best explained by the consideration of a series of examples.

There is increasing interest in the production of synthetic fuels from coal, and whilst the technology for doing this is well advanced, the same cannot be said for the treatment of the effluents produced by the process. In general, the wastes from any coal refinery producing synthetic fuels contain a wide range of phenols, heterocyclic nitrogen compounds and polynuclear aromatics. They also contain high concentrations of ammoniacal nitrogen. The result is an effluent with a high oxygen demand; typically with COD values of up to 30000 mg l⁻¹ (Neufeld, 1984). The pretreatment stages that have been proposed for these effluents are:

(a) *Ammonia removal.* This would be achieved by air-stripping to remove free ammonia followed by lime addition to pH 10.5–11 and then a further air-stripping stage to remove the saline ammonia. Steam-stripping could be used as an alternative. It should be remembered that the first stripping stage will also remove other dissolved gases or volatile material (e.g. hydrogen sulphide).

(b) *Phenol removal.* This would be accomplished by solvent extraction and to minimise costs solvent recovery would probably be practised. This would also enable potentially useful organics to be recovered. A solvent extraction stage would also reduce the level of polynuclear aromatics in the effluent.

These two stages would produce a wastewater which was capable of being treated by standard biological methods, which would remove up to 95 per cent of the soluble COD (Neufeld, 1984). If further treatment were required the most probable method would be an activated carbon treatment.

Phenols, which it must be remembered are toxic to bacteria at high concentrations, are also a major component of the liquors resulting from the production of coke for the steel industry. The other constituents of any significance are ammoniacal nitrogen, cyanides and thiocyanates. A review of treatment options for these wastes made in 1973 concluded that biological treatment was not only as efficient but also as economical as any other method (BCRA, 1973). A decade later the situation would not appear to have changed (Hofstein & Kohlmann, 1985). In some parts of the world ammonia removal and de-phenolation are used, partly as a pretreatment to reduce the load on the bio-oxidation stage and partly to recover by-products; however these processes tend to be the exception rather than the rule.

The bio-oxidation can be achieved either by trickling filters or more usually by the activated sludge process and, as can be seen from Table 12.11, a high degree of removal can be effected by either of these systems. An interesting modification to the activated sludge method of treatment is the use of 'growth factors' (Catchpole & Stafford, 1977). These are simple chemicals which are intermediates in the biodegradation pathways (e.g. glucose) and which, when added to the process in what amounts to trace quantities, enhance the rate of the overall oxidation.

The manufacture of synthetic resins also produces an effluent

Table 12.11. *Concentration of pollutants (mg l⁻¹) in raw (R) and treated (T) coking plant wastes*

Source	Cyanide R	Cyanide T	Phenol R	Phenol T	Amm. N R	Amm. N T	Aeration time (h)
Hofstein & Kohlmann, 1985	13	< 1	900	18	140	51	24
	98	1	510	2	1010	1010	24
Biczysko & Suschka, 1967	16	1	650	< 1	—	—	60
Ganczarczyk & Elion, 1978	—	—	288	3	97	125	13.8
	—	—	219	2	123	162	24

contaminated with phenols. However, in this case formaldehyde, which is also potentially toxic to bacteria, is also present. The treatment of this type of waste is best considered by the performance of an operational plant which has previously been discussed in detail (e.g. Housden, 1981). The raw process water (1200–1400 m³ d⁻¹) is first pumped to a balancing lagoon. This has a retention time of about 4 days. The first stage in the biological treatment sequence is an activated sludge unit. Operated at about half its design load of 4.5 kg BOD m⁻³ d⁻¹, the plant has achieved high BOD removal rates (80–90 per cent). A particular feature of this underloading has been the ability of the plant to operate with high mixed liquor solids. This, in turn, has enabled the plant to absorb shock loads of formaldehyde without complete de-activation. The effluent from this plant is given secondary treatment partly by trickling filters (60 per cent) and partly by a second activated sludge plant (40 per cent). The average loading rates for the two systems were reported as being 0.057 and 2.09 kg BOD m⁻³ d⁻¹ respectively. The effluents then flow into a balancing pond (the activated sludge effluent passing first through two small filters which are really surplus to the overall requirements of treatment but which were part of the original plant and therefore might as well be used) and thence through a long outfall ditch, where they are diluted with spent cooling water, to river. The performance of the overall system (Table 12.12) shows that potentially toxic effluents can be treated successfully. Obviously this is a plant which has evolved over a long period and it is unlikely that its somewhat convoluted sequence of operation would be copied in a green field situation. However, its basic philosophy, flow balancing followed by two-stage biological treatment, could be used and in fact has been (Table 12.13).

Although these examples have shown the versatility of biological treatment processes, it is sometimes necessary to use either a supplementary system or an alternative approach if a high quality

Table 12.12. *Average performance data (expressed as mg l⁻¹) for the treatment of a resin manufacture effluent*

Treatment stage	BOD	Formaldehyde	Phenol
Raw process water	1498	332	123
After primary	178	18.6	6
After secondary			
Activated sludge	39	9.7	1.5
Trickling filter	23	8	0.7
After balancing pond	28	7.5	0.5

From Housden, 1981.

Table 12.13. *Operational criteria for the biological treatment of effluents from the organic chemical industry*

Source of effluent	Method of treatment	Initial loading rate (kg m⁻³ d⁻¹)	BOD reduction (%)
Resin manufacture	2-stage filtration (plastic)	3.36	78.6
Plastic manufacture	2-stage activated	3.85	99.5

effluent is required. The same situation may apply if the removal of specific recalcitrant chemicals is necessary.

Activated carbon is a well established adsorbent for organic molecules and its potential for removing either non-biodegradable or toxic (e.g. pesticides) organics from wastewaters is well established (e.g. Holiday & Hardin, 1981; Saleh, Lee & Wolf, 1982). In most cases granular carbon is used in a packed bed. However, an alternative approach is to combine the adsorption and bio-oxidation processes within a single reactor by using powdered activated carbon (PAC) (Frost, 1979). The advantage of using carbon in this way is that it enables the activated sludge to cope with the fluctuations, both in the strength of the wastewater and the chemical composition, that can result from a modern chemical complex manufacturing a diversity of products. This is particularly true if the effluent is coloured.

An examination of the flow diagram for a typical PAC treatment system shows that the carbon (around 200 mg l⁻¹) is added to the wastewater immediately prior to the aeration tank. Flocculants are usually added to the flow before it enters the settlement tank so as to

Table 12.14. *The effect of adding PAC on the performance of an activated sludge system*

	Influent	Effluent	
		With PAC (157 p.p.m.)	Without PAC
Soluble BOD (mg l⁻¹)	197	6.6	8.7
Soluble COD (mg l⁻¹)	458	91.7	149
Colour (APHA)	2452	504	1347

From Flynn & Stadnik, 1979.

Table 12.15. *Performance of PACT plants*

Determinand		Plant				
		Chambers	Vernon	East Burlington	Sauget[a]	Kalamazoo[a]
BOD (mg l⁻¹)	*In*	182	200	93	114	200
	Out	12	4	2	3	3
COD (mg l⁻¹)	*In*	169[b]	840	471	323	455
	Out	31[b]	73	63	63	65
Colour (APHA)	*In*	1450	150–500	85	—	—
	Out	476	20–40	35	—	—

[a] Pilot-plants.
[b] TOC data.
From Dunn, 1981.

ensure an effective removal of carbon fines which have not become incorporated into the floc structure and carbon regeneration is practised. The effectiveness of this type of treatment can be seen from the data in Tables 12.14 and 12.15 which show that a high removal of organic matter is achieved, the removal rates being better than those achieved by other options (Dunn, 1981).

An alternative way of dealing with refractory organics is to effect a degree of oxidation, using chemical means, before the bio-oxidation stage. The oxidants that have been examined include hydrogen peroxide, sodium hypochlorite and ozone. An examination of the treatability of the effluent from the manufacture of herbicides (Myers, Mayes & Englande, 1977) shows that an improved reduction in both BOD and TOC could be achieved by the treatment with peroxide and ferrous ions at 90 °C (Table 12.16). These results show that although

Table 12.16. *Effect of chemical pretreatments on the reduction (%) of BOD and TOC using a loading rate of 0.1 kg BOD kg⁻¹ MLSS d⁻¹*

	BOD	TOC
Untreated	70	13
Hypochlorite	59	33
Peroxide	80	52

Table 12.17. *Effect of anaerobic digestion on the PCB content in sludge*

Period of digestion (d)	1	10	20	30	40
PCB concentration (mg l⁻¹)	0.031	0.032	0.033	0.032	0.036

From Kaneko *et al.*, 1976.

the improvement in BOD reduction was only marginal, there was a significant improvement in the TOC reduction, the latter showing that refractory organics were made more degradable by the chemical oxidants.

Despite the success of these supplementary (or alternative) techniques there is still the hope that biological systems alone will eventually be able to treat 'hard' organics either by using a properly acclimatised flora or possibly by the use of genetic engineering. However, on the basis of current information, this may be a vain hope. Consider, for example, the case of residues from the manufacture of polychlorinated biphenyls (PCB). Primary settlement has been shown to remove more than 50 per cent of the PCB material present in the raw sewage feed (Garcia-Gutierrez *et al.*, 1982). Similarly, activated sludge will remove between 50 and 80 per cent (Kaneko, Morimoto & Nambu, 1976). However, all the evidence would indicate that both these removal processes are due to absorption and not degradation. Indeed the work by Kaneko and his co-workers even examined the anaerobic treatment of the activated sludge which had absorbed PCB. The results showed that no degradation was occurring (Table 12.17). This is perhaps not surprising when the degradation of PCB by pure cultures is examined. A typical study (Baxter *et al.*, 1975) showed that although low chlorine molecules ($\leqslant 3$ per molecule) can be degraded, compounds with a larger chlorine content are not (Table 12.18).

If, therefore, only limited degradation can be achieved by

Table 12.18. *Degradation (% removal) of PCB compounds*

Compound	Degradation (%)	Reaction time (d)
2,4'-dichlorobiphenyl	70	7
3,4-dichlorobiphenyl	80	8
2,3,2'-trichlorobiphenyl	50	7
3,4,3'-trichlorobiphenyl	76	12
2,4,2',4'-tetrachlorobiphenyl	Nil	9
2,4,6,2'-tetrachlorobiphenyl	Nil	9

From Baxter *et al.*, 1975.

acclimatised microbes functioning in a carefully controlled and optimal environment, what hope is there for the flora of an effluent treatment plant? It could be argued that the flora could, and should, be built up from a specialised seed culture. However, such a flora would need the ability not only to degrade PCB but also to withstand competition (e.g. for oxygen, nitrogen or phosphorus) from those species growing on less exotic carbon sources. The problems of not only obtaining but also maintaining a culture capable of degrading PCBs to a high degree under effluent plant conditions are such that physico-chemical treatment, operated either alone or as a supplement to biological systems, will be the only acceptable method for refractory and toxic organics (e.g. see Monnig & Zweidinger, 1981; Saleh *et al.*, 1982).

12.4 **Oil**

12.4.1 *Introduction*

Although oil is not generally thought of as a material which is discharged into inland rivers, it can and does reach these waters; not only as thin coloured films but also in sufficient volume to necessitate the closing of abstraction points. It is therefore essential (a) that the potential danger from oil pollution is fully appreciated, (b) that the proper treatment techniques are used to minimise the risk of pollution, and (c) that, if 'accidents' do occur, the emergency procedures are quick and efficient.

12.4.2 *Oil users*

Industry is a fairly obvious and major user of oil, and as such may be expected to generate a certain amount of oil-containing wastes. However, the amount of oil involved (0.5×10^6 tonnes per year; Illsley, 1982) indicates the scope of the problem and although most of these wastes are subjected to a degree of treatment, interceptors can be

Table 12.19. *Comparison of oil incidents in England and Wales during three surveys*[a]

	1966/7	1968/9	1973
Pollution due to storage and associated pipeworks and fittings	109	172	479
Pollution from pipelines (local and major)	4	8	38
Spillage from delivery pipe of tanker	5	12	58
Pollution from garages, boats, vehicle depots, air	31	65	83
Road tanker accidents	16	20	92
General incidents	98	148	411
Total	263	425	1161

[a] This table does not take into account the oil incidents which could not be traced.
R. G. Toms, personal communication.

neglected and lagoons can leak. In addition, wherever oil is used, oil must be stored, and an examination of oil pollution incidents in England and Wales shows that not only are the number of incidents increasing but also that the majority stem from oil storage systems (Table 12.19). This means that farmers, horticulturists and even private homes must also be considered as potential polluters.

Most spillages could be avoided. Toms (1971) estimated that this figure was about 90 per cent and suggested that the most effective way to prevent pollution by spillages would be to require that all storage tanks be surrounded by an oil-tight compound (bund). The capacity of the bunded area should be equivalent to 110 per cent of the volume of oil being stored, in the case of a single tank, or 110 per cent of the largest tank volume if a number of tanks are contained within the bund. The area should also be large enough to collect spillages from drainage valves and overflows (see Fig. 12.3), and whilst it must be capable of being drained, the system should be a manual one to ensure that the liquors are treated after removal. Although this, like most measures to combat pollution, is the application of common-sense, there are many 'horror-stories' relating to oil installations – the plastic hose fixed with a jubilee clip to a 64 m^3 tank; pipes laid in surface water drains – but even if these can be eradicated there is still the vandal. It is essential therefore that measures are taken to minimise this type of risk (e.g. the use of tamper-proof valves).

A facility for the treatment of oil-contaminated waters is also essential for any site using large amounts of oil or any site where

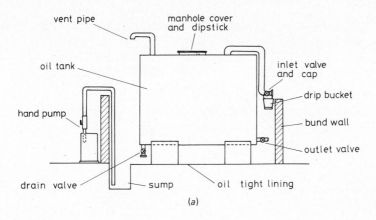

vent pipe

manhole cover
and dipstick

oil tank

inlet valve
and cap

drip bucket

hand pump

bund wall

outlet valve

drain valve

sump

oil tight lining

(a)

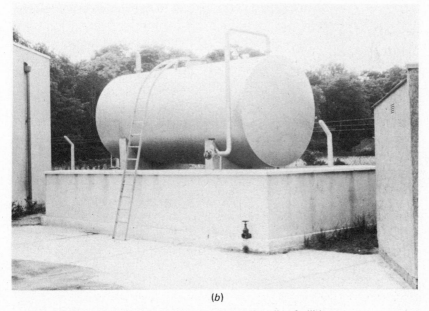

(b)

Fig. 12.3. Oil storage tank showing proper bunding facilities.

surface water run-off could become contaminated with oil. Probably the simplest form of treatment is the oil interceptor. This is a simple tank having at least two compartments (the first chamber being 3–4 times the volume of the second) and being fitted with oil booms. Interceptors for large flows or heavily contaminated waters should incorporate the means for oil removal.

An alternative, or even additional, technique is to use a tilted plate separator (Fig. 12.4). The flow of contaminated water is distributed so

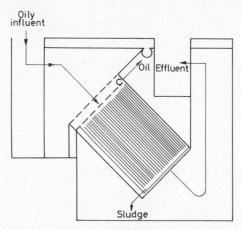

Fig. 12.4. Schematic diagram of a tilted-plate oil separator.

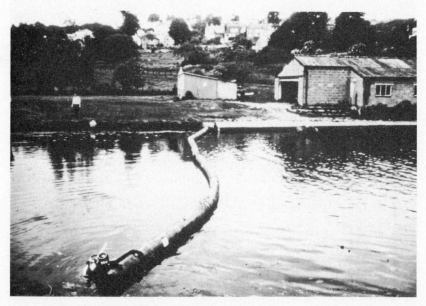

Fig. 12.5. Boom used for oil retention on a river.

that there is a uniform, laminar flow through the plate pack. Under these conditions, the oil droplets only have to rise a short distance before they are trapped by one of the plates. Coalescence occurs and the resultant film moves up the plate to the surface where it can be removed.

If a spillage does in fact reach a watercourse, the first action should be to install a boom to retain the oil (Fig. 12.5). To be effective, these

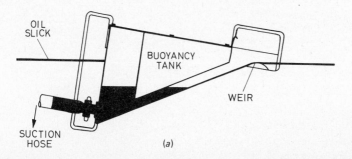

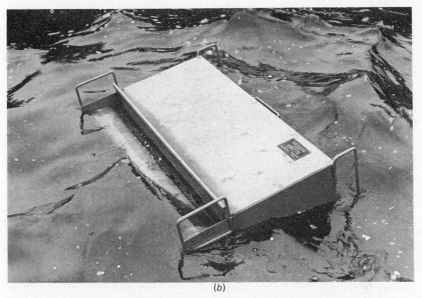

Fig. 12.6. Oil 'slurper' used for the removal of retained oil (by courtesy of Ambler Engineering).

need to extend both well above and well below the water level. However, it is important that the boom is not too close to the river bed in case the increased flow draws oil under the baffle; ideally the immersion should be no greater than half the water depth. The type of boom, the way in which it is moored and the best location for the boom system will depend on the river system, its depth and velocity. A detailed assessment of this can be found in the manual produced by CONCAWE (1974).

Having restrained the oil, it must be removed. There are various methods for doing this. These range from suction systems which remove oil and surface water (Fig. 12.6) to continuous absorption systems (rope mops) made of, for example, polypropylene. In the former case the oil is ultimately recovered by gravity separation, in the

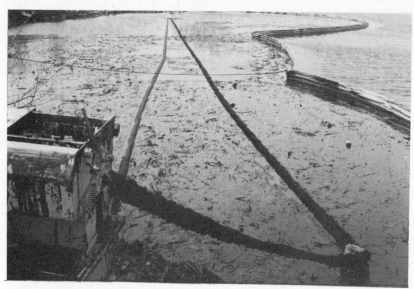

Fig. 12.7. Oil mop recovery of oil (by courtesy of OMI Ltd).

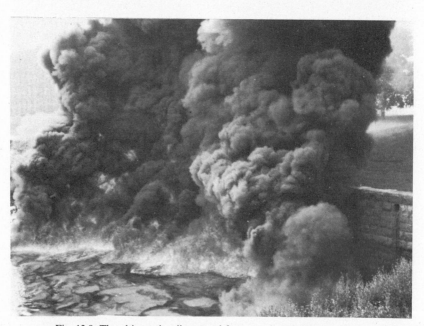

Fig. 12.8. The ultimate in oil removal from a polluted river.

latter by squeezing the absorbant (CONCAWE, 1974; Illsley, 1982; Fig. 12.7). The use of dispersants, whilst being an acceptable technique for marine pollution, is generally not one which should be considered for inland waters, except in very extreme cases. This is because of the harmful effects that the dispersive agents themselves can have on the river eco-systems. Of course the oil can be burnt (Fig. 12.8), but this should only be undertaken with very great care.

12.4.3 *Oil producers*

The characteristics of wastewaters discharged from a refinery will depend on the process on the site, the lay-out of the site drainage (both surface and foul water) and the way in which the cooling water systems are operated. In general, it is the process water which will be of greatest concern and it is usual to consider its treatment as beginning after passage through an oil separator system (Vernick *et al.*, 1984). The quality of the water at this stage is shown in Table 12.20. The volume of process water will depend on the size of the refinery but for the average plant in the EEC (handling some 4750 m^3 of crude oil per day), process water would be produced at about 2000 $m^3 d^{-1}$.

The treatment processes that can be used to reduce the residual contamination are those which are used to remove organic pollutants in general (e.g. chemical flocculation, dissolved air flotation, bio-oxidation, activated carbon). A typical process stream is shown in Fig. 12.9 (Meiners & Mazewski, 1979). This system was designed to treat a maximum flow of 1900 $m^3 d^{-1}$. The main features of this process were (a) the need for nutriment addition (0.01 kg P per kg BOD) and (b) the flexibility inherent in using a roughing filter in conjunction with a concentric channel oxidation ditch (retention time 1.01; loading rate 0.14–0.41 kg BOD per kg MLSS). The performance figures for the overall process, which are shown in Table 12.21, demonstrate that high quality effluents can be produced by a suitable combination of processes (see also Table 12.20).

An alternative approach to the treatment of refinery effluents is that developed by BP International Ltd. This process, which again

Table 12.20. *Typical refinery wastewater quality (mg l^{-1}) after various treatments*

Process	BOD	COD	Oil	Phenol	Ammonia
Oil separator	250–350	260–270	20–100	6–100	15–150
Activated sludge	5–50	30–200	1–15	0.01–2	1–100
Granular carbon	3–10	30–100	0.8–2.5	NIL–0.1	1–100

From Vernick *et al.*, 1984.

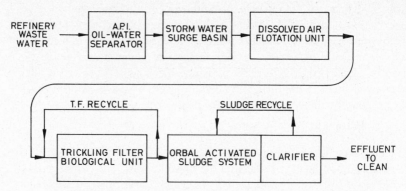

Fig. 12.9. Treatment stream for a refinery waste water. (From Meiners &
Mazewski, 1979.)

Table 12.21. *Performance data for refinery
effluent treatment*

Determinand (mg l⁻¹)	DAF feed	Final effluent
BOD	510	6
COD	1600	200
SS	28	21
Phenol	17	0.2
Amm. N.	22	53
Oil	160	8.6

From Meiners & Mazewski, 1979.

commences after primary treatment in an API separator, consists of a
granular filter followed by a conventional trickling filter. If necessary,
oil emulsions are cracked by the addition of polyelectrolytes
(< 1 mg l⁻¹) prior to the granular filter. The purpose of the granular
bed is to remove any residual oil which would otherwise coat the
biofilm and, because some 80 per cent of it (saturated ring compounds
and branched chain aliphatics) will be non-biodegradable, would thus
prevent the free sloughing of the film. The backwashings from this unit
are returned to the API separator. A trickling filter was chosen in
preference to activated sludge because, in the experience of BP, the
BOD of refinery effluents was generally low (50–100 mg l⁻¹), and as
such was on the lower limit of what was acceptable for the successful
operation of an activated sludge system. The trickling filter can be
packed either with conventional stone media or with random-fill
plastics (Oldham, 1980). Normally such a filter would be followed by a
humus tank. However, with the low influent BOD values biological

Table 12.22. *Performance data (mg l⁻¹) for two plants using the BP process*

		Plant A	Plant B
Influent BOD	max.	135	222
	min.	68	33
	mean	109	81
Effluent BOD	max.	18	22
	min.	8	2
	mean	14	7
Influent oil	max.	163	120
	min.	37	13
	mean	108	44
Effluent oil	max.	10	6.4
	min.	5	1.6
	mean	8	3.8
Influent phenols	mean	—	1.45
Effluent phenols	mean	—	0.28
Influent Amm. N	mean	—	6.4
Effluent Amm. N.	mean	—	2.8

solids are likely to be formed at a concentration less than the consent conditions. It is therefore possible to omit the final clarifier and, where possible, balance the discharge of solids. This is best done in a shallow tank, ditch or lagoon in which the flow regime is such that settlement produces an equilibrium layer of solids near the bottom surface. This then gives a more or less constant discharge concentration. In practice, this solids balancing zone can be improvised from existing tanks or even a drainage ditch. The success of this relatively simple approach can be seen from the performance data in Table 12.22.

12.5 Reactable inorganic wastes

12.5.1 *Plating wastes*

Not all effluents can be treated by biological methods; either their toxicity dictates an alternative technique or it is simply easier to remove the polluting matter by some other route. The effluents from plating works fall into this category. The main pollutants are cyanide, chromate and metal ions (see Lowe, 1970), and one of the commonest methods of treating these wastes is to use chlorine and sulphur dioxide under carefully controlled conditions of pH and redox potential. A typical flow diagram for this type of treatment is shown in Fig. 12.10.

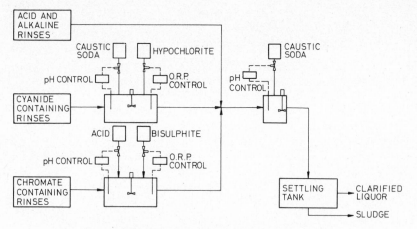

Fig. 12.10. Treatment stream for a typical metal plating waste.

The chlorine oxidises the cyanide to cyanate; this is then compatible with sewer discharge conditions. However, if necessary the cyanates can be reacted with additional quantities of chlorine resulting in the formation of carbon dioxide and nitrogen. The oxidation of cyanide to cyanate takes place in two stages:

$$CN^- + Cl_2 \rightarrow Cl^- + CNCl$$
$$CNCl + OH^- \rightarrow CNO^- + HCl$$

The second stage is dependent on both pH and the presence of free chlorine, and only above a pH of 10 can it be considered as being particularly rapid. Since the cyanogen chloride is both toxic and gaseous it is essential that the overall reaction is carried out at a high pH. This is usually achieved by the addition of sodium hydroxide with pH electrodes controlling the rate of addition. The theoretical amount of chlorine needed to complete the oxidation to cyanate is 2.73 and very frequently little more than this stoichiometric amount is needed. The chlorinators are similar to those described in Chapter 9 and their operation is controlled automatically by redox electrodes (~ 400 mV). The total reaction time for this stage would be 30–40 minutes.

Alkaline chlorination will also degrade most of the complexed cyanide in these effluents (usually zinc, cadmium and copper). Nickelocyanides, which only degrade slowly, are unlikely to be present as nickel plating does not require the use of a cyanide bath. Any nickel-bearing effluents should therefore be segregated from the main stream until the cyanide oxidation is complete. Ferrocyanides are not degraded to any appreciable extent. However, unless the final effluent is being discharged to river, their concentration is usually sufficiently low for them to be ignored. At this high pH value, the metal ions present in

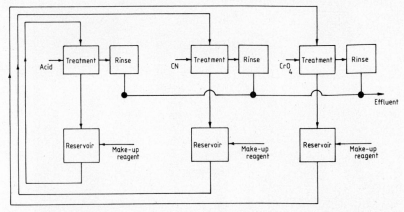

Fig. 12.11. 'Integrated' treatment stream for a plating shop effluent. (From Curry, 1976.)

the waste form insoluble hydroxides. These can be removed by sedimentation or flotation.

Chromium residues, which result either from chromium plating or the use of chromic acid in metal finishing, are present as chromates (hexavalent chromium). This form is considerably more toxic to biological systems than trivalent chromium. The usual method of treating chromates is to use sulphur dioxide (or bisulphite) to reduce the Cr^6 to Cr^3:

$$2H_2CrO_4 + 3SO_2 = Cr_2(SO_4)_3 + 2H_2O$$

For this reaction to be achieved rapidly, the pH needs to be maintained below a value of 2.5. Again pH and redox electrodes are used to control and automate the process which typically would take 15–20 minutes. The trivalent chromium is then precipitated as an insoluble hydroxide by raising the pH to 8.5. Some of this pH adjustment can be achieved by mixing the waste streams. The residual adjustment is made by the addition of either lime or caustic soda.

The combined process produces an effluent which conforms to the more usual conditions for discharge to sewer (see Chapter 11) and which, by very careful attention to pH control, reaction times and the solids separation system, can conform to more stringent conditions. It does, however, produce a sludge which is highly toxic. The disposal of this sludge is an additional and often significant part of the treatment costs. In most cases, the sludge from the settlement or flotation unit would be de-watered by filtration and disposed of to a licenced tip. An alternative could be to contemplate the recovery of specific metals from the sludge, possibly by microbial leaching. If these options are impractical or unduly expensive other options exist – for example, the

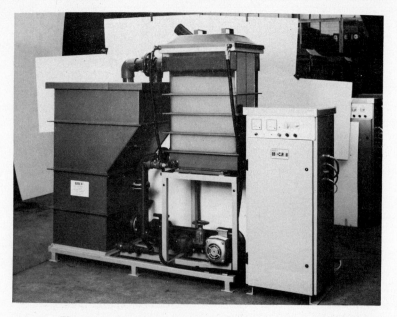

Fig. 12.12. 'Chemelec' system for metal recovery (by courtesy of BEWT (Water Engineers) Ltd).

so called 'integrated system' which is designed to achieve both metal recovery and water re-circulation (Curry, 1976; Crowle, 1972). With this process (Fig. 12.11) the effluent treatment takes place within the metal finishing sequence. As a result of the metal sludges being kept separate, a degree of recovery is possible. This method also means that the rinse waters contain no toxic impurities and the majority (80–90 per cent) can therefore be re-circulated within the works. Although this method increases the actual treatment costs, the overall cost, allowing for water recovery, is reduced (Curry, 1976).

There are, of course, other methods for treating the wastes generated by the metal-finishing industries (Wilde, 1985). For the removal of metal ions, these include ion exchange, reverse osmosis, liquid–liquid extraction and electrochemical methods. The treatment of cyanides can also be achieved by the use of ozone, ion exchange or even by biological reactors. Two of these methods are worth discussing briefly.

The Chemelec process (Fig. 12.12) is an electrolytic method developed by the UK Electricity Research Council. It consists of a fluidised bed of glass beads (500–700 μm) surrounded by expanded mesh electrodes. The anodes are usually coated (platinum or ruthenium dioxide) titanium and the cathodes, steel or titanium. The flow of wastewater through the cell fluidises the beads (80–100 per cent expansion). This combination of a fluidised bed and open mesh

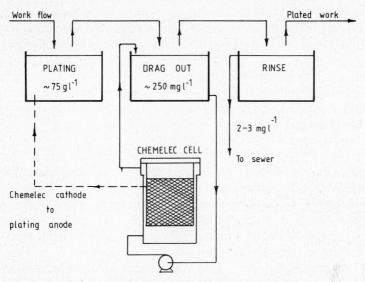

Fig. 12.13. Operation of Chemelec cell on a typical nickel plating line (by courtesy of BEWT (Water Engineers) Ltd).

Table 12.23. *Typical performance data for Chemelec cell operation*

| Metal | Effluent quality (mg metal l^{-1}) | | Mass metal recovered (kg week^{-1}) |
	With Chemelec	Without	
Cadmium	< 1	10	2–3
Nickel (site A)	< 1	> 1	20–30
Nickel (site B)	< 1.5	> 100	≤ 8
Silver	ND	150	2

By courtesy of BEWT (Water Engineers) Ltd.

electrodes results in the formation of smooth deposits and a more efficient utilisation of the applied current. A typical treatment sequence is shown in Fig. 12.13 and performance data are given in Table 12.23. If the recovered metal is of a sufficiently high quality the cathode from the Chemelec cell may be used as the anode in the main plating tank.

Although cyanide has a high toxicity to most biological species, it can be degraded biologically. Acclimatisation of activated sludge has been used and genetic engineering has been suggested. However, the former is likely to be too cumbersome for the treatment of cyanide in an exclusively inorganic wastewater and the latter is still speculation. A process which could well find an application in the metal-finishing industry is that based on immobilised enzymes/cells (Nazley & Knowles, 1981). Many fungi are able to degrade cyanide to formamide using the enzyme, cyanide hydratase, which can be induced in both spores and mycelia. The enzyme itself, spores or the mycelia can be immobilised, and although the philosophy still has to be translated into commercial reality, the preliminary data presented by Nazley & Knowles suggest that this could be a process of considerable potential.

12.5.2   *Residues from the chloro-alkali industry*

This industry produces caustic soda, sodium carbonate and chlorine by the electrolysis of sodium chloride. Three types of cell are used: the diaphragm cell, the membrane cell and the mercury cell. Only one of these, the mercury cell, produces wastes that require treatment of a more sophisticated nature than pH control and settlement. The problem with the effluents from a plant using the mercury cell is the presence of mercury and inorganic mercury compounds which have the potential of being converted into the highly toxic alkyl mercury compounds. Following the Minamata disaster the controls on the levels of mercury leaving chloro-alkali plants were increased. For example, in Canada the limit became 0.0022 kg per tonne of chlorine produced and in the United States the industry was required to achieve 'a zero discharge of pollutants' by 1983 (see Soothill, Barnes & Cook, 1985).

A variety of methods have been developed to achieve this. The most common of these relies on the formation of the highly insoluble mercuric sulphide. This is removed by filtration and the filtrate is polished by passage through an activated carbon bed. It has been reported that this type of process has produced an effluent containing 0.029 mg Hg l^{-1} (Soothill *et al.*, 1985). However, treatments of this type merely transfer the problem from one of liquid disposal to one of solid disposal and even compounds whose solubility coefficient is as low as that of mercuric sulphide are susceptible to leaching given sufficient time and the conditions normally prevalent within a land-fill site. Before disposal can be tolerated therefore, it is necessary to render the wastes as inert as possible. This can be achieved by either encapsulation or chemical fixation. Both methods depend on the attachment of the waste particles to a stable inert solid. In the case of encapsulation (see Mahalingham *et al.*, 1981), the attachment is the result of physical attachment and the inert matrix is a thermoplastic (e.g. bitumen) or a resin (e.g. urea-formaldehyde). Fixation achieves a chemical bonding of the waste to the inert solid, such as cement (Portland or pozzolanic) (see Zech, 1981). Each method has advantages and disadvantages. These, together with the standard of performance (in relation to stability) required of solidified residues, the tests used to assess the performance and the overall legal requirements for disposal both in Japan and the USA, have been reviewed in detail by Soothill and his co-workers (1985).

12.6 Pollution from cooling water

12.6.1 Thermal pollution

Although cooling water may be discharged from almost any industrial site, by far the biggest volume originates from the generation of electricity. Generating stations can be thought of as falling into one of two categories: those which re-circulate cooling water and those which do not. The former are typical of the more modern inland station which merely discharges purge water. This amounts to about 1 per cent of the total water being circulated and would be discharged at a temperature of perhaps 6–10 °C higher than that of the receiving stream. If the generating station is located at a coastal or estuarine site, re-circulation need not be used. In these cases, very large volumes of water are abstracted and discharged, the temperature increase being about 8–10 °C (Howells, 1983).

The major question that needs to be answered is whether these discharges constitute a major ecological threat. Certainly if the discharges were not well dispersed and resulted in a significant increase in the temperature of the receiving water biological activity would be increased; the potential for eutrophication could be enhanced and both the diversity and the balance of the natural species altered. Concern about the potential risks of thermal pollution has led to legislation being introduced in various parts of the world to control the temperature of discharges (e.g. US Federal Water Quality Act, 1969; EEC directive on Water Quality).

However, the evidence for problems originating from thermal pollution is limited. Indeed, it has been estimated that, on a global basis, the total area where detectable biological change can be said to occur is of the order of 1200 ha and that in many cases the changes are beneficial (Langford, 1977). It can be argued therefore that it is not cost beneficial to allocate financial resources either to detailed research into the problem of thermal pollution or to meeting over-stringent legislative controls.

What is probably of greater concern is the fact that most cooling systems (either from generating stations or other industrial sites), whether operating on a once-through basis or as a re-circulating arrangement, will contain additives to minimise: (a) corrosion, (b) scale formation and (c) biological fouling, even when the recommended quality of water (Table 12.24) is being used. These additives, albeit in trace concentration, will enter the river or coastal systems and their

Table 12.24. *Quality requirements ($mg\ l^{-1}$) for water to be used for cooling*

	Once-through		Makeup for re-circulation	
	Fresh	Brackish[a]	Fresh	Brackish[a]
Silica (SiO_2)	50	25	50	25
Aluminium (Al)	b	b	0.1	0.1
Iron (Fe)	b	b	0.5	0.5
Manganese (Mn)	b	b	0.5	0.02
Calcium (Ca)	200	420	50	420
Magnesium (Mg)	b	b	b	b
Ammonia (NH_3)	b	b	b	b
Bicarbonate (HCO_3)	600	140	24	140
Sulphate (SO_4)	680	2700	200	2700
Chloride (Cl)	600	19000	500	19000
Dissolved solids	1000	35000	500	35000
Copper (Cu)	b	b	b	b
Zinc (Zn)	b	b	b	b
Hardness ($CaCO_3$)	850	6250	650	6250
Alkalinity ($CaCO_3$)	500	115	350	115
pH	5–8.3	6–8.3	b	b
COD	75	75	75	75
DO	present	present	b	b
Temperature	b	b	b	b
Suspended solids	5000	2500	100	100

[a] Dissolved solids greater than 1000 mg l^{-1}.
[b] Acceptable as received.
From US EPA, 1972.

effect on these eco-systems must be considered. This is of particular relevance when considered in the light of the EEC lists of dangerous substances and the fact that some 63600 Ml d^{-1} of cooling water are discharged to tidal and non-tidal watercourses in England and Wales.

12.6.2 Contaminants

When metal is immersed in a conducting liquid, any dissimilarity in the metal surface (e.g. cracks in a protective oxide film) that result in potential differences on the surface can cause corrosion. The differences in potential establish an electrochemical cell in which metal ions are released at the anode (an area of low potential), and oxygen is reduced, provided the water is neutral or alkaline, at the cathode (Fig. 12.14). Corrosion inhibitors therefore act so as to modify the surface of the metal in such a way that one or both of the electrochemical reactions are blocked (e.g. Comeaux, 1967). A broad generalisation of the types

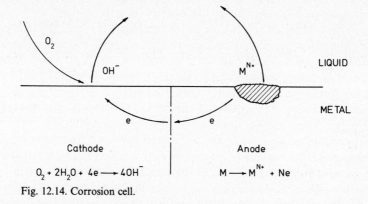

Fig. 12.14. Corrosion cell.

Table 12.25. *Classification of corrosion inhibitors*

Anodic	Usage level	Limitations
Anodic		
Sodium nitrite	400 p.p.m. to 1000 p.p.m. $NaNO_2$	Concentration required depends on chloride level. Maintain at least 2:1 nitrite/chloride, pH 7–9 bacterial nutrient
Sodium chromate	500 p.p.m. to 5000 p.p.m. CrO_4	Chloride dependent. Sodium chloride, dangerous inhibitor at low concentration, used only above pH 7.
Sodium silicate	20–40 p.p.m.	pH 6.5–7.5
Sodium borate	200 p.p.m.	pH is buffered to 8–9.5. Used with nitrite in small closed systems
Cathodic		
Zinc salts	500 p.p.m. min.	pH 6.5–7.0
Polyphosphates	10/25 p.p.m.	pH 6.5–7.5
Tannins	100 p.p.m. to 300 p.p.m.	Sludge problems in hot water. Most effective when pH = 8
Mixed inhibitors		
Zinc chromate	15–20 p.p.m. as CrO_4	Toxic. pH 6.0–7.5
Chromate/Phosphate	15–20 p.p.m. as CrO_4	Toxic. pH 6.0–7.5
$Cr/Zn/PO_4$	15–20 p.p.m. as CrO_4	Toxic. pH 6.0–7.5
Zinc/Phosphonate	3 p.p.m. as Zn	Toxic to fish. pH 7.0–8.5
Zinc polyphosphate	8–15 p.p.m. PO_4	Nutrient to micro-organisms. pH 6.0–7.0
Filming amines	Up to 100 p.p.m.	Absorption inhibitor – protects by film formation

From Cooling Water Association, 1973.

of compound used is given in Table 12.25. For the majority of discharges, either to surface waters or to sewers, it is the presence of zinc and chromium that would be of most concern. However, the Cooling Water Association's Code of practice (1973) does make the point that during the selection of an inhibitor the possible restrictions on the discharge of wastewater should be taken into consideration. This recognition of potential toxicity has led to the development of scale inhibitors which require lower levels of corrosion inhibition. Experimental work is being carried out to develop a non-toxic inhibitor which would be capable of operation over a wide pH band. However no information is available as to the progress of this work or the possible type of molecule that might be suitable for such a specification.

In the meantime therefore, the removal of the residual concentrations of inhibitors is worthy of consideration. For example, chromates can be removed either by reduction to chromium hydroxide (at alkaline pH), which is then taken off as a precipitate, or by recovery on anionic exchange resins (Kelly, 1968). Neither of these processes will affect the concentrations of phosphate but the reduction process will result in the precipitation of some zinc.

Scale in this context is normally taken to mean the deposition of calcium carbonate. Within the pH range of 5.5 to 8.5, the solubility of calcium carbonate depends on the equilibrium situation existing between the carbonate, carbon dioxide and the bicarbonate:

$$Ca(HCO_3)_2 \rightleftharpoons CaCO_3 + CO_2 + H_2O.$$

The Langelier Saturation Index (LSI) is used to indicate the scaling potential of waters and is based on the concept of a saturation pH value (pHs). This is the pH value at which a water, defined in terms of its composition (e.g. alkalinity, dissolved solids, calcium concentration), is just saturated with calcium carbonate at any given temperature. The LSI is the difference between the actual pH and the pHs: LSI = pH − pHs. Thus if the Index is positive, there will be a tendency for carbonate to be precipitated and a scale to be formed. In the past, scale formation has been overcome by the addition of polyphosphates or sulphuric acid (see for example Capper, 1974). The action of polyphosphates depends on their ability to delay the precipitation of calcium carbonate. However, polyphosphates are hydrolysed to orthophosphates which have no capacity for affecting the carbonate precipitation. If acid dosing is used, sufficient acid must be used to destroy the alkaline hardness. The resultant water is aggressive and requires the addition of high levels (e.g. 15–30 mg l^{-1} CrO_4) of corrosion inhibitors. Modern control, however, relies either on the use of: (a) dispersants, which minimise scale deposition, used in waters with positive Langelier indices, or (b) the use of polyolesters or

Table 12.26. *Typical microbial species found in cooling systems*

Algae	Fungi	Bacteria	
Chlamydomonas	*Aspergillus*	Slime-forming	Corrosive
Chorococcus	*Alternaria*	*Aerobacter*	*Desulphovibrio*
			desulphuricans
Volvex	*Penicillium*	*Bacillus mycoides*	
Spirogyra	*Trichoderma*	*Bacillus subtilis*	Iron depositing
Ulothrix	*Torula*	*Pseudomonas*	*Gallinonella*
Scenedesmus	*Monilia*	*Flavobacter*	*Crenothrix*
Navicula			

From Atkinson, 1974.

Table 12.27. *Typical biocides used in cooling water*

Oxidising types	Non-oxidising types
Chlorine	Acrolein
Sodium hypochlorite	Phenates/chlorinated phenates
Chlorine dioxide	Quaternary ammonium salts
	Organo-sulphur compounds
	(e.g. thiocyanates; dithiocarbamates; sulphones)
	Organo-nitrogen compounds
	(e.g. substituted morpholines/guanidines)
	Organo-metallic compounds
	(e.g. tributyl tin oxide)

phosphonates as scale inhibitors. These do not exacerbate the natural corrosivity in the same way as acid dosing so that lower levels (e.g. 5–7 mg l^{-1} CrO$_4$) of the potentially toxic corrosion inhibitors can be used.

Cooling water provides a good supply of the nutriments required for microbial growth. Not only does the raw water contain nutrient material, but also most of the additives used to control scale formation and corrosion are organic or contain nitrogen or phosphorus. The microbial species that cause the most nuisance are algae, fungi and bacteria (Table 12.26). Algae and fungi, in the main, are liable to cause physical blockages. Bacteria, as well as producing slime deposits, can give rise to corrosion, iron deposition and, in some cases, the very specific degradation of additives (e.g. nitrite oxidation by *Nitrobacter* spp.). There is a wide range of biocides which can be added to cooling waters (e.g. Table 12.27) – some are relatively specific in their action, while others are effective against a wide range of microbes. The choice,

Table 12.28. *Typical 'target levels' for microbial concentrations in treated cooling water*

Microbial type	Number ml^{-1}
Slime-forming bacteria	10^4
Sulphate-reducing bacteria	None
Total bacteria	10^5
Fungi	None

Table 12.29. *Approximate dosages of biocides*

Type	Dose^a (mg l^{-1})
Chlorophenate	200–400
Organo-metallic	125–200
Di-amine	50–200
Organo-sulphur	25–120
Quaternary ammonium	150
Thiocyanates	10

^{a} Based on the formulation not the active component.

therefore, depends on the precise nature of the problem to be corrected – typical control levels are shown in Table 12.28 – but, as microbes can develop resistant strains, users are advised to change the type of biocide periodically. Similarly the method, the frequency of dosing and the dose required will depend both on the severity of the problem, the physical characteristics of the individual cooling water systems, and the biocide being used (e.g. Table 12.29). The formulations which will be of most importance, as far as proscription by the EEC is concerned, are those containing organo-tin compounds or halogenated hydrocarbons.

Despite the development of these more exotic biocides, chlorine is, and will probably continue to be, the most widely used biocide. It is therefore the ecological effects of chlorinated discharges that must be of most concern. These are well documented (see Chapter 9), but it must be emphasised that whenever a new discharge is being planned it is essential to carry out a full ecological survey of the area likely to be affected by the discharge well before the discharge commences, so that the 'base-line' can be properly established.

References

Chapter 1

Atkinson, B. & Howell, J. A. (1975). Slime hold-up, influent BOD and mass transfer in trickling filters. *American Society of Civil Engineers Journal, Environment Engineering Division*, **101**, 585–605.

Clarke, A. R. & Forster, C. F. (1983). The significance of ATP in the settlement of activated sludge. *Journal of Chemical Technology and Biotechnology*, **33B**,127–35.

Cornish-Bowden, A. (1976). *Principles of Enzyme Kinetics*. London: Butterworth Press.

Curds, C. R. (1971). Computer simulations of microbial population dynamics in the activated sludge process. *Water Research*, **5**, 1049–66.

Curds, C. R. (1975). Protozoa. In *Ecological Aspects of Used-water Treatment*, vol. 1, ed. Curds, C. R. & Hawkes, H. A., pp. 203–68. London: Academic Press.

Curds, C. R. & Cockburn, A. (1970). Protozoa in biological sewage treatment processes; 2. Protozoa as indicators in the activated-sludge process. *Water Research*, **4**, 237–49.

Eikelboom, D. H. (1975). Filamentous organisms observed in activated sludge. *Water Research*, **9**, 365–88.

Gaudy, A. F. & Gaudy, E. T. (1980). *Microbiology for Environmental Scientists and Engineers*. New York: McGraw-Hill Book Co.

Hawkes, H. A. (1977). Eutrophication of rivers – effects, causes and control. In *Treatment of Industrial Effluents*, ed. Callely, A. G., Forster, C. F. & Stafford, D. A., pp. 159–92. London: Hodder & Stoughton.

Mah, R. A. (1983). Interactions of methanogens and non-methanogens in microbial ecosystems. In *Proceedings 3rd International Symposium on Anaerobic Digestion*, pp. 13–22. Massachusetts.

Owens, M., Edwards, R. W. & Gibbs, J. W. (1964). Some reaeration studies in streams. *International Journal of Air and Water Pollution*, **8**, 469–86.

Pike, E. B. & Carrington, E. G. (1972). Recent developments in the study of bacteria in the activated-sludge process. *Water Pollution Control*, **71**, 583–605.

Williamson, K. & McCarty, P. L. (1976). Verification studies of the biofilm model for bacterial substrate utilisation. *Journal of the Water Pollution Control Federation*, **48**, 281–96.

Zehnder, A. J. B., Ingvorsen, K. & Marti, T. (1982). Microbiology of methane bacteria. In *Anaerobic Digestion 1981*, ed. Hughes, D. E. *et al.*, pp. 45–70. Amsterdam: Elsevier Biomedical Press.

Chapter 2

Aziz, J. A. & Tebbutt, T. H. Y. (1980). Significance of COD, BOD and TOC correlations in kinetic models of biological oxidation. *Water Research*, **14**, 319–24.

Brown, V. M. (1968). The calculation of the acute toxicity of mixtures of poisons to rainbow trout. *Water Research*, **2**, 723–33.

Casapieri, P., Fox, T. M., Owers, P. & Thomson, G. D. (1978). A mathematical deterministic river-quality model. Part 2. Use in evaluating the water-quality management of the Blackwater catchment. *Water Research*, **12**, 1155–61.

Chandler, J. R. (1970). A biological approach to water quality management. *Water Pollution Control*, **69**, 415–22.

Cluckie, I. D. & Forster, C. F. (1982). Observations on a statistical approach to the setting of discharge consent conditions. *Environmental Technology Letters*, **3**, 111–16.

Davies, E. M. (1971). BOD *vs* COD *vs* TOC *vs* TOD. *Water Wastes Engineering*, **8**, 32–8.

Department of the Environment. (1972). *Analysis of Raw, Potable and Waste Waters*. London: HMSO.

Downing, A. L. (1971). Forecasting the effects of polluting discharges on natural waters. 1. Rivers. *International Journal of Environmental Studies*, **2**, 101–10.

Ellis, J. C. & Lacey, R. F. (1980). Sampling: Defining the task and planning the scheme. *Water Pollution Control*, **79**, 452–67.

European Inland Fisheries Advisory Commission. (1970). Water quality of European freshwater fish. *EIFAC Technical Paper No. 11*.

Hellawell, J. M. (1978). *Biological Surveillance of Rivers*. London: Water Research Centre.

Holmes, P. R. (1982). The mathematical modelling of water quality with particular reference to the industrial rivers of Yorkshire. *Water Pollution Control*, **81**, 45–58.

Ministry of Technology. (1967). *Water Pollution Research, 1966*. London: HMSO.

National Water Council. (1977). *River Water Quality, the Next Stage. Review of Consent Conditions*. London: NWC.

National Water Council. (1981). *River Quality – the 1980 Survey and Future Outlook*. London: NWC.

Scottish Development Department. (1976). Development of a water quality index, *Report No. ARD 3*.

Solbe, J. F. de L. G. (1973). The relation between water quality and the status of fish populations in Willow Brook. *Water Treatment and Examination*, **22**, 41–61.

Tebbutt, T. H. Y. (1979). A rational approach to water quality control. *Water Supply and Management*, **3**, 41–53.

Tebbutt, T. H. Y. (1982). A microcomputer program for dissolved oxygen predictions. *Public Health Engineer*, **10**, 87–9.

US Environmental Protection Agency. (1981). *Centre for water quality modelling user's manual for stream quality model* (QUAL II), *EPA Report 600/9-81-015*. Athens, Georgia: US EPA.

Warn, A. E. & Brew, J. S. (1980). Mass balance. *Water Research*, **14**, 1427–34.

Woodiwiss, F. S. (1964). The biological system of stream classification used by the River Trent Board. *Chemistry and Industry*, **11**, 443–7.

Chapter 3

Anderson, G. K., Donnelly, T. & McKeown, K. (1984). The application of anaerobic packed bed reactors to industrial wastewater treatment. *Water Pollution Control*, **83**, 491–8.

Anon. (1983). Deep Shaft II. *World Water*, September, 50–51.

Antonie, R. H. (1978). Design criteria for application of the rotating biological contactor to domestic and industrial wastewater treatment. Paper presented at the International Environment Colloquium, Liege, 1978.

Bailey, D. A. & Thomas, E. V. (1975). The removal of inorganic nitrogen from sewage effluents by biological denitrification. *Water Pollution Control*, **74**, 497–515.

Barnes, D. & Bliss, P. J. (1983). *Biological Control of Nitrogen in Wastewater Treatment*. London: E. & F. N. Spon Ltd.

Barnes, D., Forster, C. F. & Johnstone, D. W. M. (1983). *Oxidation Ditches in Wastewater Treatment*. London: Pitman Books Ltd.

Bolton, D. H. & Ousby, J. C. (1977). The ICI deep shaft effluent treatment process and its potential for large sewage works. *Progress in Water Technology*, **8**, 265–73.

Bosman, J. & Hendricks, F. (1981). The technology and economics of the treatment of a concentrated nitrogenous industrial effluent by biological denitrification using a fluidised-bed reactor. In *Biological Fluidised Bed Treatment of Water and Wastewater*, ed. Cooper, P. F. & Atkinson, B., pp. 222–33. Chichester: Ellis Horwood Ltd.

British Standards Institute. (1972). Code of basic data for the design of buildings: Chapter 5, Part 2, *Wind Loads*. CP3. London: BSI.

British Standards Institute. (1983). *Design and installation of small sewage treatment works and cesspools*. CP6297. London: BSI.

Bruce, A. M. & Merkens, J. C. (1973). Further studies of partial treatment of sewage by high-rate biological filtration. *Water Pollution Control*, **72**, 499–527.

Bruce, A. M. & Merkens, J. C. (1975). Developments in sewage treatment for small communities. *Proceedings of the Eighth Public Health Engineering Conference*, pp. 65–96. Loughborough University of Technology.

Cillie, G. G., Henzen, M. R., Stander, G. J. & Baillie, R. D. (1969). Anaerobic digestion – IV. The application of the process in waste purification. *Water Research*, **3**, 623–43.

Collins, O. C. & Elder, M. D. (1980). Experience in operating the deep-shaft activated sludge process. *Water Pollution Control*, **79**, 272–81.

Cooper, P. F. & Atkinson, B. (1981). *Biological Fluidised Bed Treatment of Water and Wastewater*. Chichester: Ellis Horwood Ltd.

Cooper, P. F. & Wheeldon, D. H. V. (1980). Fluidised and expanded bed reactors for waste-water treatment. *Water Pollution Control*, **79**, 286–306.

Cooper, P. F. & Wheeldon, D. H. V. (1982). Complete treatment of sewage in a two-stage fluidised-bed system. *Water Pollution Control*, **81**, 447–64.

Cooper, P. F., Wheeldon, D. H. V., Ingram-Todd, P. E. & Harrington, D. W. (1981). Sand/biomass separation with production of concentrated sludge. In *Biological Fluidised Bed Treatment of Water and Wastewater*, ed. Cooper, P. F. & Atkinson, B., pp. 361–7. Chichester: Ellis Horwood Ltd.

Cox, G. C., Lewin, W. H., West, J. T., Brignal, W. J., Redhead, D. L., Roberts, J. G., Shah, N. K. & Waller, C. B. (1980). Use of the deep-shaft process in uprating and extending existing sewage-treatment works. *Water Pollution Control*, **79**, 70–86.

Doman, J. (1929). Results of operation of experimental contact filter process with partially submerged rotating plates. *Sewage Works Journal*, **1**, 555–60.

Eckenfelder, W. W. & O'Connor, D. J. (1961). *Biological Waste Treatment*. London: Pergamon Press.

Forster, C. F. (1980). Aeration in fluidised beds. *Biotechnology Letters*, **1**, 253–8.

Forster, C. F. (1984). The potential of anaerobic digestion for treating liquid wastes. *Water Pollution Control*, **83**, 484–90.

Fullen, W. J. (1953). Anaerobic digestion of packing plant wastes. *Sewage and Industrial Wastes*, **25**, 576–85.

Gauntlett, R. B. & Craft, D. G. (1979). Biological removal of nitrate from river water. *Technical Report TR98*. Water Research Centre.

Guarino, C. F., Nelson, M. D., Lozanof, M. & Wilson, T. E. (1980). Uprating activated-sludge plants using rotary biological contactors. *Water Pollution Control*, **79**, 255–71.

Hanbury, M. J., Rachwal, A. J., Johnstone, D. W. M., Critchard, D. J. & Cox, G. C. (1978). Evaluation of the Carrousel system and its potential for denitrification. Paper presented to Institute of Water Engineers and Scientists, Aldershot, 1978.

Hemmings, M. L., Ousby, J. C., Plowright, D. R. & Walker, J. (1977). 'Deep shaft' – Latest position. *Water Pollution Control*, **76**, 441–51.

Hickey, R. & Owens, R. W. (1978). *Excess Growth Control System for Fluidised Bed Reactors.* US Patent No. 4177144.

Hines, D. A., Bailey, M., Ousby, J. C. & Roesler, F. C. (1975). The ICI deep shaft aeration process for effluent treatment. *Institution of Chemical Engineers Symposium Series*, **No. 41**, D1–D10.

Hobson, P. N. (1984). Anaerobic digestion of agricultural wastes. *Water Pollution Control*, **83**, 507–13.

Hoyland, G. & Robinson, P. J. (1983). Aerobic treatment in 'Oxitron' BFB plant at Coleshill. *Water Pollution Control*, **82**, 479–93.

Hutchinson, E. G. (1975). A comparative study of biological filter media. Paper presented at the Biotechnology Conference, Massey University, May 1975.

Institute of Water Pollution Control. (1972). *Manuals of British Practice – Preliminary Processes.* Maidstone, Kent: IWPC.

Institute of Water Pollution Control. (1973). *Manuals of British Practice – Primary Sedimentation.* Maidstone, Kent: IWPC.

Jank, B. E. & Bridle, T. R. (1983). Principles of carbonaceous oxidation, nitrification and denitrification in single-sludge activated sludge plants. In *Oxidation Ditches in Wastewater Treatment*, ed. Barnes, D. *et al.*, pp. 16–40. London: Pitman Books Ltd.

Johnstone, D. W. M., Rachwal, A. J. & Hanbury, M. J. (1983). General aspects of the oxidation ditch process. In *Oxidation Ditches in Wastewater Treatment*, ed. Barnes, D. *et al.*, pp. 41–74. London: Pitman Books Ltd.

Lettinga, G., van Velsen, A. F. M., Hobma, S. W., de Zeeuw, W. & Klapwijk, A. (1980). Use of the upflow sludge blanket (USB) reactor concept for biological waste treatment, especially for anaerobic treatment. *Biotechnology and Bioengineering*, **22**, 699–734.

Lumbers, J. P. (1983). Rotating biological contactors: Current problems and potential developments in design and control. *Public Health Engineer*, **11**, 41–5.

McHarness, D. D. & McCarty, P. L. (1973). Field study of nitrification with the submerged filter. *Environmental Protection Agency Report EPA-R2-73-158.*

Ministry of Housing and Local Government. (1969). *Technical memorandum on activated sludge sewage treatment installations providing for a long period of aeration.* London: HMSO.

Ministry of Housing and Local Government. (1970). *Technical Committee on Storm Overflows and the Disposal of Storm Sewage: Final Report.* London: HMSO.

Morris, G. G. & Burgess, S. (1984). Two phase anaerobic wastewater treatment. *Water Pollution Control*, **83**, 514–20.

National Research Council. (1946). Sewage treatment at military installations. *Sewage Works Journal*, **18**, 787–1028.

Pike, E. B. (1978). The design of percolating filters and rotary biological contractors, including details of international practice. *Technical Report TR 93.* Water Research Centre.

Rockey, J. S. & Forster, C. F. (1982). The use of an anaerobic fluidised bed reactor for the treatment of domestic sewage. *Environmental Technology Letters*, **3**, 487–96.

Stander, G. J. (1967). Treatment of wine distillery wastes by anaerobic digestion. *Proceedings 22nd Industrial Waste Conference*, pp. 892–907. Purdue University.

Steels, I. H. (1974). Design basis for the rotating disc process. *Effluent and Water Treatment Journal*, **14**, 431–45.

Tebbutt, T. H. Y. (1971). *Principles of Water Quality Control.* Oxford: Pergamon Press.

Wilson, F. (1981). *Design Calculations in Wastewater Treatment.* London: E. & F. N. Spon Ltd.

Wu, Y. C. & Smith, E. D. (1982). Rotating biological contactor system design. *American Society of Civil Engineers, Journal of Environmental Engineering Division*, **108**, 578–88.

Young, J. C. & McCarty, P. L. (1967). The anaerobic filter for waste treatment. *Proceedings 22nd Industrial Waste Conference*, pp. 557–74. Purdue University.

Chapter 4

Aiba, S., Humphrey, A. E. & Millis, N. F. (1973). *Biochemical Engineering*. University of Tokyo Press.

Badger, R. B., Robinson, D. D. & Kiff, R. J. (1975). Aeration plant design: Derivation of basic data and comparative performance studies. *Water Pollution Control*, **74**, 415–29.

Bell, G. H. & Gallo, M. (1971). Effect of impurities on oxygen transfer. *Process Biochemistry*, **6 (4)**, 33–5.

Bennett, C. & Shell, G. (1976). Submerged static aerators: What are they all about? *Water and Wastes Engineering*, May, 37–40.

Blachford, A. J., Tramontini, E. M. & Griffiths, A. J. (1982). Oxygenated activated sludge process: Evaluation at Palmersford. *Water Pollution Control*, **81**, 601–18.

Boon, A. G. (1976). Technical review of the use of oxygen in the treatment of wastewater. *Water Pollution Control*, **75**, 206–13.

Boon, A. G. (1983). Aeration methods. In *Oxidation Ditches in Wastewater Treatment*, ed. Barnes, D. *et al.*, pp. 173–87. London: Pitman Books Ltd.

Boon, A. G. & Chambers, B. (1984). Full scale evaluation of aerators. *Water Pollution Control* (in press).

Boon, A. G., Chambers, B. & Collinson, B. (1982). Energy saving in the activated sludge process. In *Effective Use of Energy in the Water Industry*, pp. 1–30. Maidstone, Kent: The Institute of Water Pollution Control.

Boyes, A. P., Forster, C. F., Kelly, A. J. & Maroglou, A. (1982). Design and operational features of an anaerobic fluidised bed. *Institution of Chemical Engineers Symposium Series*, **76**, 369–81.

Casey, T. J. & Karmo, O. T. (1974). The influence of suspended solids on oxygen transfer in aeration systems. *Water Research*, **8**, 805–11.

Clough, G. F. G. (1974). Physical characteristics of mechanical aerators. *Water Pollution Control*, **73**, 564–75.

Clough, G. F. G. (1982). Implications and further applications. In *Sewage Treatment: Optimisation of Fine-bubble Aeration in Activated Sludge Plant*. Project Profile No. 79, Department of Energy.

Dijkstra, F., Jennekens, H. F. & Nooren, P. A. (1978). The development and application of water jet aeration for wastewater treatment. In *International Association Water Pollution Research Conference on Aeration*, Amsterdam, 1978.

Eckenfelder, W. W. & O'Connor, D. J. (1961). *Biological Waste Treatment*. London: Pergamon Press.

Ettlich, W. F. (1978). A comparison of oxidation ditch plants to competing processes for secondary and advanced treatment of municipal wastes. *US National Technical Information Service Report No. PB 281380*.

Forster, C. F. (1984). Aerator performance. *Water Pollution Control* (in press).

Ganczarczyk, J. (1972). The influence of simple phenolics on water aeration kinetics. *Canadian Journal of Chemical Engineering*, **50**, 185–8.

Houk, D. H. & Boon, A. G. (1981). Survey and evaluation of fine-bubble dome-diffusor aeration equipment. *U.S. Environmental Protection Agency Report No. EPA-600/2-81-222*.

Hoyland, G. H. & Robinson, A. O. (1983). Aerobic treatment in 'Oxitron' BFB plant at Coleshill. *Water Pollution Control*, **82**, 479–93.

Johnstone, D. W. M. (1984). Oxygen requirements, energy consumption and sludge production in extended aeration systems. *Water Pollution Control*, **83**, 100–115.

Johnstone, D. W. M. & Carmichael, W. F. (1982). Cirencester Carrousel plant: some process considerations. *Water Pollution Control*, **81**, 587–600.

Kite, O. A. & Garrett, M. E. (1983). Oxygen transfer and its measurement. *Water Pollution Control*, **82**, 21–8.

Lewin, V. H. & Henley, J. R. (1972). Automation of an activated sludge plant. *Process Biochemistry*, **7**, 17–20.

Lewin, V. H. & West, J. T. (1978). Operating experience of oxidation systems. *Proceedings of Symposium: The Use of Oxygen in Public Health Engineering*, J1–J26. Cranfield Institute of Technology.

Lister, A. R. & Boon, A. G. (1973). Aeration in deep tanks: An evaluation of a fine-bubble diffused-air system. *Water Pollution Control*, **72**, 590–605.

Pacz, I. G. & Wassnik, J. G. (1976). Plant design aspects of surface aerators. *H₂O*, **9**, 113–16.

Pells, M. A. (1983). Construction of oxidation ditches. In *Oxidation Ditches in Wastewater Treatment*, ed. Barnes, D., Forster, C. F. & Johnstone, D. W. M., pp. 188–231. London: Pitman Books Ltd.

Rachwal, A. J. & Waller, C. B. (1982). Towards greater efficiency. In *Proceedings of Conference on Oxidation Ditch Technology*, pp. 151–60. Edinburgh: CEP Consultants.

Rees, J. T. & Skellett, C. F. (1974). Performance of a Passavant Mammoth aeration plant. *Water Pollution Control*, **73**, 608–20.

Riet, K. van't. (1979). Review of measuring methods and results in non-viscous gas–liquid mass transfer in stirred vessels. *Industrial Engineering Chemistry (Process Design Development)*, **18**, 357–64.

Schmidt, F. L. & Redmon, D. T. (1975). Oxygen transfer efficiency in deep tanks. *Journal of the Water Pollution Control Federation*, **47**, 2586–98.

Schmidtke, N. W. & Horvath, I. (1977). Scale-up methodology for surface aerated reactors. *Progress in Water Technology*, **9**, 477–93.

Speece, R. E., Madrid, M. & Needham, K. (1971). Downflow bubble contact aeration. *Journal Sanitary Engineering Division Proceedings ASCE*, **97**, 433–42.

Stalzer, W. & von der Emde, W. (1972). Tanks with turbulent flow generated by Mammoth rotors. *Water Research*, **6**, 417–21.

Stanton, P. J. & Hargreaves, D. W. (1979). Aspects of the design and operation of the Market Drayton WRW. *Journal of the Institution of Water Engineers and Scientists*, **33**, 336–42.

Tewari, P. K. & Bewtra, J. K. (1982). Alpha and beta factors for domestic wastewater. *Journal of the Water Pollution Control Federation*, **54**, 1281–7.

Zlokarnik, M. (1979). Scale-up surface aerators for wastewater treatment. *Advances in Biochemical Engineering*, **11**, 157–80.

Chapter 5

Anon. (1977). Cost information for water supply and sewage disposal. *Technical Report TR61*. Water Research Centre.

Anon. (1981). Sewage treatment optimisation model. User manual and description. *Technical Report TR144*. Water Research Centre.

Chambers, B. (1982). Effect of longitudinal mixing and anoxic zones on settleability of activated sludge. In *Bulking of Activated Sludge: Prevention and Remedial Methods*, ed. Chambers, B. & Tomlinson, E. J., pp. 166–83. Chichester: Ellis Horwood Ltd.

Forster, C. F. (1982). Microbial aspects of oxidation ditch operation. In *Proceedings of Conference on Oxidation Ditch Technology*, pp. 57–66. Edinburgh: CEP Consultants.

James, A. (ed.) (1978). *Mathematical Models in Water Pollution Control*. Chichester: J. Wiley & Sons.

Middlebrooks, E. J. & Garland, C. F. (1968). Kinetics of model and field extended aeration wastewater treatment units. *Journal of the Water Pollution Control Federation*, **40**, 586–612.

Miscellaneous Authors. (1975). *Progress in Water Technology*, **7 (1)**.

Rensink, J. H., Donker, H. J. G. W. & Ijwema, T. S. J. (1982). The influence of feed pattern on sludge bulking. In *Bulking of Activated Sludge: Prevention and Remedial Methods*, ed. Chambers, B. & Tomlinson, E. J., pp. 147–65. Chichester: Ellis Horwood Ltd.

Tomlinson, E. J. (1982). The emergence of the bulking problem and the current situation in the UK. In *Bulking of Activated Sludge: Prevention and Remedial Methods*, ed. Chambers, B. & Tomlinson, E. J., pp. 17–28. Chichester: Ellis Horwood Ltd.

Tomlinson, E. J. & Chambers, B. (1979). *The Effect of Longitudinal Mixing on the Settleability of Activated Sludge*. Technical Report TR 122. Water Research Centre.

Yang, P. Y. & Chen, Y. K. (1977). Operational characteristics and biological kinetic constants of extended aeration process. *Journal of the Water Pollution Control Federation*, **49**, 678–88.

Chapter 6

Aldred, M. I. & Eagles, B. G. (1982). Hydrogen sulphide corrosion of the Baghdad trunk sewerage system. *Water Pollution Control*, **81**, 80–96.

Anderson, J. A. (1981). Primary sedimentation of sewage. *Water Pollution Control*, **80**, 413–20.

Anderson, R. & Greaves, G. F. (1983). Wet ozonation for the treatment of sewage works odours. *Water Pollution Control*, **82**, 18–20.

Ando, S. (1980). Odor control of wastewater treatment plants. *Journal of the Water Pollution Control Federation*, **52**, 906–13.

Anon. (1975). Oxygenation and wastewater treatment. *Environmental Science and Technology*, **9**, 910–15.

Anon. (1983). Deep Shaft II. *World Water*, September, 50–51.

Antonie, R. L. (1978). Design criteria for application of the rotating biological contactor to domestic and industrial wastewater treatment. *International Environment Colloquium*, Liege, 1978.

Banks, N. (1976). UK work on the use of oxygen in the treatment of wastewater associated with the CCMS advanced wastewater treatment project. *Water Pollution Control*, **75**, 214–20.

Baum, H. E. (1975). Plastic balls suppress sewage plant smells. *Water and Pollution Control*, **113 (No. 3)**, 7–8.

Bhatla, M. N. (1975). Control of odours at an activated sludge plant. *Journal of the Water Pollution Control Federation*, **47**, 281–90.

Bignal, W. J. (1982). Latest development in the Deep Shaft wastewater treatment process. *Public Health Engineer*, **10**, 159–63.

Blachford, A. J., Tramontini, E. M. & Griffiths, A. J. (1982). Oxygenated activated sludge process: Evaluation at Palmersford. *Water Pollution Control*, **81**, 601–18.

Boon, A. G. (1976). Technical review of the use of oxygen in the treatment of wastewater. *Water Pollution Control*, **75**, 206–13.

Boon, A. G. & Lister, A. R. (1975). Formation of sulphide in rising-main sewers and its prevention by injection of oxygen. *Progress in Water Technology*, **7**, 289–300.

Boon, A. G., Skellett, C. F., Newcombe, S., Jones, J. G. & Forster, C. F. (1977). The use of oxygen to treat sewage in a rising main. *Water Pollution Control*, **76**, 98–112.

Booth, M. (1984). The alternative to aeration. *Water Pollution Control* (in press).

Bosman, D. J. & Kalos, J. M. (1978). Relation between aeration rates and settling characteristics of activated sludge. *Water Pollution Control*, **77**, 101–3.

Bruce, A. M. & Merkens, J. C. (1975). Developments in sewage treatment for small communities. *Proceedings 8th Public Health Engineering Conference*, pp. 65–96. Loughborough University.

Chambers, B. & Tomlinson, E. J. (eds.) (1982). *Bulking of Activated Sludge*. Chichester: Ellis Horwood Ltd.

Cheung, P. S. & Krauth, K. (1980). The effects of nitrate concentration and retention period on biological denitrification in the rotating disc system. *Water Pollution Control*, **79**, 99–105.

Cheung, P. S. & Mack, G. (1982). The influence of organic loading and retention period on the performance of the rotating disc system. *Water Pollution Control*, **81**, 553–7.

Cole, C. A., Paul, P. A. & Brewer, H. P. (1976). Odour control with hydrogen peroxide. *Journal of the Water Pollution Control Federation*, **48**, 297–306.

Collett, D. (1972). Problems of odour. *Process Biochemistry*, **7 (11)**, 17–18.

Collins, O. C. & Elder, M. D. (1980). Experience in operating the Deep Shaft activated sludge process. *Water Pollution Control*, **79**, 272–85.

Collins, O. C. & Elder, M. D. (1982). Experience in operating the Deep Shaft activated sludge process. *Public Health Engineer*, **10**, 153–8.

Cotton, P. (1973). Automation of the control and operation of water pollution control works. *Water Pollution Control*, **72**, 635–57.

Cox, G. C., Lewin, V. H., West, J. T., Bignal, W. J., Redhead, D. L., Roberts, J. G., Shah, N. K. & Waller, C. B. (1980). The use of the Deep Shaft process in uprating and extending existing sewage treatment works. *Water Pollution Control*, **79**, 70–86.

Dhaliwal, B. S. (1979). *Nocardia amarae* and activated sludge foaming. *Journal of the Water Pollution Control Federation*, **51**, 344–50.

Dick, R. I. & Vesilind, P. A. (1969). Sludge volume index – what is it? *Journal of the Water Pollution Control Federation*, **41**, 1285–91.

Downing, A. L. (1968). Factors to be considered in the design of activated sludge plant. In *Advances in Water Quality Improvement*, ed. Gloyna, E. F. & Eckenfelder, W. W., pp. 190–202. *Water Resources Symposium No. 1*, University of Texas Press.

Eno, J. M. & Pollington, D. C. (1975). Washington sewage works: design and operation. *Water Pollution Control*, **74**, 571–83.

Eves, E. G. (1981). Hogsmill Valley works: twenty years on. *Water Pollution Control*, **80**, 453–62.

Forster, C. F. (1968). The surface of activated sludge particles in relation to their settling characteristics. *Water Research*, **2**, 767–76.

Forster, C. F. (1969). An investigation into the Lubeck process. *Water and Waste Treatment*, **12**, 166–72.

Forster, C. F. (1982). A further examination of mass flux theory as applied to activated sludge settlement. *Biotechnology Letters*, **4**, 381–6.

Forster, F. C. (1983). Continuously operated ditches. In *Oxidation Ditches in Wastewater Treatment*, ed. Barnes, D., Forster, C. F. & Johnstone, D. W .M., pp. 75–131. London: Pitman Books Ltd.

Forster, C. F. & Choudhry, N. M. (1972). Physico-chemical studies on activated sludge bioflocculation. *Effluent and Water Treatment Journal*, **12**, 127–31.

Forster, C. F. & Lewin, D. C. (1972). Polymer interactions at activated sludge surfaces. *Effluent and Water Treatment Journal*, **12**, 520–5.

Fryer, B. & Musty, P. (1983). Optimisation of Coleshill activated-sludge plant operating conditions. *Water Pollution Control*, **82**, 443–56.

Garrett, M. E. & Jeffries, C. (1983). Odour problems at effluent treatment plants – some remedies which use commercial oxygen. *Water Pollution Control*, **82**, 590.

Guarino, C. F., Nelson, M. D. & Edwards, A. B. (1974). Philadelphia pilots and builds oxygen activated sludge. *American Society of Civil Engineers, Journal of Environmental Engineering Division*, **100**, 919–35.

Guarino, C. F., Nelson, M. D., Lozanof, M. & Wilson, T. E. (1980). Uprating activated-sludge plants using rotary biological contactors. *Water Pollution Control*, **79**, 255–71.

Hao, O. & Hendricks, G. F. (1975). Rotating biological contactors remove nutrients. *Water and Sewage Works*, 48–50.

Harbott, B. J. & Penney, C. J. (1983). The efficiency of insecticide treatment of flies on biological filters. *Water Pollution Control*, **82**, 571–81.

Hawkes, H. A. & Shepherd, M. R. N. (1971). The seasonal accumulation of solids in percolating filters and attempted control at low frequency dosing. *Proceedings 5th International Water Pollution Research Conference*, ed. Jenkins, S. H., II 11–1–II 11–8. Oxford: Pergamon Press.

Hegemann, W. & Bischofsberger, W. (1976). Development in the application of oxygen in the activated sludge process in the Federal Republic of Germany. *Water Pollution Control*, **75**, 221–6.

Hemming, M. L., Ousby, J. C., Plowright, D. R. & Walker, J. (1977). Deep-Shaft – Latest position. *Water Pollution Control*, **76**, 441–51.

Hemming, M. L. & Wheatley, A. D. (1979). Low-rate biofiltration systems using random plastics media. *Water Pollution Control*, **78**, 54–68.

Henry, J. G. & Gehr, R. (1980). Odour control: an operator's guide. *Journal of Water Pollution Control*, **52**, 2523–37.

Hitdlebaugh, J. A. & Miller, R. D. (1981). Operating problems with rotating biological contactors. *Journal of the Water Pollution Control Federation*, **53**, 1283–93.

Hopwood, A. P. & Rosen, G. D. (1972). Protein and fat recovery from effluents. *Process Biochemistry*, **7 (3)**, 15–17.

Houk, D. H. & Boon, A. G. (1981). Survey and evaluation of fine-bubble dome-diffusor aeration equipment. *US Environmental Protection Agency Report No. EPA-600/2-81-222*.

Hoyland, G. & Ronald, D. (1984). Biological filtration of finely-screened sewage. *Water Pollution Control* (in press).

Huang, J. Y. C. & Wilson, G. E. (1979). Evaluation of activated carbon adsorption for sewer odor control. *Journal of the Water Pollution Control Federation*, **51**, 1054–62.

IWPC. (1974). *Manuals of British Practice in Water Pollution. Tertiary Treatment and Advanced Waste Water Treatment*. Maidstone, Kent: The Institute of Water Pollution Control.

Jank, B. E. & Bridle, T. R. (1983). Principles of carbonaceous oxidation, nitrification and denitrification in single-sludge activated sludge plants. In *Oxidation Ditches in Wastewater Treatment*, ed. Barnes, D., Forster, C. F. & Johnstone, D. W. M., pp. 16–40. London: Pitman Books Ltd.

Jenkins, D., Neethling, J. B., Bode, H. & Richard, M. G. (1982). The use of chlorination for control of activated sludge bulking. In *Bulking of Activated Sludge*, ed. Chambers, B. & Tomlinson, E. J., pp. 187–210. Chichester: Ellis Horwood.

Johnstone, D. W. M., Rachwal, A. J. & Hanbury, M. J. (1983). General aspects of the oxidation ditch process. In *Oxidation Ditches in Wastewater Treatment*, ed. Barnes, D., Forster, C. F. & Johnstone, D. W. M., pp. 41–74. London: Pitman Books.

Jones, P. H. & Sabra, H. M. (1980). Effect of systems solids retention time (SSRT or Sludge Age) on nitrogen removal from activated sludge systems. *Water Pollution Control*, **79**, 106–16.

Kashiwaya, M. & Yoshimoto, K. (1980). Tannery wastewater treatment by the oxygen activated sludge process. *Journal of the Water Pollution Control Federation*, **52**, 999–1007.

Keddie, A. W. C. (1982). The quantification of the emissions and dispersion of odours from sewage treatment works. *Water Pollution Control*, **81**, 266–79.

Kellock, R. W. (1973). The Snodland–Ightham regional drainage scheme: design and operation. *Water Pollution Control*, **72**, 658–65.

Koczkur, E. & Stone, K. R. (1974). Odour control systems for sewage treatment plants. *Water and Pollution Control*, **112 (9)**, 28–9.

Kroiss, H. & Ruider, E. (1977). Comparison of the plug-flow and complete mixed activated sludge process. *Progress in Water Technology*, **8**, 169–73.

Lehman, P. J. (1983). Start-up and operating characteristics of a rotating biological contactor facility. *Journal of the Water Pollution Control Federation*, **55**, 1233–8.

Lemmer, H. & Popp, W. (1982). Microbiological reasons for scum formation in activated sludge plants. *Korrespondenz Abwasser*, **29**, 808–11.

Lockyear, C. F. (1980). A survey of primary treatment and sludge thickenability. *Technical Report TR 133*. Water Research Centre.

Lowe, P. (1982). A decade of experience at the Calder Vale WPC works. *Water Pollution Control*, **81**, 525–39.

McNeil, K. E. (1984). The treatment of wastes from the sugar industry. In *Surveys in Industrial Wastewater Treatment*, vol. 1, ed. Barnes, D., Forster, C. F. & Hrudey, S., pp. 1–68. London: Pitman Books Ltd.

Marais, G. V. R. (1973). *The Activated-Sludge Process at Long Sludge Ages. Research Report No. W3*. Department of Civil Engineering, University of Cape Town.

Matthews, P. J. (1976). Air pollution in sewerage and sewage treatment. *Water Pollution Control*, **75** , 377–89.

Matthews, P. J. & Boon, A. G. (1978). Odour nuisance in sewerage and treatment systems: Problems and Control. *Water Pollution Control*, **77**, 248–58.

Mayman, J. L., Jehlicka, J. & Armstrong, L. (1981). Commissioning and operational experience at Great Billing sewage treatment works. *Water Pollution Control*, **80**, 102–16.

Nash, N., Krasnoff, P. J., Pressman, W. B. & Brenner, R. C. (1977). Oxygen aeration at Newton Creek. *Journal of the Water Pollution Control Federation*, **49**, 388–400.

Nelson, J. K. (1979). Start-up and operation of Denver's pure oxygen activated sludge plant. *Journal of the Water Pollution Control Federation*, **51**, 907–17.

Neufeld, R. D. (1975). Wastewater treatment plant odors: a continuing enigma. *Public Works*, **106 (3)**, 106–7.

Neufeld, R. D. (1984). The treatment of wastes from the synthetic fuels industry. In *Surveys in Industrial Wastewater Treatment*, vol. 2, ed. Barnes, D., Forster, C. F. & Hrudey, S., pp. 65–129. London: Pitman Books Ltd.

North, A. A. (1979). Odours at a sewage treatment works. *Technical Report TR 126*. Water Research Centre.

Otter, C. S. (1966). A physical method for the permanent control of *Psychoda* pests at wastewater treatment plants. *Journal of the Water Pollution Control Federation*, **38**, 156–64.

Painter, H. A. (1980). A survey of filter fly nuisances and their remedies. *Technical Report TR 155*. Water Research Centre.

Parker, D. S. & Merrill, M. S. (1976). Oxygen and air activated sludge: another view. *Journal of the Water Pollution Control Federation*, **48**, 2511–28.

Pike, E. B. (1978). The design of percolating filters and rotary biological contactors, including details of international practice. *Technical Report TR 93*. Water Research Centre.

Pike, E. B., Carlton-Smith, C. H., Evans, R. H. & Harrington, D. W. (1982). Performance of rotating biological contactors under field conditions. *Water Pollution Control*, **81**, 10–27.

Poon, C. P. C., Chin, H. K., Smith, E. D. & Mikucki, W. J. (1981). Upgrading with rotating biological contactors for BOD removal. *Journal of the Water Pollution Control Federation*, **53**, 474–81.

Price, G. J. (1982). Use of an anoxic zone to improve activated-sludge settleability. In *Bulking of Activated Sludge*, ed. Chambers, B. & Tomlinson, E. J., pp. 259–60. Chichester: Ellis Horwood.

Rachwal, A. J., Johnstone, D. W. M., Hanbury, M. J. & Critchard, D. J. (1982). The application of settleability tests for the control of activated sludge plants. In *Bulking of Activated Sludge*, ed. Chambers, B. & Tomlinson, E. J., pp. 224–44. Chichester: Ellis Horwood.

Rachwal, A. J., Johnstone, D. W. M., Hanbury, M. J. & Carmichael, W. F. (1983). An intensive evaluation of the Carrousel system. In *Oxidation Ditches in Wastewater Treatment*, ed. Barnes, D., Forster, C. F. & Johnstone, D. W. M., pp. 132–72. London: Pitman Books Ltd.

Robinson, M., Varley, R. A. & Kimber, A. R. (1982). The use of oxygen to uprate the treatment capacity of a conventional surface-aeration plant at Holdenhurst (Bournemouth) sewage treatment works. *Water Pollution Control*, **81**, 391–8.

Ruffer, H. M. & Rosenwinkel, K. H. (1984). The treatment of wastewater from the beverage industry. In *Surveys in Industrial Wastewater Treatment*, vol. 1, ed. Barnes, D., Forster, C. F. & Hrudey, S., pp. 69–127. London: Pitman Books Ltd.

Sezgin, M., Jenkins, D. & Parker, D. S. (1978). A unified theory of activated sludge filamentous bulking. *Journal of the Water Pollution Control Federation*, **50**, 362–81.

Shahalam, A. B. M. (1982). Scrubbing odors from wastewater treatment. *American Society of Civil Engineers, Journal of Environmental Engineering Division*, **108**, 785–99.

Sims, A. F. E. (1980). Odour control with hydrogen peroxide. *Progress in Water Technology*, **12**, 609–20.

Skellett, C. F. (1978). Oxygen injection into rising mains and its effect on treatment. *Proceedings of the Symposium on The Use of Oxygen in Public Health Engineering*, pp. B1–B49. Cranfield Institute of Technology.

Smith, P. B. & Yates, D. (1980). Experiences of high-rate biological filtration at Derby sewage treatment works. *Water Pollution Control*, **79**, 87–98.

Stamberg, J. B., Bishop, D. F. & Kumke, G. (1972). Activated sludge treatment with oxygen. *American Institute of Chemical Engineers Symposium Series*, **68**, 25–34.

Steels, I. H. (1974). Design basis for the rotating disc process. *Effluent and Water Treatment Journal*, **14**, 433–55.

Steen, D. & Johnson, G. R. (1978). The use of pure oxygen in wastewater and potable water treatment. *Proceedings of the Symposium on The Use of Oxygen in Public Health Engineering*, pp. G1–G47. Cranfield Institute of Technology.

Tebbutt, T. H. Y. & Christoulas, D. G. (1975). Performances relationship for primary sedimentation. *Water Research*, **9**, 347–56.

Todd, J. J. (1974). Blow your problems. *Environmental Pollution Management*, **4 (2)**, 79, 81.

Tomlinson, E. J. (1976). Bulking – a survey of activated sludge plants. *Technical Report TR 35*. Water Research Centre.

Tomlinson, E. J. & Chambers, B. (1979). The use of anoxic mixing zones to control the settleability of activated sludge. *Technical Report TR 116*. Water Research Centre.

Toms, R. & Booth, M. (1982). The use of oxygen in sewage treatment. *Water Pollution Control*, **81**, 151–65.

Water Research Centre. (1978). Tests for assessing the oxygen demand of effluents. *Notes on Water Research No. 14*. WRC.

Water Research Centre. (1981). Sewage treatment optimisation model: user manual and description. *Technical Report TR 144*. WRC.

White, M. J. D. (1975). Settling of activated sludge. *Technical Report TR 11*. Water Research Centre.

Wood, L. B., King, R. T., Durkin, M. K., Finch, H. J. & Sheldon, D. (1976). The operation of a Simplex activated sludge pilot plant in an atmosphere of pure oxygen. *Public Health Engineer*, **4**, 67–75.

Woods, D. R., Williams, J. M. & Croydon, J. (1978). Fly nuisance control in treatment systems. *Water Pollution Control*, **77**, 259–70.

Wyatt, K. L., Brown, P. & Shabi, F. A. (1977). Oxidation processes in activated sludge at high dissolved oxygen concentrations. *Water Pollution Control*, **76**, 340–54.

Chapter 7

Ahlberg, N. R. & Giffen, A. V. (1972). Field evaluation and design considerations of aerobic digestion. *Research Report W40*, Ontario Ministry of the Environment.

Anon. (1983). *Water and Waste Treatment*, **26 (8)**, 2–4.

Baskerville, R. C. & Gale, R. S. (1968). A simple automatic instrument for determining the filterability of sewage sludges. *Water Pollution Control*, **67**, 233–41.

Baskerville, R. C. & Lockyear, C. F. (1980). Activated sludge – Thickening, pumping and dewatering, Pt. 2. Paper presented to East Midlands Branch Institute of Water Pollution Control, 1980.

Berger, O. & Warren, A. V. (1966). The Rotoplug sludge concentrator: Developments in design and operation. *Journal of the Institute of Sewage Purification*, 327–36.

Booker, D. I. J. (1981). Beddington sewage-treatment works, Croydon – Some operating experiences, 1969–79. *Water Pollution Control*, **80**, 356–77.

Brade, C. E. & Noone, G. P. (1981). Anaerobic sludge digestion – need it be expensive? Making more of existing resources. *Water Pollution Control*, **80**, 70–94.

Brade, C. E., Noone, G. P., Powell, E., Rundle, H. & Whyley, J. (1982). The application of developments in anaerobic digestion with Severn–Trent Water Authority. *Water Pollution Control*, **81**, 200–19.

Bruce, A. M. & Lockyear, C. E. (1982). Uprating sludge treatment processes. *Water Pollution Control*, **81**, 425–43.

Burgess, J. V. (1968). Comparison of sludge incineration processes. *Process Biochemistry*, **3 (7)**, 27–30.

Burley, M. J. & Bayley, R. W. (1977). Sludge disposal strategy: Processes and costs. *Water Pollution Control*, **76**, 205–21.

Burton, D. & Conway, E. (1983). Early operating experiences of sludge incineration at Douglas Valley. *Water Pollution Control*, **82**, 521–34.

Calcutt, T. & Moss, J. (1983). Effective and economic sewage sludge treatment and disposal techniques. *Water and Waste Treatment*, **26 (9)**, 36–40.

Carrington, E. G. (1980). The fate of pathogenic micro-organisms during waste-water treatment and disposal. *Technical Report TR 128*. Water Research Centre.

Coakley, P. (1960). Principles of vacuum filtration and their application to sludge drying problems. In *Waste Treatment*, ed. Isaac, P. C. G., pp. 317–34. Oxford: Pergamon Press.

Cohen, D. B. (1977). A comparison of pure oxygen and diffused air digestion of waste activated sludge. *Progress in Water Technology*, **9**, 691–702.

Coker, E. G. (1965). Experiments in East Hertfordshire on the use of liquid digested sludge as a manure for certain farm crops. *Journal of the Institute of Sewage Purification*, 419–26.

Coker, E. G., Davis, R. D., Hall, J. E. & Carlton-Smith, C. H. (1982). Field experiments on the use of consolidated sewage sludge for land reclamation: Effects on crop yield and composition and soil conditions, 1976–1981. *Technical Report TR 183*. Water Research Centre.

Collinge, V. K. & Bruce, A. M. (1981). Sewage sludge disposal: A strategic review and assessment of research needs. *Technical Report TR 166*. Water Research Centre.

Davis, R. D. & Coker, E. G. (1980). Cadmium in agriculture with special reference to the utilisation of sewage sludge on land. *Technical Report TR 139*. Water Research Centre.

Department of the Environment. (1972). *Analysis of Raw, Potable and Waste Waters.* London: HMSO.

Department of the Environment. (1975). Sewage sludge dewatering by filter belt press. *Project Report No. 4, Research and Development Division, Department of the Environment.* London: HMSO.

Department of the Environment. (1978). Sewage sludge disposal data and review of disposal to sea. *Department of the Environment/National Water Council Standing Committee Report No. 8.* London: HMSO.

Department of the Environment. (1981). Report of the sub-committee on the disposal of sewage sludge to land. *Department of the Environment/National Water Council Standing Committee Report No. 20.* London: HMSO.

Dickens, R., Wallis, B. & Arundel, J. (1980). Fluidised bed incineration of sewage sludge at Esher, 1976–1978. *Water Pollution Control,* **79,** 431–41.

Dotson, G. K. (1973). Some constraints of spreading sewage sludge on cropland. In *Proceedings of the Conference on Land Disposal of Municipal Effluents and Sludges.* EPA-902/9-73-001.

Dowdy, R. H. & Larson, W. F. (1975). The availability of sludge-borne metals to various vegetable crops. *Journal of Environmental Quality,* **4,** 278–82.

Doyle, C. B. (1967). Effectiveness of high pH for destruction of pathogens in raw sludge filter cake. *Journal of the Water Pollution Control Federation,* **39,** 1403–9.

Edmondson, B. R. & Brooks, D. R. (1978). Some tests on the membrane filter plate. *Water Pollution Control,* **77,** 117–37.

Egglink, H. J. (1975). Experience in centrifugation of sewage sludge – aspects of performance and reliability. *Progress in Water Technology,* **7,** 947–58.

Eikum, H. S. & Paulsrud, D. (1974). Filtration properties of aerobic stabilised primary and mixed primary-chemical (alum) sludge. *Water Research,* **8,** 203–9.

Eves, E. G. (1981). Hogsmill Valley Works: twenty years on. *Water Pollution Control,* **80,** 453–62.

Fish, H. (1983). Sea disposal of sludge: the UK experience. *Water Science and Technology,* **15,** 77–88.

Forster, C. F. (1973). Sludge – Waste or raw material? *Effluent and Water Treatment Journal,* **13,** 697–9.

Forster, C. F. (1981). Preliminary studies on the relationship between sewage sludge viscosities and the nature of the surfaces of the component particles. *Biotechnology Letters,* **3,** 707–12.

Forster, C. F. (1982). Sludge surfaces and their relationship to the rheology of the sewage sludge suspensions. *Journal of Chemical Technology and Biotechnology,* **32,** 799–807.

Franzen, G. & Hakanson, L. (1983). Thermophilic aerobic digestion of sewage sludge. *Vatten,* **39,** 213–16.

Frost, R. C. (1982). Prediction of friction losses for the flow of sewage sludge in straight pipes. *Technical Report TR 175.* Water Research Centre.

Gale, R. S. (1972). The sludge treatment and disposal problem. Paper presented at Symposium on Incineration of Refuse and Sludge, University of Southampton.

Gale, R. S. (1975). Control of sludge filter operation. *Filtration and Separation,* **12,** 74–6, 78–83.

Garber, W. F. (1982). Operating experience with thermophilic anaerobic digestion. *Journal of the Water Pollution Control Federation,* **54,** 1170–5.

Grieve, A. (1978). Sludge incineration with particular reference to the Coleshill plant. *Water Pollution Control,* **77,** 314–23.

Gunson, H. G. & Morgan, S. F. (1982). Aerobic thermophilic digestion of sewage sludge. *Effluent and Water Treatment Journal,* **23,** 319–20.

Hamilton, D. (1969). Mechanical dewatering of mixed sludges at Andover. *Water Pollution Control,* **68,** 224–7.

Hoyland, G., Day, M. & Baskerville, R. C. (1981). Getting more out of the filter press. *Technical Report TR 173*. Water Research Centre.

Institute of Water Pollution Control. (1978–81). *Manuals of British Practice in Water Pollution Control. Sewage Sludge I, II and III*. Maidstone, Kent: IWPC.

Jank, B. E. Discussion on Thomas, J., 1975.

Jewell, W. J. & Kabrick, R. M. (1980). Autoheated aerobic thermophilic digestion with aeration. *Journal of the Water Pollution Control Federation*, **52**, 512–23.

Johnson, M. (1981). First report on the WRC sewage pumping project. *Technical Report TR 162*. Water Research Centre.

Kabrick, R. M. & Jewell, W. J. (1982). Fate of pathogens in thermophilic aerobic sludge digestion. *Water Research*, **16**, 1051–60.

Kellock, R. W. (1973). The Snodland–Ightham regional drainage scheme: Design and operation. *Water Pollution Control*, **72**, 658–65.

Kirkham, M. B. (1974). Disposal of sludge on land: Effect on soils, plants and ground water. *Compost Science*, **15**, 6–10.

Latham, L., Latham, M. & Basta, S. S. (1977). The nutritional and economic implications of *Ascaris* infection in Kenya. *World Bank Staff Working Paper No. 271*. Washington DC: The World Bank.

Linfield, R. (1977). Potato cyst eelworm studies in AWA. In *Research Seminar on Pathogens in Sewage Sludge, Research and Development Division Tehnical Note No. 7*. Department of the Environment.

Lockyear, C. F. (1977). Gravity thickening of biological sludges. *Technical Report TR 39*. Water Research Centre.

Lockyear, C. F. (1978). Pilot scale experiments on continuous gravity thickening of activated sludge. *Technical Report TR 97*. Water Research Centre.

Lockyear, C. F. & White, M. J. D. (1979). The WRC thickenability test using a low-speed centrifuge. *Technical Report TR 118*. Water Research Centre.

Lockyear, C. F., Jackson, P. J. & Warden, J. H. (1983). Polyelectrolyte users' manual. *Technical Report TR 184*. Water Research Centre.

Lowe, P. & Williamson, S. (1983). Accelerated cold digestion: A new look at an old technique. *Water Pollution Control*, **82**, 457–70.

McIntyre, A. D. (1977). A review of the effects of the disposal of sewage sludge to sea. *Technical Note No. 6*. Research and Development Division, Department of the Environment.

Maddock, J. E. L. & Tomlinson, E. J. (1980). The clarification of effluent from an activated sludge plant using dissolved-air flotation. *Water Pollution Control*, **79**, 117–25.

Mann, H. H. & Barnes, H. D. (1963). The Woburn market-garden experiment: Summary 1944–1960. *Rothampsted Experimental Station Report*.

Matsch, L. C. & Drnevich, R. F. (1977). Autothermal aerobic digestion. *Journal of the Water Pollution Control Federation*, **49**, 296–310.

Matthews, P. J. (1983). Agriculture utilisation of sewage sludge in the United Kingdom. *Water Science and Technology*, **15**, 135–50.

Mavinic, D. S. & Koers, D. A. (1979). Performance and kinetics of low-temperature, aerobic sludge digestion. *Journal of the Water Pollution Control Federation*, **51**, 2088–97.

Melbourne, J. D. & Zabel, T. F. (eds.) (1977). *Flotation for Water and Waste Treatment*. Water Research Centre.

Ministry of Housing and Local Government. (1954). *Report of an Informal Working Party on the Treatment and Disposal of Sewage Sludge*. London: HMSO.

Ministry of Housing and Local Government. (1970). *Taken for Granted. Report of the Working Party on Sewage Disposal*. London: HMSO.

Moore, J. G. (1983). The design and construction of Springfield sewage-treatment works. *Water Pollution Control*, **82**, 37–41.

Mosey, F. E. (1976). Assessment of the maximum concentration of the heavy metals in crude sewage which will not inhibit the anaerobic digestion of sludge. *Water Pollution Control*, **75**, 10–20.

Nelson, J. K. & Tavery, M. A. H. (1978). Chemical conditioning alternatives and operational control for vacuum filtration. *Journal of the Water Pollution Control Federation*, **50**, 507–17.

Nice, J., Pullen, K. G. & Robinson, J. (1978). The sludge disposal cycle. *Water Pollution Control*, **77**, 492–508.

Noone, G. P. & Brade, C. E. (1982). Low-cost provision of anaerobic digestion: II. High-rate and prefabricated systems. *Water Pollution Control*, **81**, 479–510.

Norton, M. G. (1978). The control of monitoring of sewage sludge dumping at sea. *Water Pollution Control*, **77**, 402–7.

Pietila, K. A. & Joubert, P. J. (1981). Examination of process parameters affecting sludge dewatering with a diaphragm filter press. *Journal of the Water Pollution Control Federation*, **53**, 1708–16.

Pike, E. B., Morris, D. L. & Carrington, E. G. (1983). Inactivation of ova of the parasites *Taenia saginata* and *Ascaris suum* during heated anaerobic digestion. *Water Pollution Control*, **82**, 501–9.

Pullin, C. J. (1981). Investigations into sludge dewatering using polyelectrolyte conditioners at Bybrook sewage-treatment works. *Water Pollution Control*, **80**, 95–101.

Purves, D. (1983). EC Directive on the use of sewage sludge in agriculture – Environmental implications. In *Proceedings of Conference on Heavy Metals in the Environment*, pp. 342–5. Edinburgh: CEP Consultants Ltd.

Riegler, G. (1982). Aerobic or anaerobic sludge stabilisation. *Korrespondenz Abwasser*, **29**, 790–4.

Rose-Innes, I. H. & Nossel, S. (1983). The rheology and pumping of thickening activated sludge. *Water Science and Technology*, **15**, 59–76.

Rundle, H. & Whyley, J. (1981). A comparison of gas recirculation systems for mixing of contents of anaerobic digesters. *Water Pollution Control*, **80**, 463–80.

Sidwick, J. M., Butler, B. E. & Ruscombe-King, N. J. (1975). Sludge dewatering trials at Banbury. *Water Pollution Control*, **74**, 675–87.

Sleeth, R. E. (1970). An assessment of polyelectrolytes for sludge conditioning at Worthing. *Water Pollution Control*, **69**, 31–9.

Smith, J. T., Griffin, B. G. & Grahame, A. W. (1978). Commissioning and initial operation of the Coleshill incineration plant. *Water Pollution Control*, **77**, 324–45.

Swanwick, J. D., Shurben, D. G. & Jackson, S. (1969). A survey of the performance of sewage sludge digestion in Great Britain. *Water Pollution Control*, **68**, 639–61.

Symes, G. L. & Michaelson, A. P. (1977). Sludge disposal in the North West. *Water Pollution Control*, **76**, 50–8.

Tench, H. B., Phillips, L. F. & Swanwick, K. H. (1972). The Sheffield sludge incineration plant. *Water Pollution Control*, **71**, 176–85.

Thomas, J. (1975). Sludge incineration. New aspects of multiple hearth furnace and fluidised bed incinerator. *Progress in Water Technology*, 7, 935–46.

US Environmental Protection Agency. (1974). *Process Design Manual for Sludge Treatment and Disposal*. EPA 625/1-74-006 (updated as EPA 625/1-79-011, 1979).

Vismara, R. (1983). Aerobic thermophilic autothermal digestion: Optimisation of the process. *Ingegneria Ambientale*, **12**, 155–61.

Wase, D. A. J. & Forster, C. F. (1984). Biogas – fact or fantasy? *Biomass*, **4**, 127–42.

Water Research Centre. (1979). *Utilisation of Sewage Sludge on Land*. Papers and Conference Proceedings, WRC.

Webber, J. (1972). Effect of toxic metals in sewage on crops. *Water Pollution Control*, **71**, 404–13.

Williamson, D. J. & Wheale, G. (1981). The influence of sludge storage on chemical conditioning costs. *Water Pollution Control*, **80**, 529–36.

Wood, R. (1975). The utilisation of sewage sludge. *Effluent and Water Treatment Journal*, **15**, 455–7.

Wuhrmann, K. A. (1977). A more precise method of determination of specific resistance to filtration. *Water Pollution Control*, **76**, 377–79.

Zanoni, A. E. & Muelier, D. L. (1982). Calorific value of wastewater plant sludge. *Proceedings of the American Society of Civil Engineers, Journal of the Environmental Engineering Division*, **108**, 187–95.

Chapter 8

ADAS. (1982). *An Economic Assessment of Anaerobic Digestion*. Ministry of Agriculture, Fisheries and Food.

Anderson, G. K., Donnelly, T. & McKeown, K. (1984). The application of anaerobic packed bed reactors to industrial wastewater treatment. *Water Pollution Control*, **83**, 491–8.

Anon. (1982). *Anaerobic Digestion: A Code of Practice on Safety in and around Anaerobic Digesters*. British Anaerobic and Biomass Association.

Bedogni, S., Bregoli, M. & Viglia, A. (1983). Full scale anaerobic filter treating sugar-mill anionic effluents. In *Proceedings of the Anaerobic Wastewater Treatment Symposium*, pp. 313–14. The Hague: TNO Corporate Communication Department.

Berends, J. (1983). Nitrogen removal from waste water after anaerobic digestion. In *Proceedings of the Anaerobic Waste Water Treatment Symposium*, pp. 577–93. The Hague: TNO Corporate Communication Department.

Brunetti, A., Boari, G., Passino, R. & Rozzi, A. (1983). Physico-chemical factors affecting start-up in UASB digesters. In *Proceedings of the Anaerobic Wastewater Treatment Symposium*, pp. 317–34. The Hague: TNO Corporate Communication Department.

Campbell, D. J. V. (1983). Landfill gas resources and economics in the UK. Paper presented at the Landfill Gas Workshop, Harwell and the British Anaerobic and Biomass Association, Oxford.

Cohen, A. (1983). Two phase digestion of liquid and solid wastes. In *Proceedings 3rd International Symposium on Anaerobic Digestion*, pp. 123–38. Massachusetts.

Colin, F., Ferrero, G. L., Gerletti, M., Hobson, P., L'Hermite, P., Naveau, H. P. & Nyns, E-J. (1983). Proposal for the definition of parameters and analytical measurement applicable to the anaerobic digestion processes. *Agricultural Wastes*, **7**, 183–93.

Colleran, E., Wilkie, A., Barry, M., Faherty, G., O'Kelly, N. & Reynolds, P. J. (1983). One and two-stage anaerobic filter digestion of agricultural wastes. In *Proceedings 3rd International Symposium on Anaerobic Digestion*, pp. 285–302. Massachusetts.

Forster, C. F. & Wase, D. A. J. (1983). Anaerobic digestion. *Industrial Biotechnology Wales*, **2 (1)**, 1–10.

Forster, C. F. & Wase, D. A. J. (1984). Biogas – fact of fantasy? *Biomass*, **4**, 127–42.

Ghosh, S. & Klass, D. L. (1978). Two-phase anaerobic digestion. *Process Biochemistry*, **13 (4)**, 15–20.

Godwin, S. J., Wase, D. A. J. & Forster, C. F. (1982). The use of the upflow anaerobic reactor to treat an industrial waste rich in acetate. *Process Biochemistry*, **July**, 33–4, 45.

Hall, E. R. (1983). The development and utilisation of anaerobic technology in Canada. In *Proceedings 3rd International Symposium on Anaerobic Digestion*, pp. 393–404. Massachusetts.

Hashimoto, A. G. (1983). Commercialisation of anaerobic digestion technology in the United States of America. In *Proceedings 3rd International Symposium on Anaerobic Digestion*, pp. 437–47. Massachusetts.

Hashimoto, A. G. & Chen, Y. R. (1980). The overall economics of anaerobic digestion. In *Anaerobic Digestion 1979*, ed. Stafford, D. A., Wheatley, B. I. & Hughes, D. E., pp. 449–66. London: Applied Science Publishers.

Henrich, R. A. & Phillips, C. (1983). Purification of digester gas into saleable natural gas or vehicle fuel. Paper presented at 56th Annual Water Pollution Control Federation Conference, Atlanta, Georgia.

Henze, M. & Harremoës, P. (1983). Anaerobic treatment of wastewater in fixed film reactors – a literature review. *Water Science and Technology*, **15 (8/9)**, 1–101.

Hobson, P. N. (1984). Anaerobic digestion of agricultural wastes. *Water Pollution Control*, **83**, 507–13.

Hobson, P. N., Bousfield, S. & Summers, R. (1981). *Methane Production from Agricultural Wastes*. Barking: Elsevier Applied Science Publishers Ltd.

Hulshoff Pol, L. W., de Zeeuw, W., Dolfing, J. & Lettinga, G. (1983). Start-up and sludge granulation in UASB-reactors. In *Proceedings of the Anaerobic Wastewater Treatment Symposium*, pp. 40–3. The Hague: TNO Corporate Communication Department.

Huss, L. (1977). the Anamet process for food and fermentation industry effluent. *Tribune de CEBEDEAU*, **30**, 390–6.

Huss, L. (1982). Applications of the Anamet process for waste water treatment. In *Anaerobic Digestion 1981*, ed. Hughes, D. E. *et al.*, pp. 137–50. Amsterdam: Elsevier Biomedical Press.

Jewell, W. J. (1982). Anaerobic attached film expanded bed fundamentals. In *Proceedings 1st International Conference on Fixed Film Biological Processes*, pp. 17–42. Ohio.

Lettinga, G., Hulshoff Pol, L. W., Wiegant, W., de Zeeuw, W., Hobma, S., Grin, P., Roersma, R., Sayed, S. & van Velsen, A. F. M. (1983). Upflow sludge blanket processes. In *Proceedings 3rd International Symposium on Anaerobic Digestion*, pp. 139–58. Massachusetts.

Lettinga, G., van der Geest, A. Th., Hobma, S. & Laan, J. V. D. (1979). Anaerobic treatment of methanolic waste. *Water Research*, **13**, 725–37.

Lettinga, G., van Velsen, A. F. M., Hobma, S., de Zeeuw, W. & Klapwijk, A. (1980). Use of the upflow sludge blanket reactor concept for biological wastewater treatment, especially for anaerobic treatment. *Biotechnology and Bioengineering*, **22**, 699–734.

Maaskant, W. & Zeevalkink, J. A. (1983). First full-scale anaerobic treatment plant for dairy wastewater in the world. In *Proceedings of the Anaerobic Wastewater Treatment Symposium*, pp. 442–5. The Hague: TNO Corporate Communication Department.

Meynell, P. J. (1983). Use of landfill gas – scrubbing. Paper presented at the Landfill Gas Workshop, Harwell and the British Anaerobic and Biomass Association, Oxford.

Morfaux, J. N., Touzel, J-P. & Albagnac, G. (1982). Anaerobic digestion of vegetable canning wastewaters. In *Anaerobic Digestion 1981*, ed. Hughes, D. E. *et al.*, pp. 185–99. Amsterdam: Elsevier Biomedical Press.

Nyns, E-J., Naveau, H. P. & Demuynck, M. (1983). Biogas plants in the European Community and Switzerland, status – bottlenecks – future prospects. In *Proceedings 3rd International Symposium on Anaerobic Digestion*, pp. 429–36. Massachusetts.

Parker, J. & Lyons, B. (1983). Anaerobic digestion of high strength food processing wastes. In *Proceedings of the Anaerobic Wastewater Treatment Symposium*, p. 469. The Hague: TNO Corporate Communication Department.

Pette, K. C. & Versprille, A. I. (1982). Application of the UASB-concept for wastewater treatment. In *Anaerobic Digestion 1981*, ed. Hughes, D. E. *et al.*, pp. 121–36. Amsterdam: Elsevier Biomedical Press.

Pipyn, P. & Verstraete, W. (1979). A pilot scale anaerobic upflow reactor treating distillery wastewater. *Biotechnology Letters*, **1**, 495–500.

Richards, K. M. (1983). Landfill gas: the Department of Energy R and D programme. Paper presented at the Landfill Gas Workshop, Harwell and the British Anaerobic and Biomass Association, Oxford.

Ross, W. R., Smollen, M. & Alberts, P. S. (1981). The technological application of the anaerobic digestion process for the purification of spent wine residue. *CSIR Contract Report C WAT 43*. Pretoria: National Institute for Water Research.

Ross, W. R. & Smollen, M. (1982). Engineering problems with the anaerobic digestion of soluble organic wastes. In *Anaerobic Digestion 1981*, ed. Hughes, D. E. *et al.*, pp. 89–106. Amsterdam: Elsevier Biomedical Press.

Salkinoja-Salonen, M. S., Nyns, E-J., Sutton, P. M., van den Berg, L. & Wheatley, A. D. (1983). Starting-up of an anaerobic fixed-film reactor. *Water Science and Technology*, **15 (8/9)**, 305–8.

Seyfried, C. F., Bode, H. & Saake, M. (1983). Anaerobic treatment plant for the industrial effluent of a pectin producing company. In *Proceedings of the Anaerobic Wastewater Treatment Symposium*, p. 468. The Hague: TNO Corporate Communication Department.

Shore, M., Broughton, N. W. & Bumstead, N. (1984). Anaerobic treatment of wastewaters in the beet sugar industry. *Water Pollution Control*, (in press).

Sidwick, J. M. (1983). *Environmental Biotechnology: Future Prospects. FAST Occasional Papers No. 50*. Directorate General for Science, Research and Development, Commission of the European Communities.

Speece, R. E. & Parkin, G. F. (1983). The response of methane bacteria to toxicity. In *Proceedings 3rd International Symposium on Anaerobic Digestion*, pp. 23–36. Massachusetts.

Stafford, D. A. & Etheridge, S. P. (1982). Farm wastes, energy production and the economics of farm anaerobic digesters. In *Anaerobic Digestion 1981*, ed. Hughes, D. E. *et al.*, pp. 256–70. Amsterdam: Elsevier Biomedical Press.

Stewart, D. J., Badger, D. M. & Bogue, M. J. (1982). Crops and energy production. In *Anaerobic Digestion 1981*, ed. Hughes, D. E. *et al.*, pp. 237–55. Amsterdam: Elsevier Biomedical Press.

Sullivan, J. L., Petters, N. & Ostrovski, C. M. (1981). A methane production feasibility model for central anaerobic digesters. *Resource Recovery and Conservation*, **5**, 319–31.

Sutton, P. M. & Evans, R. R. (1983). Anaerobic system designs for efficient treatment of industrial wastewaters. Poster paper presented at the 3rd International Symposium on Anaerobic Digestion, Massachusetts.

Szendrey, L. M. (1983). Start-up and operation of the Bacardi Corporation anaerobic filter. In *Proceedings 3rd International Symposium on Anaerobic Digestion*, pp. 365–378. Massachusetts.

Taylor, D. W. & Burm, R. J. (1973). Full-scale anaerobic filter treatment of wheat starch plant wastes. *American Institute of Chemical Engineers Symposium Series*, **129**, 30–7.

Van den Berg, L. & Kennedy, K. J. (1983). Comparison of advanced anaerobic reactors. In *Proceedings 3rd International Symposium on Anaerobic Digestion*, pp. 71–90. Massachusetts.

Verrier, D., Moletta, R. & Albagnac, G. (1983). Anaerobic digestion of vegetable canning wastewater by the anaerobic contact process. In *Proceedings 3rd International Symposium on Anaerobic Digestion*, pp. 303–14. Massachusetts.

Wilkie, A., Reynolds, P. J. & Colleran, E. (1983). Media effects in anaerobic filters. In *Proceedings of the Anaerobic Wastewater Treatment Symposium*, pp. 242–58. The Hague: TNO Corporate Communication Department.

Witt, E., Humphrey, W. J. & Roberts, T. E. (1979). Full-scale anaerobic filter treats high strength wastes. In *Proceedings 34th Industrial Waste Conference*, pp. 229–34. Purdue University.

Young, J. C. (1983). The anaerobic filter – past, present and future. In *Proceedings 3rd International Symposium on Anaerobic Digestion*, pp. 91–106. Massachusetts.

Young, J. C. & Dahab, M. F. (1983). Effect of media design on the performance of fixed-bed anaerobic filters. *Water Science and Technology*, **15 (8/9)**, 321–35.

Young, J. C. & McCarty, P. L. (1969). The anaerobic filter for waste treatment. *Journal of the Water Pollution Control Federation*, **41**, R160–71.

Conference Proceedings, 1979–1983.
Anaerobic Digestion 1979, ed. Stafford, D. A. *et al.* London: Applied Science Publishers (1980).
Anaerobic Digestion 1981, ed. Hughes, D. E. *et al.* Amsterdam: Elsevier Biomedical Press (1982).
Anaerobic Digestion 1983. Proceedings 3rd International Symposium on Anaerobic Digestion, Boston, Massachusetts.
Anaerobic Wastewater Treatment. Proceedings of the European AWWT Symposium. The Hague: TNO Corporate Communication Department (1983).
Anaerobic Treatment of Wastewater in Fixed Film Reactors. Proceedings 1981 IAWPR Specialised Seminar, Water Science and Technology, 1983, 15(8/9).
Energy from Biomass. EC Conferences: Applied Science Publishers (1980, 1982).

Chapter 9

Bennett, J. E. (1974). Non-diaphram electrolytic hypochlorite generators. *Chemical Engineering Progress*, **70**, 60–3.
Benzina, A., Lin, S. & Wang, R. L. (1974). Counter jet and hydraulic blockage theory applications to mixing. *Journal of the Water Pollution Control Federation*, **46**, 2719–31.
Bradley, R. M. (1973). Chlorination of effluents and the Italian concept. *Effluent and Water Treatment Journal*, **13**, 683–9.
Bruce, A. M., Havelaar, A. H. & L'Hermite, P. (eds.) (1982). *Disinfection of Sewage Sludge: Technical, Economic and Microbiological Aspects*. London: D. Reidal Publishing Co.
Collins, H. F., Selleck, R. E. & White, G. C. (1971). Problems in obtaining adequate sewage disinfection. *American Society of Civil Engineers Journal Sanitary Engineering Division*, **97**, 549–62.
Culp, R. L. (1974). Breakpoint chlorination for virus inactivation. *Journal American Water Works Association*, **66**, 699–703.
Englmann, E. & Wizigmann, E. (1979). Disinfection of sewage sludge by treatment with gamma rays. *Gas und Wasserfach*, **120**, 481–7.
Geisser, D. F., Garver, S. R. & Murphy, C. B. (1979). Design optimisation of high-rate disinfection using chlorine and chlorine dioxide. *Journal of the Water Pollution Control Federation*, **51**, 351–7.
Hansen, J. A. & Tjell, J. C. (1979). Guidelines and sludge utilisation practice in Scandinavia. In *Proceedings of the Conference on Utilisation of Sewage Sludge on Land*, pp. 317–39. Water Research Centre.
Hart, F. L. & Vogiatzis, Z. (1982). Performance of modified chlorine contact chamber. *Journal American Society of Civil Engineers, Environmental Engineering Division*, **108**, 549–61.
Homann, P. S., Hartwigsen, C. C. & Zak, B. D. (eds.) (1982). Bibliography of the beneficial uses of sewage sludge irradiation project, 1974–1982. *Report SAND 82-1550*. Sandia Research Laboratories, Albequerque.
Hrudey, S. E. (1984). The management of wastewater from the meat and poultry products industry. In *Surveys in Industrial Wastewater Treatment*, ed. Barnes, D., Forster, C. F. & Hrudey, S. E., pp. 128–207. London: Pitman Publishing Ltd.
Irving, T. E. (1980). Sewage chlorination and bacterial regrowth. *Technical Report TR 132*. Water Research Centre.
Irving, T. E. & Solbe, J. F. de L. G. (1980). Chlorination of sewage and effects on marine

First published in Great Britain in 2010 by
Bantam Press
an imprint of
Transworld Publishers, London

First Charnwood Edition
published 2012
by arrangement with
Transworld Publishers
A Random House Group Company, London

British Library CIP Data

Steel, Danielle.
   Legacy.
   1. Genealogy- -Fiction. 2. Family secrets- -Fiction.
   3. Indians of North America- -South Dakota- -
   History- -18th century- -Fiction. 4. Indian women
   - -Fiction. 5. France- -Court and courtiers- -History
   - -18th century- -Fiction. 6. Large type books.
   I. Title
   813.6–dc23

   ISBN 978–1–4448–1018–9

Published by
F. A. Thorpe (Publishing)
Anstey, Leicestershire

Set by Words & Graphics Ltd.
Anstey, Leicestershire
Printed and bound in Great Britain by
T. J. International Ltd., Padstow, Cornwall

This book is printed on acid-free paper

disposal of chlorinated sewage: A review of the literature. *Technical Report TR 130.* Water Research Centre.

Joshi, M. G. & Shambaugh, R. L. (1982). The kinetics of ozone-phenol reaction in aqueous solution. *Water Research*, **16**, 933–8.

Kinman, R. M. (1972). Ozone in water disinfection. In *Ozone in Water and Waste Water Treatment*, ed. Evans, F. L., pp. 123–43. Michigan: Ann Arbor Science Publishing Inc.

Leeuwen, J. van & Prinsloo, J. (1980). Ozonation at the Stander water reclamation Plant. *Water SA*, **6**, 96–102.

Legeron, J. P. (1982). Experimental data about waste-water tertiary treatment with ozone. *Water Pollution Control*, **81**, 166–76.

Longley, K. E., Moore, B. E. & Sorber, C. A. (1980). Disinfection efficiencies of chlorine and chlorine dioxide in a gravity flow contactor. *Journal of the Water Pollution Control Federation*, **54**, 140–5.

McCarthy, J. J. & Smith, C. H. (1974). A review of ozone and its application to domestic wastewater treatment. *Journal American Water Works Association*, **66**, 718–25.

Majumdar, S. B., Ceckler, W. H. & Sproul, O. J. (1973). Inactivation of poliovirus in water by ozonation. *Journal of the Water Pollution Control Federation*, **45**, 2433–43.

Majumdar, S. B. & Sproul, O. J. (1974). Technical and economic aspects of water and wastewater ozonation: A critical review. *Water Research*, **8**, 253–60.

Marson, H. W. (1967). Electrolytic sewage treatment: The modern process. *Water Pollution Control*, **66**, 109–24.

Melmed, L. M. & Comninos, D. K. (1979). Disinfection of sewage sludge with gamma radiation. *Water SA*, **B**, 153–9.

Nebel, C., Unangst, P. C., Gottschling, R. D., Hutchinson, R. L., McBride, T. J. & Taylor, D. M. (1972). Ozone disinfection of combined industrial and municipal secondary effluents. In *Proceedings 27th Industrial Waste Conference*, pp. 1056–70. Purdue University.

Ogden, M. (1970). Ozonation to-day. *Industrial Water Engineering*, 36–40.

Osborn, D. W. & Hattingh, W. H. J. (1978). Disinfection of sewage sludge: a review. *Water SA*, **4**, 169–78.

Poon, C. P. C. & Brueckner, T. G. (1975). Physicochemical treatment of wastewater–seawater mixture by electrolysis. *Journal of the Water Pollution Control Federation*, **47**, 66–78.

Rakness, K. L. & Hegg, B. A. (1980). Full-scale ozone disinfection of wastewater. *Journal of the Water Pollution Control Federation*, **52**, 502–11.

Rice, R. G., Evison, L. G. & Robson, C. M. (1981). Ozone disinfection of municipal wastewater – current state-of-the-art. *Ozone Science and Technology*, **3**, 239–72.

Roberts, K. J. & Vanjdic, A. H. (1974). Alternative methods of disinfection: How effective? *Water and Sewage Works*, **121**, 72–5.

Roberts, P. V., Aieta, E. M., Berg, J. D. & Chow, B. M. (1981). Chlorine dioxide for wastewater disinfection. A feasibility evaluation. *US EPA Report EPA-600/2-81-092.*

Sepp, E. (1981). Optimisation of chlorine disinfection efficiency. *American Society of Civil Engineers Journal Environmental Engineering Division*, **107**, 139–53.

Sproul, O. J., Pfister, R. M. & Kim, C. K. (1982). The mechanism of ozone inactivation of water borne viruses. *Water Science and Technology*, **14**, 303–14.

Stover, E. L. & Jarnis, R. W. (1981). Obtaining high-level wastewater disinfection with ozone. *Journal of the Water Pollution Control Federation*, **53**, 1637–47.

Suss, A. (1980). Irradiation of sludge. *Korrespondenz Abwasser*, **27**, 142–6.

Thalhamer, M. G. (1981). A site specific design of chlorination facilities. *American Society of Civil Engineers Journal Environmental Engineering Division*, **107**, 473–80.

Toms, R. G., Saunders, C. L. & Hodges, E. (1981). The control of bacterial pollution caused by sea discharges of sewage. *Water Pollution Control*, **80**, 204–20.

US Department of Energy. (1981). *Executive Strategy Plan for Beneficial Uses Program Cesium-137 Sewage Sludge Irradiation.*

Venosa, A. D. (1972). Ozone as a water and wastewater disinfectant: A literature review. In *Ozone in Water and Waste Water Treatment*, ed. Evans, F. L., pp. 83–100. Michigan: Ann Arbor Science Publishing Inc.

Venosa, A. D. (1983). Current state-of-the-art of wastewater disinfection. *Journal of the Water Pollution Control Federation*, **55**, 457–66.

Ward, P. S. (1974). Carcinogens complicate chlorine question. *Journal of the Water Pollution Control Federation*, **46**, 2638–40.

Wei, N. S. & Heinke, G. W. (1974). Sewage electrolysis. *Water and Pollution Control*, **112**, 31–6.

White, G. C. (1972). *Handbook of Chlorination.* New York: Van Nostrand Reinhold Co.

White, G. C. (1974*a*). Disinfecting wastewater with chlorination/dechlorination, Part 1. *Water and Sewage Works*, **121**, 70–1.

White, G. C. (1974*b*). Disinfection practices in the San Francisco Bay area. *Journal of the Water Pollution Control Federation*, **46**, 89–101.

White, G. C. (1974*c*). Disinfecting wastewater with chlorination/dechlorination, Part 3. *Water and Sewage Works*, **121**, 100–1.

Whitlock, E. A. (1953). The application of chlorination in the treatment of water. *Water and Wastes Engineering*, **57**, 12–22.

Yeager, J. G. & O'Brien, R. T. (1983). Irradiation as a means to minimise public health risks from sludge-borne pathogens. *Journal of the Water Pollution Control Federation*, **55**, 977–83.

Chapter 10

Antani, S. H. (1972). Experiences in the operation of BOD Moderator treatment of domestic sewage and industrial wastes. In *Proceedings Symposium on Low Cost Waste Treatment*, pp. 183–93. Nagpur: CPHERI.

Arceivala, S. J. & Alagarsamy, S. R. (1972). Design and construction of oxidation ditches under Indian conditions. In *Proceedings Symposium on Low Cost Waste Treatment*, pp. 172–82. Nagpur: CPHERI.

Arceivala, S. J., Bhalerao, B. B. & Alagarsamy, S. R. (1972). Cost estimates for various waste treatment systems in India. In *Proceedings Symposium on Low Cost Waste Treatment*, pp. 239–54. Nagpur: CPHERI.

Bradley, R. M. (1983). BOD removal efficiencies in two stabilization lagoons in series in Malaysia. *Water Pollution Control*, **82**, 114–22.

Bradley, R. M. & da Silva S. A. (1977). Stabilization lagoons including experiences in Brazil. *Effluent and Water Treatment Journal*, **17**, 21–9.

Ettlich, W. F. (1978). A comparison of oxidation ditch plants to competing processes for secondary and advanced treatment of municipal wastes. *US National Technical Information Service Report No. PB 281380.*

Gunn, I. W. (1976). Wastewater treatment in New Zealand. *Water Pollution Control*, **75**, 448–56.

Handa, B. K. (1972). Preliminary studies on the performance of oxidation ditches at Nagpur. In *Proceedings Symposium Low Cost Waste Treatment*, pp. 194–99. Nagpur: CPHERI.

Lumbers, J. P. (1979). Waste stabilization ponds: Design considerations and methods. *Journal of the Institute of Public Health Engineers*, **7**, 70–9.

McGarry, M. G. (1977). Domestic wastes as an economic resource. In *Water, Wastes and Health in Hot Climates*, ed. Feacham, R. G., McGarry, M. & Mara, D., pp. 347–64. Chichester: John Wiley & Sons.

McGarry, M. G. & Pescod, M. B. (1970). Stabilization pond design criteria for tropical Asia. In *2nd International Symposium for Waste Treatment Lagoons*, Kansas, 1970.

Mara, D. (1977). Sewage treatment in hot countries. *Overseas Building Notes, No. 174*. Department of the Environment.

Mara, D. (1976). *Sewage Treatment in Hot Countries*. Chichester: John Wiley & Sons.

Pineo, C. S. & Subrahmanyam, D. V. (1975). Community water supply and excreta disposal: A commentary. *Offset Publication No. 15*. Geneva: WHO.

Polprasert, C. (1979). A low-cost biogas digester. *Appropriate Technology*, **6**, 22–4.

Simpson, J. R. & Bradley, R. M. (1978). The environmental impact of water in overseas countries. *Water Pollution Control*, **77**, 222–47.

Suwanarat, K. (1972). Cost of waste treatment in Thailand. In *Proceedings Symposium on Low Cost Waste Treatment*, pp. 260–4. Nagpur: CPHERI.

Chapter 11

ATV. (1980). Hinweise für das Einleiten von Abwasser on eine offentliche Abwasserlage. *Abwassertechnische Vereinigung Arbeitsblatt A 115 (Entwurf)*.

Barth, E. F., Ettinger, M. B., Salotto, B. V. & McDermott, G. N. (1965). Summary report on the effects of heavy metals on the biological treatment processes. *Journal of the Water Pollution Control Federation*, **37**, 86–96.

Burgess, S. G. (1957). The analysis of trade-waste waters. In *The Treatment of Trade Waste Waters and the Prevention of River Pollution*, ed. Isaac, P. C. G., pp. 65–84. University of Durham.

Burrows, M. C. (1969). Inhibition of aeration process – a quantitative assessment of some toxic materials. *Water Pollution Control*, **68**, 457.

Catchpole, J. R. & Stafford, D. A. (1977). The biological treatment of coke-oven liquors. In *Treatment of Industrial Effluents*, ed. Callely, A. G., Forster, C. F. & Stafford, D. A., pp. 258–72. London: Hodder & Stoughton Ltd.

Dart, M. C. (1977). Industrial effluent control and charges. *Water Pollution Control*, **76**, 192–204.

Fassbender, H. (1967). Effluent pre-treatment and biological effluent treatment in the oil industry. *Chemistry and Industry*, 1539–46.

Hunter, M. T., Painter, J. C. & Eckenfelder, W. W. (1983). The effects of sludge age and metal concentration on copper equilibrium in the activated sludge process. *Environmental Technology Letters*, **4**, 475–84.

Jackson, S. & Brown, V. M. (1970). Effect of toxic wastes on treatment processes and watercourses. *Water Pollution Control*, **69**, 292–303.

Lawson, H. M. & Fearn, R. J. (1970). Further throughts on trade effluent charges. *Water Pollution Control*, **69**, 436–44.

Lockett, W. T. (1952). The discharge of trade effluents into sewers. *Surveyor (London)*, **111**, 285–6.

Luthy, R. G. (1981). Treatment of coal coking and coal gasification wastewaters. *Journal of the Water Pollution Control Federation*, **53**, 325–39.

McDermott, G. M., Moore, W. A., Post, W. A. & Ettinger, M. B. (1963). Copper and anaerobic sludge digestion. *Journal of the Water Pollution Control Federation*, **35**, 655–62.

Mattock, G. (1968). The problems of industry in trade waste treatment. *Water Pollution Control*, **67**, 295–300.

Mattock, G. (1969). Effluent standards from the viewpoint of the industrialist. *Water Pollution Control*, **68**, 339–46.

Moore, W. A., McDermott, G. M., Post, M. A., Mandia, J. W. & Ettinger, M. B. (1961). Effects of chromium on the activated sludge process. *Journal of the Water Pollution Control Federation*, **33**, 54–72.

Mosey, F. E., Swanwick, J. D. & Hughes, D. A. (1971). Factors affecting the availability of heavy metals to inhibit anaerobic digestion. *Water Pollution Control*, **70**, 668–80.

Sherrard, J. H. (1983). The effects of nickel on organic removal and nitrification in the completely mixed activated sludge process. In *Proceedings of the International Conference on Heavy Metals in the Environment*, pp. 385–8. Edinburgh: CEP Consultants.

Simpson, J. R. (1970). The effects of oil on sewers and treatment plants. *Water Pollution Control*, **69**, 593–5.

Stones, T. (1960). The fate of lead during the treatment of sewage. *Journal Proceedings of the Institute of Sewage Purification*, 221–3.

Water Pollution Research Laboratory. (1971). *Notes on Water Pollution No. 53*. WPRL.

Chapter 12

An Foras Taluntais. (1974). Methods of treatment of milk processing wastes. *An Foras Taluntais*, Dublin.

Ashworth, D. R. & Tristram, G. R. (1973). The application of ultrafiltration to the treatment of a bone degreasing effluent. *Water Pollution Control*, **72**, 94–9.

Atkinson, A. (1974). Biocides in cooling systems. *Process Biochemistry*, **9 (8)**, 31.

Baxter, R. A., Gilbert, P. E., Lidgett, R. A., Mainprize, J. H. & Vodden, H. A. (1975). The degradation of polychlorinated biphenyls by micro-organisms. *The Science of the Total Environment*, **4**, 53–61.

BCRA. (1973). *Methods for Treating Carbonisation Effluents: a Critical Review.* Chesterfield, Derbyshire: British Coke Research Association.

Biczysko, J. & Suschka, J. (1967). Investigations on phenolic waste treatment in an oxidation ditch. *Advances in Water Pollution Research*, **Part 2**, 285–308.

Brown, H. B. & Pico, R. F. (1980). Characterization and treatment of dairy wastes in the municipal treatment system. In *Proceedings 34th Purdue Industrial Waste Conference*, pp. 326–34. Ann Arbor Science.

Capper, C. B. (1974). The protection of open recirculating cooling systems. *Effluent and Water Treatment Journal*, **14**, 577–83.

Catchpole, J. R. & Stafford, D. A. (1977). The biological treatment of coke-oven liquors. In *Treatment of Industrial Effluents*, ed. Callely, A. G., Forster, C. F. & Stafford, D. A., pp. 258–72. London: Hodder & Stoughton.

Chambers, J. V. (1980). Cost of dairy wastewater disposal and management. *American Dairy Review*, **42 (11)**, 27, 28, 32, 36, 40.

Chipperfield, P. N. J. (1968). The development, use and future of plastics in biological treatment. In *Effluent and Water Treatment Manual*, pp. 60–74. London: Thunderbird Enterprises Ltd.

Comeaux, R. V. (1967). Basic cooling water inhibitor guide. *Hydrocarbon Processing*, **46 (12)**, 129–32.

CONCAWE Secretariat. (1974). *Inland Oil Spill Clean-up Manual*. The Hague: Stichting CONCAWE.

Cooling Water Association. (1973). *Cooling Water Treatment – A Code of Practice*. London: CWA.

Crowle, V. A. (1972). Effluent treatment and materials recovery from the metal finishing industry using the integrated method of treatment. *Water Pollution Control*, **71**, 636–45.

Curry, R. W. (1976). Treatment of metal-finishing effluents. In *Industrial Pollution Control Yearbook*, pp. 181–7. Fuel and Metallurgical Journals Ltd.

Dearborn Environmental Consulting Services. (1978). Disinfection of poultry packing effluents containing *Salmonella*. *Report EPS 3-WP-78-9*. Ottawa: Environmental Protection Service, Environment Canada.

Dunn, G. F. (1981). PACT – An improvement in wastewater treatment. Paper presented at the 54th Annual Conference of the Water Pollution Control Federation.

Flynn, B. P. & Stadnik, J. G. (1979). Start-up of a powdered activated carbon–activated sludge treatment system. *Journal of the Water Pollution Control Federation*, **51**, 358–69.

Forster, C. F. (1974). The biological treatment of food industry wastes. *Proceedings of the Institute of Food Science and Technology*, **7**, 227–36.

Forster, C. F. (1983). Continuously-operated ditches. In *Oxidation Ditches in Wastewater Treatment*, ed. Barnes, D., Forster, C. F. & Johnstone, D. W. M., pp. 75–131. London: Pitman Books Ltd.

Frost, R. C. (1979). The use of powdered activated carbon in the activated-sludge process: a technical and economic assessment. *Technical Report TR 124*, Water Research Centre, 1979.

Galpin, D. B. & Parkin, M. F. (1981). Estimating the yield of butter by the measurement of losses. *New Zealand Journal of Dairy Science and Technology*, **16**, 231–41.

Ganczarczyk, J. & Elion, D. (1978). Extended aeration of coke-plant effluents. In *Proceedings 33rd Industrial Waste Conference*, pp. 895–902. Purdue University.

Garcia-Gutierrez, A., McIntyre, A. E., Perry, R. & Lester, J. N. (1982). The behaviour of polychlorinated biphenyls in the primary sedimentation process of sewage treatment. A pilot-plant study. *Science of the Total Environment*, **22**, 243–52.

Harper, W. J., Blaisdell, J. L. & Grosskopf, J. (eds.) (1971). Dairy food plant waste treatment practices. *US EPA 12060 EGU 03/71*. Washington DC: US Environmental Protection Agency.

Harrison, J. R., Licht, L. A. & Peterson, R. R. (1984). The treatment of waste from the fruit and vegetable processing industries. In *Surveys in Industrial Wastewater Treatment*, vol. 1, ed. Barnes, D., Forster, C. F. & Hrudey, S. E., pp. 209–95. London: Pitman Books Ltd.

Hofstein, H. & Kohlmann, H. J. (1985). The treatment of wastewaters from steel plants. In *Surveys in Industrial Wastewater Treatment*, vol. 3, ed. Barnes, D., Forster, C. F. & Hrudey, S. E., London: Pitman Books Ltd.

Holdsworth, S. D. (1970). Effluents from fruit and vegetable processing. *Effluent and Water Treatment Journal*, **10**, 265–8.

Holiday, A. D. & Hardin, D. P. (1981). Activated carbon removes pesticides from waste water. *Chemical Engineering*, **88 (6)**, 88–9.

Housden, A. J. (1981). Operational experiences in the effective treatment of effluents from synthetic resin manufacture. *Water Pollution Control*, **80**, 490–6.

Howells, G. D. (1983). The effects of power station cooling water discharges on aquatic ecology. *Water Pollution Control*, **82**, 10–17.

Hrudey, S. E. (1984). The management of wastewater from the meat and poultry products industry. In *Surveys in Industrial Wastewater Treatment*, vol. 1, ed. Barnes, D., Forster, C. F. & Hrudey, S. E., pp. 128–208. London: Pitman Books Ltd.

Illsley, P. (1982). Oil spill clean up and waste oil recovery. *Water and Waste Treatment*, **25 (9)**, 43–4.

Kaneko, M., Morimoto, K. & Nambu, S. (1976). The response of activated sludge to polychlorinated biphenyls. *Water Research*, **10**, 157–63.

Kelly, B. J. (1968). Cooling tower chromates – recovery and disposal. *Oil and Gas Journal*, **66 (43)**, 77–9.

Langford, T. (1977). Biological problems with the use of sea water for cooling. *Chemistry and Industry*, **No. 14**, 612–16.

Lowe, W. (1970). The origin and characteristics of toxic wastes, with particular reference to the metal industries. *Water Pollution Control*, **69**, 270–80.

Lunt, J. & Hemming, M. L. (1979). The treatment of effluents from the palm oil industry. *Environmental Pollution Monitor*, 175–9.

Mahalingham, B., Jain, P. K., Biyani, R. K. & Subramanian, R. V. (1981). Mixing alternatives for the polyester microencapsulation process for immobilization of hazardous residues. *Journal of Hazardous Materials*, **5**, 77–91.

Marshall, K. R. & Harper, W. J. (1984). The treatment of wastes from the dairy industry. In *Surveys in Industrial Wastewater Treatment*, vol. 1, ed. Barnes, D., Forster, C. F. & Hrudey, S. E., pp. 296–376. London: Pitman Books Ltd.

Meiners, H. & Mazewski, G. (1979). Design, start-up and operation of a refinery treatment system with muscle. In *Proceedings 34th Industrial Waste Conference*, pp. 710–18. Purdue University.

Monnig, E. & Zweidinger, R. A. (1981). Treatability studies of pesticides manufacturing waste waters: dinoseb and atrazine. Springfield: *US National Technical Information Service, Report PB81-178840*.

Myers, W. A., Mayes, J. H. & Englande, A. J. (1977). Pretreatment of a biorefractory herbicide waste stream to enhance biodegradability. In *Proceedings 32nd Industrial Waste Conference*, pp. 450–3. Purdue University.

Nazley, N. & Knowles, C. J. (1981). Cyanide degradation by immobilized fungi. *Biotechnology Letters*, **3**, 363–8.

Neufeld, R. D. (1984). The treatment of wastes from the synthetic fuels industry. In *Surveys in Industrial Wastewater Treatment*, 2, ed. Barnes, D., Forster, C. F. & Hrudey, S. E., pp. 65–129. London: Pitman Books Ltd.

Oldham, G. F. (1980). Oily effluent treatment by the BP treatment process. *Water Pollution Control*, **79**, 236–43.

Parkin, M. F. & Marshall, K. R. (1976). Spray irrigation disposal of dairy factory effluent – a review of current practice in New Zealand. *New Zealand Journal of Dairy Science and Technology*, **11**, 196–205.

Saleh, F. Y., Lee, G. F. & Wolf, H. W. (1982). Selected organic pesticides; behaviour and removal from domestic wastewater by chemical and physical processes. *Water Research*, **16**, 479–88.

Scheltinga, H. M. J. (1972). Measures taken against water pollution in dairies and milk processing industries. *Pure and Applied Chemistry*, **29**, 101–11.

Sheehan, G. J. & Greenfield, P. F. (1980). Utilisation, treatment and disposal of distillery waste water. *Water Research*, **14**, 257–77.

Soothill, R., Barnes, D. & Cook, D. (1985). Chloroalkali wastewater treatment. In *Surveys in Industrial Wastewater Treatment*, vol. 3, ed. Barnes, D., Forster, C. F. & Hrudey, S. E., London: Pitman Books Ltd.

Tinker, J. (1975). River pollution: the Midlands Dirty Dozen. *New Scientist*, **65**, 551–4.

Toms, R. G. (1971). The threat to inland waters from oil pollution. In *Water Pollution by Oil*, pp. 13–20. London: The Institute of Petroleum.

US EPA. (1972). *Water Quality Criteria*. Washington DC: US Government Printing office.

US EPA. (1974). Treatment of cheese processing wastewaters in aerated lagoons. *Environmental Protection Technology Series, EPA-660/2-74-012*, Washington DC: US Environmental Protection Agency.

Vernick, A. S., Lanik, P. D., Langer, B. S. & Hrudey, S. E. (1984). The management of wastewater from the petroleum refining industry. In *Surveys in Industrial Wastewater Treatment*, vol. 2, ed. Barnes, D., Forster, C. F. & Hrudey, S. E., pp. 1–64. London: Pitman Books Ltd.

Wilde, J. (1985). Liquid wastes from the metal finishing industry. In *Surveys in Industrial Wastewater Treatment*, vol. 3, ed. Barnes, D., Forster, C. F. & Hrudey, S. London: Pitman Publishing Ltd.

Zech, A. F. (1981). Solidification of wastes. The Petrifix process. *Eau et Industrie*, **No. 60**, 65–8.

Index

374

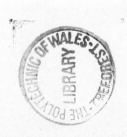